CLINICAL PSYCHIATRY

CLINICAL PSYCHIATRY

HOWARD S. SUDAK, M.D., EDITOR

Associate Editors
RICHARD B. CORRADI, M.D.
GLENN C. DAVIS, M.D.
STEPHEN B. LEVINE, M.D.
T. REEVES WARM, M.D.

WARREN H. GREEN, INC.
St. Louis, Missouri, U.S.A.

Published by

WARREN H. GREEN, INC.
8356 Olive Blvd.
St. Louis, Missouri 63132, U.S.A.

All rights reserved

© 1985 by WARREN H. GREEN, INC.

ISBN No. 0-87527-333-5

LIST OF CONTRIBUTORS

Agle, David P., M.D.
Professor of Psychiatry
Department of Psychiatry
Case Western Reserve University
School of Medicine
Cleveland, Ohio

Althof, Stanley E., Ph.D.
Assistant Professor of Psychology
Department of Psychiatry
Case Western Reserve University
School of Medicine
Cleveland, Ohio

Arison, Zipora, M.D.
Assistant Professor of Psychiatry
Department of Psychiatry
Case Western Reserve University
School of Medicine
Cleveland, Ohio*

(*Now in private practice
   in Ft. Lauderdale, Florida)

Clemens, Norman A., M.D.
Associate Clinical Professor of Psychiatry
Department of Psychiatry
Case Western Reserve University
School of Medicine
Cleveland, Ohio

Corradi, Richard B., M.D.
Assistant Professor of Psychiatry
Department of Psychiatry
Case Western Reserve University
School of Medicine
Cleveland, Ohio
Staff Psychiatrist
Cleveland Veterans Administration
   Medical Center

Davis, Glenn C., M.D.
Associate Professor of Psychiatry
Department of Psychiatry
Case Western Reserve University
School of Medicine
Cleveland, Ohio
Assistant Chief of Staff
Staff Psychiatrist
Cleveland Veterans Administration
   Medical Center

Dogin, Judith W., M.D.
Assistant Clinical Professor of Psychiatry
Department of Psychiatry
Case Western Reserve University
School of Medicine
Cleveland, Ohio

Foster, Dodi, PA-C
Coordinator of Psychiatric Emergency
   and Consultation Team
Brecksville Veterans Administration Hospital
Brecksville, Ohio

Freedheim, Donald K., Ph.D.
Associate Professor of Psychology
Department of Psychology
Case Western Reserve University
Cleveland, Ohio

Klonoff, Elizabeth A., Ph.D.
Assistant Professor of Psychology
Department of Psychiatry
Case Western Reserve University
School of Medicine
Cleveland, Ohio

Levine, Stephen B., M.D.
Associate Professor of Psychiatry
Department of Psychiatry
Case Western Reserve University
School of Medicine
Cleveland, Ohio

Lothstein, Leslie M., Ph.D.
Associate Professor of Psychology
Department of Psychiatry
Case Western Reserve University
School of Medicine
Cleveland, Ohio

Macklin, Martin R., M.D.
Assistant Clinical Professor of Psychiatry
Department of Psychiatry
Case Western Reserve University
School of Medicine
Cleveland, Ohio

Martin, Ruth S., M.D.
Assistant Professor of Psychiatry
Department of Psychiatry
Case Western Reserve University
School of Medicine
Cleveland, Ohio
Staff Psychiatrist
Cleveland Veterans Administration
   Medical Center

McCormick, Richard A., Ph.D.
Assistant Chief, Psychology Service
Brecksville Veterans Administration Hospital
Brecksville, Ohio

Moir, Robin N., M.D.
Assistant Clinical Professor of Psychiatry
Department of Psychiatry
Case Western Reserve University
School of Medicine
Cleveland, Ohio

Resnick, Phillip J., M.D.
Associate Professor of Psychiatry
Department of Psychiatry
Case Western Reserve University
School of Medicine
Cleveland, Ohio
Staff Psychiatrist
Cleveland Veterans Administration
   Medical Center

Rosenthal, Miriam, M.D.
Assistant Professor of Psychiatry
Department of Psychiatry
Case Western Reserve University
School of Medicine
Cleveland, Ohio

Rothchild, Ellen N., M.D.
Associate Clinical Professor of Psychiatry
Department of Psychiatry
Case Western Reserve University
School of Medicine
Cleveland, Ohio
Staff Psychiatrist
Cleveland Veterans Administration
   Medical Center

Simpson, Dale M., M.D., Ph.D.
Assistant Professor of Psychiatry
Department of Psychiatry
Case Western Reserve University
School of Medicine
Cleveland, Ohio
Staff Psychiatrist
Cleveland Veterans Administration
   Medical Center

Sudak, Howard S., M.D.
Professor of Psychiatry
Department of Psychiatry
Case Western Reserve University
School of Medicine
Cleveland, Ohio
Chief, Psychiatry Service
Cleveland Veterans Administration
   Medical Center

Warm, T. Reeves, M.D.
Assistant Professor of Child Psychiatry
Department of Psychiatry
Case Western Reserve University
School of Medicine
Cleveland, Ohio

Wasman, Marvin, Ph.D.
Assistant Professor of Psychology
Department of Psychiatry
Case Western Reserve University
School of Medicine
Cleveland, Ohio

Zinn, Stephen B., M.D.
Assistant Professor of Psychiatry
Department of Psychiatry
Case Western Reserve University
School of Medicine
Cleveland, Ohio

ACKNOWLEDGMENTS

The editors wish to acknowledge the extensive editorial assistance provided by Mrs. Barbara Juknialis and are particularly grateful for the formidable coordinating and clerical services of Mrs. Myrna Andell.

Howard S. Sudak, M.D.

CONTENTS

CLINICAL PSYCHIATRY

Chapter 1

INTRODUCTION
HOWARD S. SUDAK, M.D.

PART I
DESCRIPTION OF THIS TEXT

Every psychiatric textbook has its own strengths and weaknesses, and is oriented toward specific audiences. The present work is intended as an introduction to clinical psychiatry for students of medicine and allied health professions. Much of the book is derived from "The Mind Committee Syllabus," used in teaching psychiatry to second year medical students at Case Western Reserve University. Some specific features of that course are detailed in Part III of this chapter.

This book is divided into six sections. The Introduction (I) is followed by sections on Psychoses (II) and Development Throughout the Life Cycle (III). The developmental sequence includes material on child pathology; it seems more relevant to include it with child development than with adult pathology. Very little space is devoted to developmental tasks in the middle years of adulthood—mostly because they are not well understood. A list of additional readings is included in the chapter on Older Age. Section IV addresses Non-Psychotic Problems, such as neuroses, character disturbances, suicide, and substance abuse. Section V focuses on Human Sexuality Throughout the Life Cycle. The concluding section (VI) is devoted to Psychiatric Therapies.

There are many approaches to the study of human behavior. Psychiatrists focus on the individual, rather than society, i.e., how the individual relates to, and copes with, the powerful forces in his or her external and internal worlds. To a lesser degree, we are interested in extrapolating a group psychology from experience with individuals. This book reflects a psychodynamic theoretical framework, which we believe offers the most comprehensive approach to "mental" phenomena. A minimum of psychoanalytic theory per se will be presented. Instead, we will attempt to acquaint readers with a small portion of the data which were important to the development of analytic theory, i.e., material gathered by observation and therapy of normal and abnormal children and adults. Although certain basic psychodynamic concepts, e.g., the unconscious, psychic determinism, the theoretical agencies of the mind (id, ego, superego), the role of defense mechanisms, childhood sexuality, will be considered "givens," there is nothing sacred about these orientations. We ask only that the reader try to keep as open a mind as possible. The book's objectives are to:

1. Present an approach to observing and understanding behavior;
2. Impart a body of knowledge about:
    a. Normal behavioral landmarks and characteristics—i.e., cognitive, social, psychosexual, for the entire life cycle;
    b. The influences of these landmarks and characteristics on physical illness, and vice versa;
    c. Common conflicts and problems which physicians should recognize as part of normal growth;
    d. Psychopathology and its treatment.

PART II
INTRODUCTION TO PSYCHIATRY
AND PSYCHODYNAMIC CONCEPTS

Psychiatry has made enormous progress in the past few decades. More objective data have been gathered about the probable neurochemical bases of the major mental disorders, and our pharmacological weapons have become more potent and specific. Nevertheless, students may be initially disconcerted by the lack of precision in the "softer" behavioral and social sciences.

The natural inclination to identify with whatever pathological syndrome is being studied is another source of student anxiety. This is, of course, similar to what happens with any medical areas being studied—e.g., when students first study hematology, they may worry about leukemia and begin to palpate their own axillae or cervical areas for lymphadenopathy. It is not difficult to identify with patients with psychiatric problems—particularly those whose problems are not blatant. Although not all of us have neurotic disorders, we all have some quirks or hangups—areas in which our functioning is impaired by some idiosyncrasy. Similarly, the study of character disorders reminds us that we too are character types. Many readers, for example, may find descriptions of the obsessive-compulsive personality a little too close for comfort. However, this is not all negative; some obsessive-compulsive tendencies can help us master repetitive tasks, keep our noses to the grindstone, etc.

The next few paragraphs will detail other ways in which students may be confused by the interplay of social, biological, and psychological forces and their effects on diagnosis.

Defining the category of "patienthood" may appear more nebulous in psychiatry than in other areas of medicine. Psychoses are easier to recognize than neuroses or character disorders, since they are similar to other pathological states in medicine. The psychotic disorders are relatively well-delineated syndromes, probably with organic causes, which respond to medication, and have a well-defined onset, temporal course, etc. The identification of those with psychoses is thus rather straightforward. On the other hand, just how neurotic does one have to be before one qualifies as having a "Neurosis?" People have vastly different tolerances for psychic pain or anxiety. Some seek out intensive types of therapy to alleviate minimal psychic distress. Time and economic factors may preclude others from availing themselves of such therapies. People who are biased against being labelled as "abnormal" or receiving psychiatric treatment may tolerate an enormous amount of psychic disturbance without seeking help. For those whose largely subjective levels of stress do not prevent them from functioning and behaving in a "reasonable" manner, patienthood may be more a matter of "attitude" than of "pathology."

Identifying patients with characterological problems poses another dilemma. For instance, a person who fears flying, but transfers to a job which requires a lot of flying, is apt to wind up in a psychiatrist's office complaining of an airplane phobia. Such a person becomes a self-labelled "neurotic." Patients with character or personality disturbances rarely identify themselves as disordered (i.e., having character or personality disturbances). This is particularly true of psychopathic (also known as antisocial, dyssocial, or character defect) personality disorders in which the label "psychopath" is generally appended to an individual who has run afoul of the law. Patients with characterological disturbances are generally comfortable "the way they are," and do not seek change.

The convergence of sociological and biopsychological factors can result in misleading statistics. For example, how can we explain the apparent discrepancy in the prevalences of male and female neuroses? Are women intrinsically more neurotic than men? It is possible that merely being a woman in a male-dominated society predisposes to neuroses (as some recent epidemiologic studies of depression have indicated) (1). There are, however, reasons to suspect the influence of potent sociological forces. Is the admission to being "weak, dependent, sick, neurotic" more acceptable to a woman's self-image? Having more time available for treatment is also a factor, particularly in an era when fewer women were working. Social class differences pose a related issue. Prevalence data indicate that neuroses occur proportionately more often in middle and upper social classes. However, the considerable amount of time and money necessary to obtain treatment certainly might prevent the disadvantaged from getting both the treatment and the label. It seems ludicrous to assume that being poor affords some protection against being neurotic. Those factors which would cross-correlate with being poor, e.g., broken homes, less education, more social chaos, should, if anything, foster the development of psychopathology. On the other hand, one could argue that the factors associated with poverty predispose toward character disturbances (i.e., acting-out disturbances); while "better," "more advantaged" childhood development would be more apt to cause sexual and aggressive inhibitions with resultant intrapsychic, neurotic-style problems, rather than disinhibition. Nonetheless, it appears, at least to some degree, that having a clinical neurosis is a luxury the poor can ill-afford.

The interaction among individual and sociological factors is also illustrated by the prevalence differences of character problems among males and females, blacks and whites, etc. Does the smaller prevalence of psychopathic character disorders in women mean that their superegos (consciences) are superior to those of men? This does not seem probable. To use anti-social personality disorders (psychopaths) as an example: the label "psychopath" is frequently applied to persons in trouble with the law. Since female psychopaths are apt to be the consorts or "hangers-on" of male psychopaths, rather than the ones who actually commit the crimes, they are less likely to be arrested and assigned such labels. Some of the same reasoning may be applied to the black-white disparity. Being black is associated with being socioeconomically disadvantaged, which further correlates with having a less intact family. Although these factors may increase the likelihood of having a defective superego and developing character pathology, it is likely that other factors are present. For instance, whites, or socioeconomically advantaged groups in general, may find more socially acceptable channels for acting-out some of their aggressive impulses than blacks or those of lower socioeconomic status. Undoubtedly, the reader can think of various methods for "burying" personal psychopathology in socially acceptable ways. In addition, our double standard of justice makes the economically advantaged lawbreaker less likely to be arrested, arraigned, convicted, sentenced, etc.

Treatment considerations may also be confusing. The appropriate treatment for a given condition is often a matter of opinion. Because the guidelines for treating neurosis or character problems, are less clear than those for the psychoses, individual biases are more evident. Proponents of analytically oriented therapy will claim that their treatments are the most effective. Similar claims are made by those who endorse behavioral, pharmacological or other psychological approaches, such as Gestalt, Rogerian, Rankian, and Jungian. No wonder patients and beginning therapists are often confused about choosing therapies. It is only fair to note that every area in medicine has its own internal disputes, waged by vocal proponents of every persuasion.

According to psychodynamic principles, mental functioning represents the balance among various theoretical aspects (constructs) of the mind and external reality. The therapist attempts to assess the individual's strengths and weaknesses, coping and defense mechanisms, and general adaptation to present and past life situations. The concepts of "psychic determinism" and an "active unconscious" are basic to this approach.

The concept of psychic determinism is based upon the assumption that mental events do not occur at random or by chance. This does not mean that accidents do not occur. It means that chance is never the sole determinant of our feelings, thoughts, or actions. Every mental event is influenced by antecedent events; it then becomes part of the basis for subsequent events. Thus, the past is always a part of the present. The fact that we are frequently unaware of these influential antecedents does not detract from their importance; a great deal of mental function is not under our conscious control or awareness.

Although it originally met with considerable resistance, Freud's concept of an unconscious mental life is now widely accepted by behavioral scientists. However, since most people prefer to view themselves as totally rational and in firm control of their thoughts and feelings, the general public has not fully accepted Freud's concepts. Skeptics are rarely convinced by the usual "proofs," e.g., dreams, slips of the tongue, posthypnotic suggestions. However, a modest amount of introspection leads most of us to acknowledge our lack of complete rational control. We all have feelings for which we can't account, e.g., anxiety, sadness; forget things we ought to have remembered, e.g., appointments with the dentist; and make decisions for obscure reasons.

The Id

The concept "id" refers to mental activities associated with instincts and their drive-derivatives, particularly sexual (libidinal) and aggressive. The other drives, e.g., hunger, thirst, etc., ordinarily undergo less complex vicissitudes, except when they become intertwined with the sexual or aggressive drives. The id is essentially unconscious. Its goal is to reduce tension through gratification of its drives. This goal is also referred to as the "pleasure principle," i.e., the attempt to obtain pleasure and avoid pain. In its search for immediate gratification, the id operates on a "primary process" level. Thus, if one means of discharge is blocked or unavailable, substitute pathways will be utilized, e.g., thumb-sucking when the breast or bottle is unavailable.

A newborn infant has many innate drives. Although we formerly thought of the mental life of infants as mostly "id," recent physiological and psychological studies have revealed that infants have remarkably sophisticated and advanced perceptual and cognitive abilities. As the infant matures, parental expectations result in certain frustrations—particularly in relation to the delay of drive gratification. The child gradually differentiates him or herself from the environment and forms an early concept of self. As the brain matures and perceives the environment in increasingly complex ways, the child attempts to control and master it through the "ego."

The Ego

The concept "ego" refers to that mental activity which perceives and organizes memories and thoughts into logical relationships. Its function is to integrate the inner drives with realistic goals.

The ego includes all conscious and unconscious psychological functions concerned with the individual's relationship to the environment: perception; motility; memory; judgment; reasoning; language; thought; control over consciousness. As the ego matures, the "reality principle" gradually begins to replace the "pleasure principle." The child now operates on a more "secondary process" level, i.e., he or she learns that alternate pathways are not always preferable or readily available; this necessitates learning to delay gratification. Emotional involvement with specific persons and objects also complicates the attainment of gratification. The desire to please his parents, i.e., earn their love or avoid their displeasure, helps motivate the child to learn to postpone immediate, automatic attempts to gain pleasure. Such early hesitations, or delays, between impulses and action are one of the preconditions for "thought," i.e., a mental trial action which helps us decide what course to follow. Thus, the ego mediates between the person and the external world, between drives and conscience; it also serves as the medium through which we view ourselves and the world around us.

The Superego

The "superego" is a concept which comprises the moral precepts of a person's mind, e.g., conscience; guilt; ideal self-aspirations. With the exceptions of "ideals" or standards of self-assessment, the operations of the superego are essentially unconscious. The superego is not established until the child begins latency, around age 6; it is not fully consolidated until adulthood. Prior to its establishment, the child feels little, if any, guilt. He may "behave" himself to avoid *external* disapproval, e.g., not sneak an extra cookie to avoid being scolded. The internalization of parental standards causes the child to refrain from an act because it will cause guilt, even if the external world was not aware of the act.

It is important to realize that all development is gradual. Reality principles do not suddenly supplant pleasure principles, nor does a superego dramatically crystallize out of an ego solution. These changes occur simultaneously along many different dimensions, at varying rates, and with varying degrees of success, e.g., motor development; ego skills and patterns of defenses; instinctual foci. A focus on only one dimension or agency of the mind may seem artificial, but it is necessary for illustrative purposes.

The child's ego, superego, and perceptions of the external world shape the ultimate character structure, defensive patterns, and personality. Basic personality structure is largely dependent upon the resolution of these various critical pivotal issues. The developmental changes in the libidinal and aggressive sides of the child's instinctual life will be covered in greater detail in the section on child development.

Role of Anxiety

According to a unitary view of psychologic phenomena, the individual's primary methods of coping with anxiety account for all psychological manifestations. If anxiety is handled "internally" through excessive defense mechanisms, "neurotic" or "psychoneurotic" problems will result. For example, suppose a 5-year-old boy becomes both excited and fearful after witnessing his parents having intercourse. His (oedipal) wishes to be the one his mother loves best arouse his anxiety; gratification would place him in direct competition with his father, and he fears retaliation. In addition, he may misconstrue intercourse as a battle between his parents. Resolving such libidinal and aggressive wishes by possessing the mother and eliminating the father as a rival would be both unrealistic and unacceptable to his ego and superego. Defense mechanisms provide one method of resolution, e.g., displacement and symbolization might cause the child to develop a simple phobia. The fear of his father's retaliation (through castration) might be displaced to big, scary animals like horses. The child might also worry about horses falling down in the street and kicking their legs (symbolizing the parents' legs during intercourse). This paradigm is contained in Freud's *An Analysis of a Phobia in a 5-Year-Old Boy* (2). It represents an internal resolution (that is, one which employs intrapsychic defense mechanisms) to a conflict between the id and the ego.

There are alternative ways to decrease anxiety by preventing an unacceptable libidinal or aggressive wish from reaching consciousness. The individual may opt for an "external" or characterological resolution, rather than the "internal" means described above. In such an instance, "Little Hans" (the child in the above-mentioned paper) might have elected to develop a lifestyle in which he handled his aggressive excitement by beating up some littler Hans in the neighborhood. Such a child could thus develop a life-style in which he was always acting-out his conflicts with the outside world. Note that a neurotic individual is in pain; the conflict is resolved by a dystonic or ego-alien solution, and the individual suffers. In a characterological resolution, the conflict is not between two intrapsychic agencies (his ego and his id) but between the individual and the world around him. It is "external" to the individual, and is acted-out with society. In a characterologic resolution, society tends to suffer, e.g., the smaller boy down the street who got socked. Since persons who resolve their conflicts characterologically are either in less pain or less aware of psychic pain, these are known as ego-syntonic, rather than ego-dystonic, resolutions.

A third method of attempting to cope with anxiety is to channel it directly through the autonomic nervous system. Some individuals, when anxious, are prone to have their anxiety manifested by gastrointestinal symptoms (such as diarrhea, nausea, etc.), neurodermatological conditions, respiratory symptoms, etc. Although everyone, at times, expresses some anxiety through autonomic pathways, some individuals seem particularly predisposed to such routes. A psychophysiological symptom does not entirely dissipate the anxiety, per se, but does express some of it through such routes.

Defense Mechanisms

While there are many sources of anxiety, we shall only consider that which arises from a conflict between an id wish and the ego and/or superego. If the child wants to gratify a wish, e.g., to smear or otherwise play with his feces, which would be unacceptable to his ego (and/or his developing superego), the ego may unconsciously react by producing a small amount of anxiety ("signal anxiety"). One of the ego's unconscious defense mechanisms may then be called upon, both to prevent an undisguised expression of the unacceptable wish, and to allow some partial gratification. In the example cited, the defense mechanism of "reaction-formation" might be employed, i.e., the impulse would be turned into its opposite (in this example, the child might become inordinately clean). Although certain defense mechanisms or patterns are characteristic of certain developmental stages or conflicts, this is by no means invariably true, e.g., projection and introjection in the one-year-old; reaction formation in the anal period; displacement and repression in the phallic/oedipal period. Moreover, certain kinds of anxiety are associated with specific periods in the child's life, e.g., separation anxiety or anxiety over losing the loved-object in the "oral" period, anxiety over loss of parental love in the "anal" phase; castration anxiety in the phallic/oedipal period; "moral anxiety" (guilt) after the establishment of the superego.

Symptom Formation

Exclusive reliance upon selected defense patterns may account for specific symptoms, e.g., a phobic symptom results from the excessive use of symbolization and displacement; conversion hysteria results from excessive repression. Since a given defense does not invariably produce a specific symptom, this simplification is misleading. It would be more accurate to say that when defenses work well, they do not result in symptoms. True neurotic symptoms only occur when excessive defensive or regressive means are employed to compensate for ineffective defenses. Defenses fail for a number of reasons: a particular defense may be incapable of warding off the impulse; the ego, in general, may be weak and less able to cope (e.g., during physical illness); the id impulse may increase, throwing the instinct vs. defense equilibrium out of balance (e.g., at puberty). Symptoms represent compromise formations between the id and the ego. They represent both sides of the conflict —the wish and the defense against it. For example, the patient with an obsessive-compulsive neurosis may wash his hands fifty times per day as a defense against the wish to be dirty; yet, this constant preoccupation with issues of dirt and contamination also unconsciously gratify the interest and wishes pertaining to dirt. Psychoneurotic symptoms are "multiply determined," i.e., they are composed of determinants related to both conscious and unconscious levels of awareness, all three agencies of the mind (id, ego, superego), and all libidinal and aggressive aspects of psychosexual development (oral, anal, phallic, Oedipal); They have present, past, and often future relevance.

Neither defense mechanisms nor anxiety per se (particularly "signal," as opposed to "traumatic," anxiety) are pathologic in and of themselves. If defenses were not called into action by anxiety, we would be unable to learn and grow. We would have to gratify every instinct and partial instinct that arose in our ids, even those with conflicting aims and objects. We would ultimately be overwhelmed by both our instincts and anxiety.

Though simplified and sketchy, this introduction should acquaint you with some of the basic psychiatric concepts which will be developed in this course. The Brenner (3) reference in the Suggested Reading List provides a much more comprehensive summary.

PART III
THE PSYCHIATRY COURSE
AT CASE WESTERN RESERVE UNIVERSITY:
A DESCRIPTION AND SOME PEDAGOGICAL SUGGESTIONS

The psychiatry course at CWRU has evolved over the past twenty years. It is given to second year medical students over a three-week period: 4 hours every morning, with options from 12 to 1 nearly every day; plus 4 afternoon sessions, from 1 to 5 p.m. for clinical interviewing. Other teachers may find it instructive to understand how we arrived at our present system of teaching.

The course was originally organized in chronological order. Childhood development was followed by milder mental disorders (such as neuroses and character problems), more severe syndromes (psychoses), and therapies. It soon became clear, however, that students did not respond well to this sequencing of material. Learning about childhood development after studying about the cardiovascular system, for instance, seemed too soft and nebulous; they were either bored or amused. We next attempted to interdigitate adult-pathological sequelae with their relevant preceding stages of childhood psychosexual development, hoping to enhance child development by showing its role in the later pathological syndromes of adulthood. This worked out relatively well when trying to relate adult neuroses to the appropriate childhood stage (e.g., obsessive-compulsive neurosis to the anal stage of toddler development), and reasonably well when trying to explain certain aspects of hysteria (relating it to the oedipal stage development). However, a neat correspondence between childhood developmental stages and later psychopathology is very difficult to illustrate when one leaves neuroses and character development. This proved to be clumsy and resulted in confusing the students.

The current course starts with psychoses, in order to gain the students' attention and interest and imprint upon them the relevance of psychiatry. Students start to wonder about the workings of the mind and become more curious about normal psychological development. This method seems to make students much more receptive to the material on childhood development. Consequently, this text follows the same sequence in the hope that others will also find it a useful way to approach this body of data.

Daily small group discussions are an important aspect of the psychiatry course at CWRU. We utilize twenty small group leaders who attend the entire 72-hour course. Each small group leader meets with approximately eight medical students for one hour every day to discuss the lecture or demonstration material in more detail. The small groups afford a little more time for students to explore areas of particular interest. Also, the subject matter lends itself to small groups, where questions can be raised in an atmosphere which is less threatening than a large classroom; it may also be possible to overcome some student resistances which might never be manifested in a larger setting. Much of the small group time is spent discussing the audiovisual materials, particularly videotapes, and live patient presentations used in the lectures. We highly recommend enhancing this text with such illustrative material. Tapes such as *The Electronic Textbook of Psychiatry,* produced by Dr. James Ryan at Columbia University, are invaluable resources.

Interviewing of psychiatric patients is another important part of the course. Under the supervision of the small group leaders, each student interviews two patients at a psychiatric hospital. Students find it fascinating to work with patients; the experience deepens their understanding of, and interest in, the course material.

Lunch hour electives usually deal with topics which are not part of the core-curriculum. Typical electives include: The Changing Roles of Women and Men; Working Mothers and the Problems of Raising Young Children; Management of Grief in Pediatric and Family Practices; Psychology of Rapists; videotapes illustrating Group Therapy or Family Therapy, etc.

We have experimented with a number of different examination systems over the years. An optional oral examination is usually offered midway through the course. It generally consists of 10 or 15 minutes of general questions, and is administered in the small groups. The course final is generally a written multiple choice examination. Although we are fond of essay-type, subjective examinations, grading them is a grueling experience. Also, "scientifically-oriented" students often complain that "humanistic-literary" students have an advantage in such subjective exams. (On the other hand, multiple choice exams may give the former group an advantage.) One year the students were given paperback copies of John Knowles' *A Separate Peace* (4). The book was distributed early in the course, and students were permitted to discuss the book with one another. The examination had questions about the concepts of adolescent development illustrated in the book, the possible unconscious homosexual feelings between the two boys (Gene and Phineas) and the defenses against them. While both faculty and students enjoyed this examination, it proved difficult to grade.

While this teaching format may not be totally compatible with those of other schools, some may wish to utilize the CWRU model in conjunction with our text. More detail regarding the CWRU course can be found elsewhere (5).

REFERENCES

1. Weissman MM, Myers JK, Thompson WD: Depression and its treatment in a U.S. urban community: 1975-1976. *Arch Gen Psychiatry* 1981;38:417-421.
2. Freud S: 1909, An analysis of a phobia in a 5 year old boy, in Strachey J (ed): *The Complete Psychological Works of Sigmund Freud,* st'd ed. London, Hogarth Press, vol 10, 1955, pp 3-149.
3. Brenner C: *An Elementary Textbook of Psychoanalysis.* Garden City, New York, Doubleday Anchor, 1957.
4. Knowles J: *A Separate Peace.* New York, Bantam Books, 1966.
5. Sudak H: En-bloc psychiatry teaching. *Br J Med Ed* 1974;8:279-286.

Chapter 2

THE PSYCHIATRIC CASE STUDY
NORMAN A. CLEMENS, M.D.

This chapter deals with an intense, emotional experience between two people. In order to avoid being impersonal, the author addresses the chapter to "you," the beginning interviewer.

THE INITIAL INTERVIEW

Few experiences in psychiatry are more challenging and interesting than the initial interview with a new patient. You are getting to know a new person in a very searching way and establishing a new relationship. All of your clinical skills are brought into play, and you may have to make some crucial decisions in a short period of time. While maintaining a relaxed and unhurried atmosphere in which the patient may feel free to elaborate his or her difficulties, you must use time wisely to obtain the most relevant information—always a limited amount selected from a mass of detail.

The relationship you establish now will set the tone for what could be many hours of future work between you (or other psychiatric treatment personnel) and the patient. As the patient attempts to articulate concerns and relate them to life events, he or she will often see them more clearly and experience more focused emotional responses. Thus, psychotherapy begins. The emphasis on restoring health, which is the essence of your clinical approach, may aid even the most disturbed psychotic patient to strengthen some slight grip on reality and accept treatment.

Flexibility must be the hallmark of your approach as you tailor your responses to the individual patient. For that reason, nothing can be unvarying in the case study approach described in this chapter. The patient and your clinical judgment will make each case a unique experience.

The purpose of the initial interview will greatly affect its course, as will the expectations of your subsequent relationship; the evaluation of a psychiatric patient brought to the emergency room by the police will differ markedly from the first session with a prospective psychoanalytic patient.

Even at the start, you and the patient will relate on many levels. As Menninger (1) put it, part of your task is "to imagine what it would be like" to be in the patient's state of mind. Despite the desire to communicate with you and establish a helpful relationship, the patient also wishes to conceal important matters and withdraw (2,3). The psychiatrist is seen as a powerful stranger who evokes both magical expectations of cure and a sense of grave danger. Aside from the conscious and realistic intentions you both bring to the encounter, powerful unconscious forces may be activated in you and the patient. In the throes of facing the damage done by a deeply gratifying behavioral pattern, the patient may not realize how reluctant he or she is to give it up. In the wee hours of the morning, you may find it tempting not to confront the evidence that a patient is suicidal, because the diagnosis will commit you to several hours' work to get the patient admitted.

These understandable conflicts in either party may be further complicated by the patient's transference responses and the therapist's counter-transference reactions. Some patients will automatically shift into a dependent mode or develop outlandish expectations of a magical cure; others will confront your authority by subtly competing, rebelling in a surly way, or fearfully acting as if you will criticize or reject them. By the same token, you will inevitably find that some patients awaken in you new versions of responses to important figures in your ancient past.

All of these developments both enrich and distort the material of the initial interview. The patient may reveal more than he or she intends, as well as omit and unknowingly conceal important data. You may overlook things or respond in a manner that is unusual for you. These elements are ubiquitous; you cannot avoid them, and they provide vital raw material for the evaluation. Your professional expertise enables you to recognize these elements, discern your part in them as much as possible, and manage them competently. In an initial session, you would not ordinarily discuss with the patient the things you perceive that he or she is not aware of; however, you should realize that this developing interaction is also the beginning of psychotherapy (3-6).

Although this chapter deals primarily with the initial interview, it should be understood that the process described here is frequently extended over several sessions. On the other hand, circumstances may sometimes limit evaluation time to less than the 45 minutes to an hour that is ordinarily desirable for an initial session.

Setting

The optimal setting is comfortable and non-threatening, with a relaxing chair for the patient and a furniture arrangement that does not emphasize the therapist's authority or distance. In an emergency room setting, there should be adequate support available to assure the patient that you and your staff will maintain control of destructive or wild behavior. The paraphernalia used in physical restraint, physical examination, and medications are put out of sight. When violence is a possibility, the room decor should be simple and free of objects that could be used destructively. All interruptions are kept to a minimum.

If it is conspicuous and laborious, *note-taking* puts a distance between you and your patient; it also distracts both of you from the flow of thought needed to do the job. You can unobtrusively jot down basic factual data and key words or phrases without significantly breaking eye contact with the patient, or making him or her feel that the notes are the main objective of the interview. If it is your responsibility to obtain essential information such as name, address, telephone number, birthdate, next of kin, names and ages of spouses and children, work place, referral source, race, religion, ethnic background, etc., do so early in the interview. This will preclude your having to interrupt the productive flow of more highly charged information later, and also gives the patient a chance to size you up before you delve into the problem together.

Getting Started

When the patient is there with family or others, it is generally a mark of respect to the patient to start with the patient's view of the situation. You should make it clear that you are there as the patient's therapist. If the patient's condition or the needs of the other people involved make it necessary to start with the others, you should later acknowledge this to the patient; make it clear that you are keeping an open mind and want to know how the patient looks at things. Even if you have advance information, as from a referring physician, suggest that the patient not assume anything about what you know already lest important material be overlooked. You want to hear the whole story from the patient.

It helps to acquaint the patient early with the *format* of the evaluation session: how much time you have together; definition of the task; the course of the evaluation; handling of confidentiality and responsibility; if appropriate, what decisions will have to be made. If you are acting for an agency other than the patient—e.g., an assessment requested by an employer, insurance company, court or other government body, etc.—this should be clear from the start, since it alters the rules regarding confidentiality and allegiance to the patient. Being straightforward about these realistic issues will help the patient to trust and be open with you.

The Interview Process

The *flow of the initial interview* is generally from the open-ended and non-directive to the specific. Your goal is to get the patient to talk freely about the reason for the evaluation. Once this is established, you will cone down on essential details, as well as eliciting sufficient background information to complete an initial evaluation. There must be time at the end for questions and feedback to the patient, as well as decisions and their implementation.

The traditional medical case evaluation calls for systematic questioning to obtain a standard, comprehensive set of information. However, much more in-depth understanding is gained by letting the patient tell the story with a minimum of interruptions or directions to alter the flow of associations. Depending upon the type of problem and the purpose of the interview, the modern psychiatric evaluation usually involves some degree of compromise between the two conflicting approaches. In any given situation, what transpires may be at one end of the spectrum or the other (1–3,5–8).

There are many ways to initiate a serious discussion of the problem. In general, you invite the patient to explain what the difficulties are in his/her own way. You may assure the patient that you will focus the discussion by asking questions as the interview goes along—but to start out, the patient's description of the problem would be more informative. If the patient finds it difficult to begin, you may comment on how hard it can be to discuss important personal problems with a stranger. Ask how the patient feels at the moment, and whether this is similar to the state of mind that has been troublesome. If so, when do they notice this problem, and can they tell you more about it? Your interest and support, as well as manifest concern with feelings, will often get things moving.

Try not to disturb the patient's *associative patterns*—i.e., linkages of thought, usually based on emotional, rather than logical or chronological connections. Besides leading to crucial revelations or giving important clues, these linkages indicate the influence of the past upon the present. If silences occur, allow the patient a little time to think before you intrude with a question or comment; keep the silence from becoming heavy by commenting on it and asking what the patient is thinking or feeling.

As the patient begins to talk more freely, ask brief questions to clarify what is being said, get the precise facts, or obtain more detail. Questions that can be answered with "yes" or "no" are much less effective in starting the flow of associations than open-ended inquiries, such as, "Tell me about . . ." "And what happened then?" "Can you expand on that?" and so forth. Repeating something that the patient has said usually elicits elaboration and more of the emotional overtones.

You may find it appropriate to acknowledge the emotional impact of the patient's words, without making assumptions beyond what has been clearly expressed. For example, "I can understand how that would bring tears to your eyes" is an acknowledgement. "You must have felt angry" is an assumption. Besides drawing out more information, these responses assure the patient that you are listening and comprehending. These restatements also help patients to view their words with more of a sense of objective reality; occasionally, patients will exclaim, "I really said that, didn't I?"

It is important to maintain a *neutral, non-judgmental attitude* toward the patient's revelations. At this stage, you do not know enough to form a judgment, even if it were appropriate. Neutrality does not mean being impassive or unempathic, nor is it expressed in silent detachment. You are placing your professional skills at the service of the patient, but you are not taking sides. The healthier part of the patient will welcome this aspect of your professional competence. In a similar vein, false reassurances or condescending support do not convince the patient that you really understand. Adroit interviewing is particularly important with the delusional patient, who may confront you by asking whether you agree with the delusions. You should give the impression of trying to understand without agreeing or disagreeing (which would be futile anyway); however, you will not permit action based on the delusions.

If the patient is merely reporting a series of facts, you may inquire about the patient's *feelings and responses,* both now and at the time when the events occurred. If the patient is evasive, or seems to have trouble describing feelings, you may comment on this and explore the issue. In other instances, the patient may have difficulty in pursuing a subject until you discuss the strong feelings (e.g., shame, guilt, sadness, anger) that cause the hesitation. Sometimes patients will give more *detail or peripheral information* than is necessary, which may be a manifestation of a circumstantial or tangential manner of expression or of defensive obfuscation. You may then have to explain that time is limited and tactfully steer the focus back to more relevant information. The management of time and detail call for the constant exercise of judgment.

Many points of inquiry concern delicate matters, involving embarrassing symptoms, socially questionable behavior, sexual dysfunctions, suicide, or violence to others. Exploring these areas will rarely present serious problems if you use an *ego-oriented* approach. An impulse-oriented question is, "Do you want to harm yourself?" An ego-oriented question is, "Are you afraid that your despair might bring you to the point of harming yourself?" By identifying the patient's own concern, which is almost never totally absent, and attempting to help deal with the problems, you will often find that the patient welcomes your inquiry with relief and eagerness for assistance.

As the interview progresses, you are both *observing* the patient and *listening* to what is said. You are collecting both objective and subjective data, by being attentive to both form and content. Your objective observations of the patient's behavior, emotions, ideas, and formal thought processes are the raw material of the mental status examination; the subjective report given by the patient becomes part of the history, often supplemented by material from other sources. Although the interview does not follow the same order as the final written accounts of history and mental status, you should be mentally categorizing the necessary data and preparing to seek what is not spontaneously offered by the patient.

You gradually become *more active* in guiding and controlling the discussion. The essential information needed to fulfill your medical-legal responsibility must be covered to the best of your ability under the circumstances. Functional psychosis and organic illness affecting mental function must be diagnosed or ruled out. A basic medical history is necessary. You are responsible for determining the presence or absence of danger through violence—either self- or other-directed. You must evaluate the patient's judgment and potential for damaging consequences through poor self-care or management of affairs. It is important to assess the patient's own level of understanding of his or her condition, expectations of what is needed, and motivation for carrying out a treatment plan. These general points apply to all new patients, although their application will vary according to the considerations mentioned earlier.

As the nature of the patient's particular problem becomes clearer, you move from the *general to the specific,* i.e., by eliciting details of the symptoms and events that are part of the present illness, as well as enough background information to assist in the diagnosis and treatment recommendations. A branching process occurs, in which the course of inquiry depends upon the major problems under investigation. For instance, evidence of impaired cognitive function calls for detailed inquiry about medical conditions and a complete examination of cognitive functions. A full evaluation of depression includes information about recent losses, current functional status, the vegetative symptoms of affective disorder, a careful investigation of suicidal risk, the past history of depressive or manic states, and the family history of affective disorders and related conditions, such as alcoholism. Indications of psychosis would lead you to a thorough exploration of delusions, hallucinations, altered thought patterns, and affective concomitants as well as appropriate past and family history. If a mixture of neurotic and characterological symptoms clearly predominate, your highest priority is the assessment of suitability for psychotherapy. You then begin to lay the foundation for possible future work together.

Closing Stages

In closing the evaluation interview, you have a number of tasks to perform. It is essential that you be in charge. You wish to communicate to the patient your view of what is wrong and what is needed. In order to assure proper follow-up, the course of action must be clear, e.g., setting and procedure of psychotherapy, the administration and effects of medication, etc. The patient needs an opportunity to respond and ask questions. It may also be helpful to ask the patient to reiterate certain main points of your instructions. Plans for seeing family members or obtaining data from other sources can be made and written permission obtained when necessary. As you part, you may think it appropriate to assure the patient that you are available by telephone before the next appointment, if new questions or concerns should arise.

THE PSYCHIATRIC CLINICAL HISTORY

The following description of the clinical history is a topical survey of the various kinds of historical data needed to reach a perceptive understanding of patients and their difficulties. Since individual patients vary widely, the relevance of individual topics to the case at hand will also vary. The sequence of topics is not intended to be a rigid formula for all case reports; it should rather remind you of meaningful areas of inquiry and act as a guide for organizing the data collected.

Psychiatric history-taking differs from other branches of medicine in the degree of emphasis on the patient's emotional, intellectual, and social transactions. This does not mean that a detailed medical history is not important. However, the bald facts of the present illness, social history, and family history are only a skeleton for the kind of information that enables understanding the subtleties of a patient's psychiatric problem. Thus, we concern ourselves with not only the events but also their meaning to the patient, his or her relationships with the key figures, and the kind and amount of emotional reaction which the patient recalls and/or now attaches to the memory of the events.

The Record

The written report of the initial history is the cornerstone of the clinical record. It documents the patient's care for medical-legal purposes; in a hospital setting, it is the central point for active daily communication among the many people who work with the patient. Write the initial clinical report as soon as possible after the evaluation of the patient—certainly the same day—and update it with each subsequent contact. Headings of various sections will aid the reader in finding selected information. As you write the report, be aware of the setting in which the record is being used; balance the desirability of recording complete data against the concern for confidentiality of very sensitive personal information. In some situations, it is best to keep some private, well-guarded notes, apart from an institutional record.

In all notes, an appropriate style, respectful of the patient's dignity, will avoid the risk of future embarrassment. Despite the need for detail, conciseness is a virtue. Technical terms for clinical observations are most valuable when you support them by using the patient's words or examples in plain English. As you record information, it may be desirable to note the source of important items, i.e., the patient or other observers.

Opening Statements

The record of the clinical history begins with *identifying data:* patient's name; age; marital status; race; religious and ethnic backgrounds; occupation; date and place of evaluation. Next are the *informants,* their relationship to the patient, how they became familiar with the situation, and how reliable they are.

The *chief complaint or presenting problem* is the headline of the history. When possible, it should be in the patient's own words. If other informants have differing ideas about what the problem is, describe these also. It may be appropriate to tell the manner in which the patient presented for evaluation.

Present Illness

The present illness is the most important part of the history and should be carefully developed. It is usually a chronological presentation of changes in behavior, emotional state, mentation, and personality, from the time the patient was last considered to be "well" up to the present time. Parallel with the changes in the patient, describe relevant environmental stresses. What efforts has the patient made to deal with the difficulties, and what strengths has he or she shown? Include earlier contacts with medical or psychiatric assistance for this problem, and their results. The history of the present illness should lead up to the events that culminated in the patient's seeking psychiatric evaluation.

Background History

The *Past Psychiatric History* documents prior episodes of mental illness, psychiatric treatment or hospitalization, use of psychotropic medications, behavioral disturbances, suicide attempts, violence, or antisocial activity.

Although you may only have time to gather limited material for the *Family History* in the initial evaluation interview, you should at least elicit the ages and states of health of parents and siblings, as well as any family background of mental and emotional illness, including alcoholism, personality problems, or major medical disorders. Later you will wish to obtain detailed information about the patient's ethnic, religious, social, and educational backgrounds. Ongoing psychotherapy will bring out important subtleties to augment your first impressions of the patient's relationships with parents, siblings, and other key figures.

The *Personal History* is the background of the patient's life and development, from prenatal time to the present. It is generally recorded chronologically within certain major categories. The initial interview usually illuminates only the major framework of the personal history; the really significant details emerge later. However, the patient's first statements about his or her past may be very revealing, including material that the patient will resist talking about in treatment for months. Learning about the patient's background, personality, and environment enables you to evaluate the intrinsic and external reality factors that set the conditions for possible therapy. The personal history starts with whatever is known of the patient's *birth* circumstances and significant prenatal influences. This is followed by any available information about the patient's *growth and development* through the major biological and psychosocial stages of childhood and adolescence or tracing out certain lines of personality development. This, in turn, leads into the complete *educational* history. Any *military service,* including combat duty and the classification of discharge, comes next. *The occupational* history traces the sequence of the patient's jobs; this includes the places of residence if the patient has moved about with job changes. Be particularly concerned with an assessment of the present job, the patient's relationships with supervisors and co-workers, working conditions, hours, income, and possible exposure to toxins or other environmental stress. This leads naturally into a description of the patient's *habitat and economic status,* i.e., the nature of the home and possessions, as well as general financial solvency. Obtaining information about income, major financial assets, and liabilities often requires considerable tact; people may be very reluctant to discuss this part of their lives. Additional information concerns the patient's *religious* affiliation, practices, and attitudes, as well as *hobbies, spare time pursuits, and social activities.*

Approach the *sexual and marital* history with tact, but with evident willingness to be frank and factual. The interaction of sexual behavior with other aspects of the relationship with the partner is often very informative. Discreet general inquiries such as, "Tell me something about your married life," "How is your sexual energy?" "What problems did you have as a teenager?" or questions about the menstrual history can, if necessary, lead into more specific questions. This makes it clear that sexual matters can be discussed as openly as anything else. It is relevant to inquire about sexual education and early sexual events, puberty and adolescence, menarche or first ejaculation. This leads to premarital relationships, courtship and marriage(s), divorce(s), extramarital living arrangements, homosexual experiences and relationships, problems with aborted pregnancies, obstetrical difficulties, menopausal or climacteric manifestations, and so forth, as appropriate. One is, of course, most concerned with the present spouse or partner—age, state of health, personality, general characteristics of home life, sexual relationship, handling of birth control, and any difficulties, including outside involvements.

Often, very significant material comes up in connection with the patient's *children*. You should carefully note their ages, the status of their psychosocial development, general personality characteristics, problems, and the particulars of their relationships with the patient.

The personal history often includes a description of the patient's *personality* as seen by others and the patient. Personality encompasses temperament, emotional control, energy level, creativity, independence, ability to form relationships, sense of humor, intellectual endowment, and attitudes towards oneself. Try to form some impression of the strength and flexibility of the patient's conscience, as well as his or her self-esteem, standards, and ideals. Is the patient unusually harsh or lax in self-evaluation? Explore assets as well as liabilities, and try to convey a sense of the patient's usual life style. Be sure to mention unusual personal *habits* concerning food and sleep, as well as the use of alcohol, drugs, tobacco, and caffeine.

In addition to the above mentioned, the *Medical History* describes current medical problems and pertinent positive or negative findings from the review of systems. It lists major past illnesses as well as all operations, and distressing childhood disorders. List the names and dosage pattern of all current medications. Describe any allergies or drug reactions that have occurred, especially those involving psychotropic or closely related medications.

Hospital Course

If the patient has already been in the hospital for a period of time prior to your evaluation, this is the appropriate place to summarize the hospital course; describe changes in clinical status and the evolution of treatment.

THE GENERAL EXAMINATION

The *physical examination* includes a thorough evaluation of all systems, especially cardiovascular status, the state of hydration and nutrition, and the signs of endocrine or metabolic dysfunction. Undiagnosed medical disorders frequently accompany or cause psychiatric symptoms in a patient who has not had medical attention. A complete neurological examination is essential, and should include carefully documented evaluation of the extrapyramidal system for involuntary movement disorders and other medication side effects. If the patient has not been on medication, this may serve as a baseline for future monitoring of medication effects. In many instances—especially with paranoid or seductive patients, or when intensive psychotherapy is contemplated—the physical examination will be performed by a physician other than the potential therapist.

Laboratory studies ordinarily include screening measures that have been determined to be cost effective in picking up unsuspected health problems or establishing a baseline for the possible use of psychotropic medication in a hospitalized patient. It is common practice to obtain a complete blood count, blood sugar, electrolytes, liver function profile, urinalysis, blood urea nitrogen or serum creatinine, thyroid function studies, and a cardiogram. If these tests have recently been performed by the patient's general physician, the cost of repeating them should be weighed against any possible advantages. Further studies commonly depend on the nature of the patient's difficulties, e.g., specialized neurological studies, such as a lumbar puncture, computerized axial tomogaphy, or electroencephalogram; psychotropic or other medication levels in blood or urine; dexamethasone suppression test. No laboratory test can be a substitute for a thorough clinical evaluation.

THE MENTAL STATUS EXAMINATION

The mental status examination is the specialized psychiatric part of the general examination; a significant portion should be included in every examination done by a physician. Mental status findings may be clues to important physiological disturbances, and enable assessment of patient's ability to cooperate with medical studies and treatment programs (8,9).

The following topics should be used only as a mental check list to ensure that each aspect of the mental status will be examined—not as the structure of the interview. You can gather a large part of the information in an informal manner while meeting the patient, taking a history, and making judicious inquiry into various remarks made by the patient. In the history you recorded the information that the patients and others chose to give you; here you record the first-hand observations you made along the way.

Since mental status may fluctuate widely, you should make serial observations of significant positive or negative findings. The initial mental status examination is especially important as a baseline. Later observations will be included in the progress notes. Be sure to note the date of the observations, as well as the time of day. Important findings should be reported in both technical terms and ordinary language, which conveys a sense of the patient as a person and supports the choice of terminology. Give examples of abnormal findings whenever possible.

Appearance and Behavior

One begins with general observations of appearance and behavior, such as habitus, state of consciousness, state of health, aging, posture, and gait. The patient's dress gives clues to the mental state, as do facial expressions. Actions should be observed for the *degree* of activity (which may be increased in mania or agitation, or decreased in the psychomotor retardation of depression), *appropriateness* (which may be altered to the point of being bizarre in schizophrenia or organic states), and repetitive or peculiar *mannerisms* (e.g., waxy flexibility). Involuntary movements should be noted here as well as in the neurological examination. You should also note the patient's general attitude and degree of *cooperation* in the evaluation, as well as the capacity to establish a *relationship* with the examiner. Be attentive to the patient's non-verbal communications to you and others.

Affect

The patient's affect or general emotional state may not appear the same as the feelings being reported by the patient; in such cases, note the discrepancy and record both views. Report the degree of *anxiety* and the *mood(s)* displayed by the patient—for example, elated, haughty, cheerful, apathetic, depressed, sad, labile, fearful, suspicious, irritable, angry, etc. Also indicate the *manner* in which the patient shows emotions, e.g., tearfulness, tremulousness, or belligerance, and whether they are *appropriate* to the patient's mental content. For example, they are inappropriate if the patient is giggling while telling about a major injury or loss.

Sometimes the beginning interviewer finds it hard to distinguish between the intense, leaden, oppressive affect of depression and the detached, wooden, so-called "flat" affect of schizophrenia. Your emotional response to the patient is often an important aspect of your observations, if you are careful to sort out personal reactions unrelated to the patient's condition. The depressed patient may communicate a feeling of depression, whereas you may have a peculiar sense of difficulty in empathizing with the schizophrenic patient.

Stream of Talk

Although stream of talk is one of the most important observations of mental function, it is frequently neglected in general medical evauations. Here one observes primarily the *formal* aspects, rather than the content of speech. These findings are crucial to the differential diagnosis of various psychiatric disorders. In trying to distinguish between schizophrenia and manic disorder, for example, records of the patient's clinical state upon first presentation may help diagnose episodes of illness that occur months or years later.

There are three main parameters to evaluate: 1. *Productivity* will be altered in depression, with impoverishment of talk, lack of spontaneity, and/or psychomotor retardation; mania is characterized by pressured speech or flight of ideas. 2. *Relevance* to the topic at hand will be affected by conscious evasiveness, by circumstantiality or tangentiality—all of which may appear with some personality disorders, as well as more serious conditions. Major irrelevancies occur in psychotic illness. Confabulation and perseveration appear in some organic disorders. 3. *Coherence and organization* of the patient's associative patterns will be disturbed by scattering of thought or loose associations, flight of ideas, distractibility, clang associations, neologisms, concreteness, and echolalia. These all indicate major mental disorder or central nervous system dysfunction.

When there is serious disruption of the stream of talk, it may be difficult to distinguish between loose associations and flight of ideas. The pressure and rapid pace of manic productions often help in diagnosis; the schizophrenic may be more conversational in tone, even if his speech is stilted, stereotyped, or agitated. It is usually easier to observe some kind of connection among the thoughts of a manic than among those of a schizophrenic with a significant associative disorder. However, many schizophrenics, particularly those who are paranoid or moving towards remission, have fairly coherent thoughts for one or two paragraphs and then abruptly change to an unrelated topic; the change may escape your notice if you are not alert. At the other extreme, loose associations may present a "word salad," a jumble of incoherent words. Blocking, in which the patient repeatedly loses the train of thought without being aware of it, may also be present.

Content of Thought

Content of thought focuses on what was said, rather than how it emerged. Note the predominant *trends and preoccupations* of the patient's thoughts—fears, hopes, ambitions, identifications, optimism, pessimism, fantasies, and described dreams. Document *neurotic symptoms* reported by the patient, such as obsessions, compulsions, phobias, and somatization, as well as related defense mechanisms evident in the interview. Another cluster of observations may center around *depressive characteristics,* such as self-deprecation, feelings of helplessness, hopelessness, worthlessness, and inappropriate guilt, nihilistic fantasies, and suicidal thoughts. If *suicidal or homicidal* impulses are present, elicit the degree to which they preoccupy the patient, the extent to which the patient has elaborated on them or considered specific actions, the modes selected, associations to past attempts by the patient or family members, and how near the patient has come to acting on them.

The *sine qua non* of evaluating thought content is to establish the presence or absence of *defects in reality testing.* Some of these will emerge in skillful open-ended interviewing; others, such as hallucinations, may be revealed only through direct questioning. Sometimes hallucinations will be evident because the patient behaves as if the apparent stimuli were real, e.g., staring at a blank spot or picking imagined bugs off the skin. *Delusions* (i.e., fixed beliefs that are not based on reality or shared religious or social doctrine) may be present in many disorders; the type of disorder determines whether they are persecutory, jealous, religious, grandiose, nihilistic, cataclysmic, self-accusatory, or somatic. Less extreme forms of the same disturbances in reality testing may occur in *ideas of reference* or *ideas of influence*. *Hallucinations* (i.e., perceptions not based on real external stimuli) may affect any of the senses—hearing, sight, touch, smell, taste, visceral sensation. Olfactory, gustatory, and tactile hallucinations should raise a high index of suspicion of structural or metabolic organic disease. *Illusions* are distorted interpretations of actual perceptions that occur in organic disorders—for instance, a patient in a hepatic stupor described a green wardrobe as a tree. *Depersonalization, derealization,* and *deja vu* phenomena may occur in major psychoses, temporal lobe pathology, or severe dissociative disorders.

Sensorium and Intellectual Functions

Although the sensorium and intellectual functions are most often disturbed in organic disorders, abnormalities may also be present with severe anxiety, depression, or amnesic and fugue states of psychic origin (10,11). All patients should be screened for these symptoms. You can unobtrusively make many observations during the general interview by noticing the patient's orientation, recent and remote memory, retention and recall, use of abstractions and figures of speech, and general level of intelligence. Pursue more formal testing with hospitalized patients or if there is any indication whatsoever of cognitive malfunction. Remember that cognitive defects may fluctuate in a diurnal pattern.

When introducing direct tests, explain to the patient that some of the tasks may seem overly simple and some quite challenging; state that they will be helpful to you in evaluating his or her difficulties. It is not a matter of passing and failing. Describe each task carefully, with illustrations if necessary. In some tests, it is appropriate to give the patient a second chance if an error is made. If the patient is too anxious to handle detailed testing in the initial interview, more accurate results may be obtained in a second session.

Orientation is evaluated for time, place, and person. Time indicators are the year, month, date, day of the week, and time of day. "Place" refers to the interview location (e.g., the hospital and its significance), as well as the city. "Person" includes the names of the interviewer and patient, as well as the identities of others known to the patient. Occasionally, delusional beliefs must be sorted out from actual disorientation, as with a patient who explained that everyone else claimed it was the current date; since he was Napoleon, however, he knew it was 1812.

Memory may be disrupted in various dimensions. The precision and consistency of answers to questions about the patient's personal history (origins, schooling, family, occupation, etc.) will indicate the intactness of *remote* memory. The patient's ability to report current life events, including those related to the illness and the community in general, will demonstrate *recent* memory function. *Immediate* memory—e.g., the events of the past few minutes or hours, may be selectively disturbed in disorders such as Korsakoff's psychosis.

There are several formal tests for evaluating *retention and recall. Digit span* is a good bedside device for serial use in documenting a fluctuating sensorium. It measures the length of a series of numbers that the patient is able to retain and repeat. Start with three digits and proceed up to six or seven digits. Be sure to use random numbers without sequences or recurring digits. State them slowly and evenly without fluctuations in inflection; in other words, avoid a telephone number format which breaks a seven-digit span into three and four. Discontinue the test after two successive failures using the same number of digits, and record the span successfully repeated. A further step is to ask the patient to repeat the digits in reverse order. You may have to illustrate the task: "Now I will say more numbers, but this time I want you to say them backwards. For instance, if I were to say 694, you would say 496." If you give the test on repeated occasions, use different series of random numbers to avoid a learning effect.

Other tests of retention and recall involve reading a *simple story* and asking the patient to repeat it to you, and giving three *test phrases or objects* (e.g., "red ball, leather shoes, Chevrolet") to be recalled after specific time periods, such as two and five minutes.

Concentration is often measured by the *serial sevens* test, in which the patient is asked to subtract from 100 in intervals of seven; a reasonable time is 25–50 seconds. Since this is an evaluation of the ability to sustain attention and perform an operation repeatedly, rather than a test of arithmetic, you may ask the patient to subtract threes from 50 or count backwards from 20 if subtracting sevens is too difficult. Note the speed with which the patient performs the operations, how well they are sustained, and the number and kinds of errors. You will, of course, also describe any difficulty the patient has in sustaining concentration during the entire evaluation interview.

The ability to *calculate* is sometimes impaired in focal cortical lesions that do not affect other functions. You may test this ability with simple calculations and story problems that progress from easy to more difficult and involve more complex operations. For example: How much are three dollars plus four dollars? If a person buys eight 20-cent stamps and gives the clerk $2.00, how much change should he or she get back? How long will it take a man to walk eleven miles at the rate of three miles per hour? Start by asking the patient to do the calculations without using pencil and paper; if the patient is unable to do so, see if it helps to write them down.

The patient's fund of *general information* may vary greatly, depending upon educational level, verbal abilities, interests, and environmental expectations. You wish to estimate the breadth of the patient's information about his or her world, and the ability to apply it to life circumstances. Again, a graded series of questions may be used:

How many things are there in a dozen?

What do we celebrate on the Fourth of July?

Name the four seasons of the year.

Name the last four Presidents.

Who is the governor of your state?

What is the capitol of Greece?

Who invented the airplane?

Why does oil float on water?

How far is it from New York to Chicago?

What is a barometer?

Who wrote *Paradise Lost?*

If the patient does poorly on these questions, you may find it illuminating to shift to topics closer to the patient's interests, such as sports, music, movies or other aspects of the entertainment world, or local or national politics. Word definitions are frequently used.

Abstract reasoning is evident throughout the interview in the patient's ability to generalize and abstract. Defects may appear in concreteness, literal interpretation of colloquial expressions or figures of speech, or personalizing of general questions and statements. Schizophrenia or organic disorders may cause impairments of abstract reasoning.

There are two categories of structured testing of abstract reasoning. *Similarities* are tested by asking how a graded series of paired objects are alike—for example, plum/peach, beer/wine, piano/violin, scissors/copper pan. *Proverb interpretation* may require more explanation and illustration; the idea is that these common sayings convey some kind of message about everyday life. One asks, "What does it mean when people use the expression, . . .?" Sample proverbs are:

People who live in glass houses should not throw stones.

Rolling stones gather no moss.

A bird in the hand is worth two in the bush.

As the twig is bent, so is the tree inclined.

The squeaking wheel gets the grease.

The final assessment of the sensorium is your global estimate of the patient's *intelligence,* based on general self-expression, vocabulary, manipulation of concepts, quickness of understanding, and so forth. State your sense of the patient's internal and external *apperception,* or grasp, of the subtleties of his or her environment. In your estimate, note the congruence of the patient's intellectual capacity with the educational and occupational backgrounds, as well as the extent of any apparent deterioration.

There are varying levels of *insight* or awareness of one's present condition. Does the patient know that he or she is ill? Is there a clear idea of the kind of problem? How much does the patient understand the cause and effect relationships involved (e.g., a recent loss causing a depression), or perceive operational psychological processes? The assessment of the patient's willingness and *motivation* to make use of therapeutic attention is also relevant. Here also one may comment on the patient's self-image and self-esteem.

Judgment

The evaluation of judgment is your global assessment of the patient's ability to care for himself or herself, manage interpersonal situations appropriately, and handle personal business matters realistically. This evaluation should be based on everything you know about the patient from all sources, but especially on your own observations. If you think the patient shows poor judgment, clearly state your reasons. Judgment used to be tested with questions such as, "What would you do if you found a stamped, sealed, addressed letter on the street?" or "What would you do if you saw smoke in a crowded theater?" These are of limited value and used infrequently.

Suicidal and Homicidal Risks

Your estimate of the risk that the patient will become violent may not always be correct, but not stating an opinion is a serious error. This estimate should be based on all available information; a supporting explanation should be included if there is significant risk. The risks of suicide and harm to others should be stated separately, and graded as none, minimal, moderate, or severe. If the patient does not volunteer thoughts about violence, it is your responsibility to ask. Such impulses are sometimes present when you might assume otherwise, e.g., a mother with small children; a patient who appears very passive. The finding of significant risk makes you responsible for taking protective measures.

FURTHER DATA

You may wish to add other information that has come to light since the initial evaluation, if the case study report is being written at some later date. Such data might include: subsequent serial observations of mental or physical states; laboratory studies; psychometric evaluation; treatment instituted and the response and/or side effects.

DISCUSSION AND WORKING HYPOTHESIS

At this point, the available data are used to construct a working hypothesis that explains what is happening to the patient. This hypothesis points the way to further investigation, immediate and long-range treatment plans, and feedback to the patient and family. It encompasses intrapsychic, interpersonal, and physiological processes in a dynamic interplay, in which multiple vector forces are almost always present. Often your understanding can be only fragmentary, and the hypothesis will be constantly readjusted as your knowledge of the patient increases. Although this hypothesis represents much more than a diagnosis, differential diagnosis should be used as a descriptive foundation; cite clinical evidence to support your conclusions.

To put it in more human terms: what sort of a person are we dealing with? How has he or she habitually handled life, and what are his or her strengths and weaknesses? Is the current crisis a result of characteristic behavioral modes? What is happening in the patient's external reality or inner emotional life that may have upset a previous homeostatic equilibrium? What psychic processes (such as impulses, defenses, self-criticism, or guilt) are activated or intensified by this disturbance? If a structural change in the brain, a metabolic imbalance, or a functional psychotic process has disrupted the patient's ego functions, how is this perceived and handled by the patient? Are the psychological symptoms somehow advantageous to the patient, even though they interfere with healthy functioning? What qualities in the patient's character, or aspects of his or her reality situation, seem particularly amenable or resistant to therapeutic work? How does all of this manifest itself in the patient's working relationship with you?

These are only a few of the possible questions that could be raised. The inquiry must be tailored to each individual; an effort must be made to bring the *central issues* into focus. It is crucial that the intellectual discussion be based on an empathic awareness of a human being coping with inner and outer worlds. This part of the case study is often referred to as the *formulation*.

DIAGNOSIS

State your diagnoses according to the standard nomenclature of DSM-III, the *Diagnostic and Statistical Manual* of the American Psychiatric Association (9). The multiaxial structure separates the categories of psychiatric symptom disorder, personality disorder, and medical diagnoses. When diagnosis is uncertain, list the major problems and the differential diagnosis of each problem grouping.

PLANS FOR FURTHER EVALUATION AND TREATMENT

Management begins with an effort to reach a *diagnosis,* if one has not been firmly established. In either the traditional or the problem-oriented format, outline a stepwise series of measures to obtain the information needed to clarify the diagnosis. Measures may include obtaining further data from the patient, family, or other informants, physical or laboratory examinations, psychological testing, in-hospital observation, etc. Consider both short- and long-term goals. Update the plan of investigation regularly as the diagnostic possibilities are refined.

Treatment plans should also be described in a systematic, orderly fashion, including both immediate and long-term approaches. Note any factors that may facilitate or interfere with implementing treatment. Indicate the manner in which you will present your impressions and plans to the patient and family to enlist their cooperation. Planning for hospital discharge should begin at the time of admission.

PROGRESS NOTES

Progress notes document the work that is under way. They are especially important when there are new observations, changes in thinking about the patient, or new treatment plans to report. Frequent, concise, and well-focused notes are the most effective means of maintaining communication. In institutional settings, notes documenting each visit with the patient are often essential to establish eligibility for third-party reimbursement.

Enter your notes under headings to highlight the problem being discussed. Separate subjective from objective findings, state your assessment, and describe your diagnostic treatment plan.

When intensive psychotherapy is being used as a primary treatment modality, the detail in progress notes will depend upon the degree of confidentiality afforded by the medical record. Psychotherapists often limit their notes in the hospital records to the general directions of treatment; specific details of the therapy are kept private. Staff observations and decisions related to the patient's management are recorded in greater detail.

DISCHARGE OR TRANSFER SUMMARY

When passing on responsibility to another therapist or service, you should convey the maximum amount of useful information about a patient in the most clear and concise manner possible. Such a summary does not generally exceed a page or two in length. Include: chief complaint; the most important aspects of the history; a summary of major findings in physical and mental status examinations; laboratory and other studies; initial diagnosis; treatment and results; new developments; final diagnoses; recommendations for future care.

REFERENCES

1. Menninger KA: *A Manual for Psychiatric Case Study,* ed 2. New York, Grune & Stratton, 1962. The Menninger Clinic Monograph Series, No 8.
2. Bird B: *Talking with Patients,* ed 2. Philadelphia, Lippincott, 1973.
3. Sullivan HS: *The Psychiatric Interview.* New York, WW Norton, 1954.
4. Colby KM: *A Primer for Psychotherapists.* New York, Ronald Press, 1951.
5. Gill MM, Newman R, Redlich FC: *The Initial Interview in Psychiatric Practice.* New York, International Universities Press, 1954.
6. MacKinnon RA, Michels R: *The Psychiatric Interview in Clinical Practice.* Philadelphia, WB Saunders, 1971.
7. Garrett A: *Interviewing: The Principles and Methods.* New York, Family Welfare Association of America, 1942.
8. Morgan WC Jr, Engel GL: *The Clinical Approach to the Patient.* Philadelphia, WB Saunders, 1969.
9. American Psychiatric Association Committee on Nomenclature and Statistics: *Diagnostic and Statistical Manual of Mental Disorders,* ed 3. Washington, DC, American Psychiatric Association, 1980.
10. Denny-Brown D: *Handbook of Neurological Examination and Case Recording,* ed 2. Cambridge, MA, Harvard University Press, 1982.
11. Keller, MB, Manschreck TC: The bedside mental status examination—reliability and validity. *Comp Psychiatry* 1981;22:500–511.

Chapter 3

DELIRIUM AND DEMENTIA

RICHARD B. CORRADI, M.D.

Organic brain syndromes are characterized by cognitive, psychological, and behavioral abnormalities associated with transient or permanent brain dysfunction. Brain dysfunction may be due to diffuse or focal primary brain disease, or a systemic illness which secondarily affects the brain. Delirium and dementia are the most important, as well as the most common, organic brain syndromes (1); both result from relatively diffuse brain damage or dysfunction. Other DSM-III (2) syndromes are either associated with focal brain lesions or produced by endogenous or exogenous chemical factors.

The Concept of Cerebral Insufficiency

The global impairment of cognitive function which characterizes delirium and dementia can be understood as the consequence of cerebral insufficiency (3). The manifestations of cerebral insufficiency are related to their organic substrate—the brain—in the same manner as is the decompensation of other organs, such as heart, kidney, or liver. Analogous to the more familiar types of organ failure, cerebral insufficiency occurs when there is interference with the function of the organ as a whole, for whatever reason. Whether it occurs in the liver, kidney, or brain, this interference can be the result of two basic processes: 1. the failure of metabolic processes to maintain the organ's function; 2. the death of enough cellular units to render organ function insufficient. In the brain, the former process (delirium) is potentially reversible; the latter (dementia) frequently is not.

Impaired cognition is the feature of cerebral insufficiency which is essential to the diagnosis of delirium and dementia. Basic cognitive functions are: orientation; memory; attention or concentration; perception; thinking. A person's intellectual capability depends upon the integrity of these cognitive functions. "Intellect" is the capacity to receive new information, compare it with past experience, apply abstract or general concepts, and synthesize appropriate responses in a coherent, logical way. Comprehension, apperception, or "grasp," i.e., the awareness of one's immediate reality, with full comprehension of its complexities and significance, is an extension of the cognitive functions. Comprehension is the basis of good judgment. These functions are impaired to varying degrees in delirium and dementia.

Cerebral insufficiency is more complicated than other organ failure because the brain is also the substrate for personality organization. The cognitive functions may also be thought of as basic "ego" functions, upon which depend other ego functions such as reality testing, appropriate discharge of emotions, repression of primitive modes of thinking, control and regulation of instinctual drives, and self-awareness. Defects in the latter ego functions frequently result from organic mental disorders. However, personality and emotional manifestations are highly variable and non-specific—i.e., similar disturbances are seen in "functional" (no demonstrable organic pathology) psychiatric disorders. Delirium and dementia, particularly in their early stages, can simulate almost any "functional" psychiatric disease, and are frequently misdiagnosed when mental status examination of cognitive functions is not performed.

Thus, *diagnosis of delirium and dementia must be based upon impairment of basic cognitive functions: disorientation; memory loss; impaired concentration; disordered perception and thinking.*

DELIRIUM

The DSM-III (2) diagnostic criteria for Delirium are:
A. Clouding of consciousness (reduced clarity of awareness of the environment), with reduced capacity to shift, focus, and sustain attention to environmental stimuli.
B. At least two of the following:
   (1) Perceptual disturbance: misinterpretations, illusions, or hallucinations.
   (2) Speech that is at times incoherent.
   (3) Disturbance of sleep-wakefulness cycle, with insomnia or daytime drowsiness.
   (4) Increased or decreased psychomotor activity.
C. Disorientation and memory impairment (if testable).
D. Clinical features that develop over a short period of time (usually hours to days) and tend to fluctuate over the course of a day.
E. Evidence, from the history, physical examination, or laboratory tests, of a specific organic factor judged to be etiologically related to the disturbance.

Nomenclature. "Delirium," the official, preferred term for this syndrome, implies that the patient's clinical state fulfills the above criteria. Much misunderstanding has resulted from the use of other terms with definitions which are frequently known only to the user (e.g., acute confusional state, toxic psychosis, metabolic encephalopathy, acute exogenous reaction type, etc.). Referring to a patient as simply "confused" is meaningless and should be avoided.

Clinical Features (2). Worsening delirium tends to cause disorientation in the sequence of time, place, and person. Disorientation may be spotty (e.g., only to certain time elements, with orientation in other spheres intact) or variable (e.g., more pronounced at certain times than at others). It is typically worse at night when visual and other cues to orientation are diminished; patients in early or mild delirium may be disoriented only at night. Disorientation to person (not knowing one's identity) is an ominous sign which usually portends stupor or coma. Disoriented patients may mistake strangers for persons familiar to them; this may represent an ego-adaptive response.

Recent memory is more impaired than remote. Historical, emotionally meaningful, and "overlearned" material may be relatively well preserved in mild delirium and dementia, while retention of recently acquired information may be severely impaired. As delirium worsens, remote memory also becomes progressively more affected. In severe delirium and some forms of dementia, retention of new information may be almost non-existent (e.g., names of three test objects may not be retained for 20–30 seconds). "Confabulation" refers to the use of fictitious or anachronistic information to fill in memory blanks. It occurs infrequently in delirium, is sometimes seen in dementia, and is probably an unconscious restitutive maneuver.

The concentration disorder in delirium usually involves difficulty in shifting, focusing, and sustaining attention. The patient is easily distracted by irrelevant external stimuli (e.g., noises and visual objects), and internal stimuli (e.g., preoccupation with one's own bewildering thoughts, perceptions, and feelings). It may be difficult or impossible to obtain a coherent history because the patient's attention wanders.

The perceptual disturbances in delirium exist on a continuum of severity, progressing from simple distortions, through illusions, to hallucinations. Although perceptual distortions are common even in mild delirium, they are often missed because the physician does not inquire about them. The patient may not volunteer this information because he thinks he's "going crazy." Motion pictures and TV simulate the perceptual distortions experienced by a delirious person when, for example, they show the subjective perceptual experiences of a person regaining consciousness after a blow to the head— visual images are blurred and out of focus for several moments, before gradually becoming more sharply "tuned in;" voices and other sounds briefly seem distant, muffled, or distorted. A bed-ridden delirious patient experiences similar perceptual distortions which frequently persist for the duration of the delirium. Illusions, or misinterpretations of actual perceptual stimuli, are also common, e.g., mistaking the sound of a door slamming for a pistol shot; perceiving folds in the bed clothes as snakes. Hallucinations are more dramatic, but less common, than perceptual distortions or illusions. A hallucination is defined as a perceptual experience that occurs in the absence of an external perceptual stimulus, e.g., perceiving a group of menacing people hovering over the bed when there is actually no one there. Visual hallucinations are the most common in delirium, although hallucinations may occur in other sensory modalities as well.

The belief in the reality of hallucinations constitutes a delusion, which is a disorder of thinking. This delusional thinking frequently leads to emotional and behavioral responses consistent with the hallucinatory content. For example, a delirious patient hallucinates people with scowling faces and menacing postures, and becomes convinced that his life is in danger (a delusion); he then either becomes panicky and flees, or takes action against his imagined tormentors. A disorder of thinking more common than delusions is the inability to maintain a coherent stream of thought. The delirious patient's thinking is fragmented and disjointed, rather than logical and goal-directed. Mild delirium may be characterized by either slowing or acceleration of thought, while thinking may be totally disorganized in more severe cases. The thinking disorder is, of course, reflected in the patient's speech, which may be slowed and underproductive, pressured and rapid-fire, or incoherent. Patients frequently make loose associations, jumping from one subject to another with no apparent logical connection between ideas. It should be recognized that the thought disorder described for delirium is sometimes similar to the formal thought disorder frequently seen in schizophrenia (See Chapter 4, Schizophrenia). Both disorders apparently represent a regression to "primary process" thinking. In delirium, the regression results from an organic insult to the brain which compromises "ego" function; the reasons for impaired "ego" function in schizophrenia are as yet unknown. The qualifying phrase, "in an intact sensorium," is, therefore, added to any definition of schizophrenia to indicate that other important cognitive functions are unimpaired.

As indicated above, DSM-III mentions "clouding of consciousness" as a cardinal sign of delirium. This is an ambiguous concept which is defined parenthetically in DSM-III as "reduced clarity of awareness of the environment," and related to the attention or concentration disorder in delirium. The concept is actually closer to the disorder of comprehension or grasp that results from global impairment of all the cognitive functions, not just attention. It is not sufficient to simply describe a patient in a mental status examination as having a "clouded consciousness;" each of the cognitive functions upon which this judgment is based should be tested and described.

The sleep-wakefulness cycle and *level* of consciousness are disturbed in delirium. Level of consciousness can vary from simple drowsiness, through increasing stages of torpor, to stupor and semicoma. At the other extreme, some delirious patients are hypervigilant and have great difficulty sleeping. Fluctuations from a depressed level of consciousness to excitement and sleeplessness may occur. Vivid dreams and nightmares may merge with hallucinations.

Psychomotor activity is usually disturbed. Many patients are agitated and restless. Common manifestations of psychomotor agitation include picking at the bedclothes, purposeless attempts to get out of bed, striking out at imaginary objects, and sudden changes of position. Some patients experience decreased psychomotor activity, with sluggishness or almost catatonic immobility. Levels of psychomotor activity often shift abruptly from one extreme to another.

Associated Emotional Features. Although various emotional disturbances always accompany the overwhelming cognitive dysfunction occurring in delirium, they are not diagnostically distinctive. They include anxiety, fear, depression, irritability, anger, euphoria, and apathy. During the course of a delirium, some patients abruptly and unpredictably shift from one of these emotional states to another; others seem to maintain the same emotional state throughout the episode. Fear, which is common, may become panic in the face of threatening hallucinations and delusions. Actions taken in response to hallucinations may be deliberately or accidentally self-injurious.

Etiological Factors. The causes of delirium usually lie outside the nervous system and include: systemic infections; metabolic disorders such as hypoxia, hypercarbia, hypoglycemia, ionic imbalances, hepatic or renal disease, or thiamine deficiency; post-operative states; and substance intoxication and withdrawal. Delirium also occurs in hypertensive encephalopathy, following seizures, and on regaining consciousness after head trauma (DSM-III) (2).

Course. Onset of delirium is usually fairly acute. It may begin abruptly, e.g., after head injury or seizure, or evolve over hours or days, e.g., secondary to systemic illness or metabolic imbalance. Slow evolution often includes prodromal symptoms, such as restlessness, insomnia, daytime somnolence, vivid dreams and nightmares, hypersensitivity to perceptual stimuli, and loss of clarity in thinking.

Symptoms of delirium typically fluctuate, becoming worse during sleepless nights. More lucid intervals may occur at any time, but are common in the morning—often precluding diagnosis during medical rounds.

Recovery from delirium is often complete, if the underlying causative disorder is either self-limited or quickly corrected. If a persistent metabolic disorder results in permanent cerebral damage, delirium can progress to dementia or coma and death.

Predisposing Factors. While delirium can occur at any age, children and the elderly are especially susceptible. Dementia and preexisting brain damage, from any cause, increase vulnerability.

In many cases of delirium, particularly in hospitalized patients, there are multiple causative factors, e.g., fever, plus electrolyte imbalance, plus hypoxia, plus prescribed drugs—any one of which may be insufficient to cause delirium by itself but does so in combination. Susceptible patients succumb to delirium under less toxic stress than others, e.g., an elderly, demented individual may become floridly delirious secondary to a moderate fever; a young adult may sustain the same temperature elevation without any cognitive impairment.

A number of clinically important *environmental stresses* predispose to delirium: sensory and sleep deprivation; sensory overload; unfamiliar or threatening surroundings; physical immobilization. These factors have become increasingly important because many modern hospital settings, such as the CCU and ICU, subject patients to just such stresses. These environmental stresses usually combine with organic factors to produce delirium; they may, however, be sufficient by themselves to cause delirium in otherwise susceptible people, such as the elderly.

Diagnosis and Treatment. Delirium is significantly underdiagnosed in the hospital setting. The agitated or psychotic delirious patient gets a psychiatric consultation, although the underlying delirium may not be identified by the referring physician; the "quietly" delirious patient, who is much more common, frequently goes unrecognized. Delirium is common in severely medically ill patients, particularly the elderly, alcoholics, and those with preexisting brain damage.

Diagnosis rests upon the physician's high level of awareness and a mental status examination to demonstrate the global impairment of cognitive function (See Chapter 2, The Psychiatric Case Study). Most deliria may be detected during history-taking, and by the routine use of a few simple tests. Defects in attention and concentration are evidenced by the patient's inability to give a logical, coherent history, loosened connections between ideas, rambling, tangential responses to questions, and frequent distractions by irrelevant stimuli. Recent memory loss may be reflected by inaccuracies in the account of the events of the present illness or the hospital course. Defects in orientation may be manifested by behaviors inappropriate to the hospital setting (e.g., the patient behaving as though he were at home or in a familiar setting; misidentification of unfamiliar people for familiar ones), or inaccurate answers to questions about the time of day, date, day of the week, month, and year. Perceptual disorders may be evidenced by the patient's attending to hallucinated sights and sounds, frequently indicated by breaks in the conversational flow. When the latter occur, the patient should be asked what he is experiencing. The physician should specifically ask about less severe perceptual disorders, such as illusory misinterpretations and perceptual distortions, since the patient may not volunteer this information.

Some simple tests should be performed routinely when delirium is suspected. Serial subtraction (asking the patient to subtract 7s or 3s from 100 down to zero) tests both concentration and memory. Asking the patient to repeat a series of numbers both forward and backwards (digit span) tests attention, registration, and recall. Short-term memory can be tested by giving the patient 3 unrelated items to repeat and then recall after several minutes of distraction. Ability to abstract is tested by interpretation of familiar proverbs. The delirious patient has difficulty with abstract concepts and frequently will give a literal, concrete response.

The delirious patient's mental status examination should be recorded and subsequently repeated in a standardized fashion, so that the course of the delirium can be followed. The patient who becomes mildly delirious during the course of his hospitalization is frequently frightened and bewildered by his experience, and may attempt to conceal it. The physician's brief, simple explanation of the phenomenon may both reassure the patient and ensure his cooperation in its assessment.

Treatment of delirium depends upon the identification and correction, if possible, of the underlying etiologic factors. Etiology usually involves a systemic process secondarily affecting cerebral metabolism, which is often readily identifiable in the hospitalized patient. Treatment of systemic infection, restoration of electrolyte or metabolic balance, appropriate management of a drug withdrawal syndrome, or removal of offending drugs may then alleviate the delirium. Causative factors are often multiple, and may include environmental stresses—which are often correctable if recognized by the physician. The patient's drug regimen should always be carefully reviewed, since prescribed medication frequently plays a primary or secondary role in the etiology of delirium. Obtaining a detailed medical history from relatives or other knowledgeable sources is essential in an Emergency Ward evaluation of delirium, and may reveal pertinent etiologic data, such as chronic medical illness, trauma, or recent drug or alcohol abuse. A delirious patient with unexplained fever should undergo lumbar puncture so the cerebrospinal fluid can be examined for CNS infection.

Management. Purely symptomatic drug treatment of delirium often does more harm than good, and may obscure etiologic factors. When agitated behavior is dangerous or interferes with medical treatment, however, the judicious use of the benzodiazepines or certain neuroleptics, such as haloperidol (4), may be indicated. Nighttime sedation may also be helpful to the sleepless delirious patient, but barbiturate-like hypnotics should be avoided. In some drug and alcohol withdrawal deliria, more specific drug management is indicated, e.g., reintoxication with barbiturates and gradual tapering of dosage in barbiturate withdrawal; benzodiazepines in delirium tremens.

Interpersonal, psychological, and environmental considerations are very important in the management of the delirious patient; this is particularly true in deliria with secondary psychotic features, such as delirium tremens. Scrupulous attention must be paid to the prevention of self-injury with patients suffering from extreme agitation and apprehension. Threatening hallucinations and misinterpretations of perceptual stimuli, combined with poor judgment and confusion, may lead to impulsive, self-destructive, or aggressive behavior, e.g., misidentifying a window for a door; striking out against hospital personnel who may be delusionally regarded as persecutors. Such patients may require removal from the multi-bed ward and constant attendance. If possible, seclusion is preferable to the use of mechanical body restraints, which may cause further agitation as a confused and excited patient struggles to release himself. In addition, these restraints may be interpreted in a delusional manner, thus confirming the patient's belief that he is in danger.

Thoughtful use of the seclusion room is important. It is often necessary to remove items of furniture to prevent injury. Personal articles which could be injurious should be removed, and smoking should not be allowed. Windows should be securely screened. The room should be quiet and lighted, with a minimum of unnecessary stimuli. A patient in seclusion should not be left unattended. The attendant preferably should be experienced in managing delirious patients and familiar with the nature of the illness. He can allay the agitated and hallucinating patient's anxiety and apprehension if he understands his role in helping the patient to "test reality." When the patient misidentifies persons or objects, the attendant can help correct his misperceptions, e.g., "No, that man is not a gangster who has come here to kill you. He is Dr. Smith. You have been ill and confused and are in University Hospitals for medical treatment. You are safe here." When the patient hallucinates threatening objects, the attendant can correct and reassure, e.g., "There are no rats in this room, so there is no reason for you to try to leave. What you seem to be seeing comes from your illness, and you will realize this when your confusion has cleared up. I will stay with you and help you to understand what is going on. I am a nurse and you are in University Hospitals for medical treatment." The patient's relatives are best suited to function in this role as "reality tester," as familiar persons are always more reassuring. If they are available, they can be encouraged to work out a regular schedule to attend the patient and should be instructed as to their function.

Knowledge of the delirious patient's need for help in ordering his sensory input and testing reality leads to other obvious measures for allaying anxiety. Delirium is usually worse at night, when visual cues to orientation are lacking; the seclusion room should, therefore, remain lighted. Any diagnostic or treatment procedures should be carefully explained to the patient. Even a procedure as routine as venipuncture can be delusionally interpreted as an assault and greatly increase agitation. Procedures which can safely wait until the acute phase of the delirium is resolved should be postponed. Unnecessary noises and activities should be avoided, as should whispered conversations which the patient can overhear and misinterpret. The behavior of those in attendance to the patient should be reassuring and anxiety-allaying.

DEMENTIA

The DSM-III (2) diagnostic criteria for dementia are:
A. A loss of intellectual abilities of sufficient severity to interfere with social or occupational functioning
B. Memory impairment
C. At least one of the following:
    (1) Impairment of abstract thinking as manifested by concrete interpretation of proverbs, inability to find similarities and differences between related words, difficulty in defining words and concepts, and other similar tasks
    (2) Impaired judgment
    (3) Other disturbances of higher cortical function, such as aphasia (disorder of language due to brain dysfunction), apraxia (inability to carry out motor activities despite comprehension and motor function), agnosia (failure to recognize or identify objects despite intact sensory function), "constructional difficulty" (e.g., inability to copy three-dimensional figures, assemble blocks, or arrange sticks in specified designs)
    (4) Personality change, i.e., alteration or accentuation of premorbid traits
D. State of consciousness not clouded (i.e., does not meet the criteria for Delirium or Intoxication although these may be superimposed).
E. Either (1) or (2):
    (1) Evidence from the history, physical examination, or laboratory tests, of a specific organic factor that is judged to be etiologically related to the disturbance
    (2) In the absence of such evidence, an organic factor necessary for the development of the syndrome can be presumed if conditions other than Organic Mental Disorders have been reasonably excluded and

if the behavioral change represents cognitive impairment in a variety of areas.

Clinical Features (2). Both delirium and dementia involve relatively global cognitive impairment. The DSM-III again refers to the vague concept of "clouding of consciousness" as a distinguishing feature, present in delirium but not in dementia. Differences in the nature of onset and adaptive personality features may be more helpful distinctions. The cognitive disorder in delirium is usually relatively acute in onset, and can produce a profound mental disorganization. When the personality is suddenly "overwhelmed" by the intellectual dysfunction, dramatic and florid symptoms often result, e.g., hallucinations; poorly-formed delusions; panic-like fear; agitation. In contrast, dementia, which is frequently slower and more progressive in onset, often causes less acute personality disruption. Since the "ego" has time to adapt to the decremental cognitive functioning, symptomatology may be less florid, although functional impairment may be just as great. In fact, when dementia is sudden in onset, as after severe head trauma, the initial clinical picture is often that of a delirium with marked behavioral disorganization. As the acute effects of cerebral trauma (e.g., edema) resolve, the patient often achieves a more stable personality adjustment to the residual cognitive loss, however severe it may be.

The orientation of mild or moderately demented patients may be dependent upon familiar environmental cues. If patients are removed from their familiar surroundings, orienting cues are lost and disorientation may be more pronounced. This may occur, for example, in a shopping mall, or during a short walk away from home; it typically occurs in the unfamiliar, anxiety-provoking hospital environment. It should be remembered that an unfamiliar and threatening environment, in addition to sensory deprivation or overload, sleep deprivation, and immobilization, is a predisposing factor to delirium in vulnerable individuals. In the elderly, mildly demented person who is hospitalized for any reason, a delirium is often superimposed upon the underlying dementia, since the hospital environment unfortunately provides most or all of these environmental stresses. The physician who forgets this will despair, along with the family, that the deteriorated delirium-plus-dementia clinical state is permanent. In fact, once the medical problem which required hospitalization is corrected and the patient returns to his familiar environment, he will probably return to his baseline level of cognitive functioning. Elderly people are sometimes moved from hospitals to nursing homes because their deteriorated mental status is regarded as permanent. This misconception is apparently confirmed by the patient's progressive deterioration in the even more stressful nursing home setting.

Memory is usually the most prominent cognitive loss in dementia. Mild memory loss may simply appear to be forgetfulness. More severe impairment may cause the individual to forget names, directions, conversations, and the day's events. He may forget to complete tasks after being interrupted, sometimes placing himself and others in danger. A severely demented person may forget the names of close relatives, his own occupation or date of birth, and even his own name. Although remote memory may be affected in a spotty fashion, it tends to be better preserved than recent memory. Short-term memory may be tested by asking the patient to remember the names of several unrelated objects after a few minutes of distraction; long-term memory can be tested by asking about past events. Some patients suffering from a fairly stable dementia "live in the past;" their conversation consists largely of rambling reminiscences about past life events. Since the past is better remembered, and presumably more pleasant than the present, this may be an ego-adaptive response to cognitive loss.

Rigidity of attention or concentration is often seen in demented patients, as opposed to the distractability of delirium. When giving their histories, demented patients may be unable to easily shift their attention from one topic to another. Once they marshall their concentration on a topic, they become "hung up" and cannot focus on new material. This frequently manifests as "perseveration," e.g., the carry-over of material, often in the form of repetitious words or phrases, from a relevant context to one in which it is either irrelevant or only peripherally relevant.

In a stable or slowly progressive dementia, perceptual disorders tend to occur, as does more severe disorientation, in situations of diminished or unfamiliar perceptual cues, i.e., at night and in strange or anxiety-provoking environments. These settings can provoke perceptual distortions and even hallucinations. However, hallucinations and delusions are more common in sudden onset or rapidly progressive dementias.

Impairment of abstract thinking is the most common disorder of thinking in dementia. (Since this is also common in chronic schizophrenia, the symptom by itself does not discriminate between the two disorders.) Demented patients have been described as "stimulus bound"—i.e., they react in a literal, concrete fashion because of their impaired ability to abstract, generalize, or symbolize. They will miss the point of a joke, and cannot cope with novel tasks that require processing of new information or abstract concepts. As a result, they may rigidly adhere to the old and familiar, avoiding new situations, tasks and ideas. When confronted with the latter, they sometimes become befuddled and panicky (Goldstein's "catastrophic reaction"). Abstractability can be tested by asking about proverb interpretations or similarities and differences between related words. Be suspicious of the patient who refuses to comply with formal mental status testing. The patient who appears "insulted" by the "easy questions," trivializes the procedure, or employs a variety of other defensive maneuvers may be hiding an inability to perform.

Some neurologic disorders which produce dementia may make speech vague, stereotyped, and circumstantial; aphasias, agnosias, and apraxias may also be present. Visual-motor organization is also impaired. It can be tested by having the patient copy three-dimensional figures, assemble blocks, or arrange objects in specific designs.

Judgment and control of impulses often suffer as a result of the global cognitive impairment. Inattention to appearance and personal hygiene, deterioration of ethical and moral standards, coarse language and vulgar jokes, imprudent business decisions, uncharacteristic sexual behavior, impulsivity, and irritability may all occur. Dementing processes that attack the frontal lobes in particular are apt to affect judgment and impulse control.

Associated Emotional Features. Personality changes are inevitable and, as with delirium, variable and non-specific. Anxiety, depression, apathy, and social withdrawal, however, are common reactions to an awareness of deterioriating intellectual functioning. Patients with mild dementia often attempt to conceal and compensate for cognitive loss. Preexisting personality traits may be altered or accentuated. In the latter case, individuals become "more like themselves": preexisting traits of suspiciousness and a tendency to project blame may evolve into frankly paranoid ideation; a propensity to depression in the face of loss may lead to severe depression; traits of excessive orderliness and attention to detail may evolve into rigidly compulsive patterns of behavior (sometimes adaptive); impulsive people may become more impulsive.

People with dementia are particularly vulnerable to physical and psychosocial stresses. While intellectual deficits may be compensated for in a well-structured routine of daily living, they are greatly aggravated by new stresses, e.g., retirement, bereavement, hospitalization.

Etiological Factors. Primary degenerative dementia of the Alzheimer type is the most common dementia. Other causes include: central nervous system infections (including tertiary neurosyphilis, tuberculous and fungal meningitis, viral encephalitis, and Jakob-Creutzfeldt disease); brain trauma (especially chronic subdural hematoma); toxic-metabolic disturbances (such as pernicious anemia, folic-acid deficiency, hypothyroidism, bromide intoxication); vascular disease (multi-infarct dementia); normal-pressure hydrocephalus; neurological diseases such as Huntington's chorea, multiple sclerosis, and Parkinson's disease; and post-anoxic or post-hypoglycemic states (DSM-III) (2).

Course. Dementia occurs primarily in the elderly, although certain of the above etiologic factors may produce dementia at any age. The nature of onset and course of the disease depends upon the underlying etiology. Dementia which results from a clearly defined episode of neurologic disease, e.g., cerebral hypoxia, encephalitis; brain trauma, is sudden in onset, but may then stabilize. Alzheimer's disease (primary degenerative dementia) is usually insidious in onset, with a slow and progressive course over several years. Gradual onset dementia may also result from brain tumors, subdural hematomas, and metabolic factors. When the etiologic disorder is treatable, e.g., hypothyroidism; subdural hematoma; normal pressure hydrocephalus; neurosyphilis, dementia may be reversed or arrested. Clinical improvement is less likely, however, if there has been widespread structural cerebral damage.

Diagnosis and Treatment. As with delirium, the diagnosis of dementia depends upon the use of the mental status examination to demonstrate the impaired cognition. However, many patients with dementia first come to physicians with personality, emotional, or behavioral problems—not with complaints of cognitive dysfunction. Frequently, initial mild intellectual deficits go unrecognized by the family, or are concealed by the patient, while the associated behavioral features are prominent and can easily be regarded as "functional." The unwary physician may be easily fooled if he does not perform a careful mental status examination. Depression is a very common presenting complaint in elderly demented individuals. Depression secondary to an evolving dementia can easily be misdiagnosed as functional. Conversely, some physicians mistakenly attribute most depressions in the elderly to an "organic brain syndrome." The differential diagnosis is sometimes difficult because the psychomotor retardation and mental slowing which accompany depression (pseudodementia) may make concentration on mental status examination tasks very difficult. The question can usually be resolved by patient, persistent efforts at having the individual participate in the mental status examination; if this cannot be accomplished, a neurological workup is essential.

Even when an affective disorder does not confound the clinical picture, the diagnosis of early dementia may be obscured by the patient's physical or functional complaints, or by the use of well-preserved social skills to conceal cognitive loss. For this reason the evaluation of an elderly person with suspected dementia should always include a careful history from informed relatives or friends, who will frequently document the patient's intellectual and functional deterioration. Additionally, any middle-aged or older patient who presents with personality changes or other recent-onset psychiatric problems, particularly in the absence of a psychiatric history, should be suspected of having an organic brain syndrome.

In addition to the history, psychiatric interview, mental status examination, and medical and neurological examinations, a standardized battery of ancillary diagnostic procedures are indicated in the diagnostic workup of dementia. Wells (5) has recommended the following diagnostic procedures to identify potentially remediable dementias: blood studies, including complete blood count, serological test for syphilis, standard metabolic screening battery (e.g., SMAC–20), thyroid function studies, vitamin B 12 and folate levels; computerized cranial tomography; urinalysis; chest x-ray. In cases of suspected dementia in which the clinical mental status examination is equivocal, neuropsychological testing may be helpful.

Potentially remediable causes are found in perhaps 15–20% (5,6) of dementias. These include normal pressure hydrocephalus, resectable mass lesions, thyroid disease, pernicious anemia, and hepatic failure. Alzheimer's disease is by far the most common cause of irreversible dementias, accounting for some 50% of all dementias. Other irreversible dementias include alcohol-related dementias, multi-infarct dementias, and Huntington's chorea. A few dementias, while not reversible, may be arrested if the etiologic factor is corrected, e.g., alcoholism; neurosyphilis; epilepsy.

Management. Careful management and supportive treatment for demented patients in whom the process is not reversible is essential, and may mean the difference between fairly successful functioning in a home environment and deterioration in a nursing home or other institutional setting. Management considerations include: environmental manipulation; supportive psychotherapy; judicious pharmacotherapy; family support and counselling. Such measures may significantly enhance the quality of life for patients with mild or stable dementias, as well as those in the earlier phases of Alzheimer's disease.

The demented person's environment should be as well-structured, familiar, and predictable as possible. He should remain in familiar surroundings, ideally in his own home with his own possessions and familiar persons, for as long as possible. Well-meaning relocations to distant retirement communities with better climates, or rotating residence in the homes of various children, can produce devastating cognitive and emotional consequences. Activities should be routinized, structured, and non-demanding. Daily living should be a well-structured routine, consistent, predictable, and without surprises. The entire day may have to be planned for some patients, with self-care activities, housekeeping, meals, and diversionary activities performed on a firmly-established rote schedule. Some demented patients who can refer to a written schedule may require less supervision and may experience a sense of greater autonomy. The degree to which environment can be controlled, of course, will vary greatly, depending upon the people and resources available, the severity of the dementia, and the patient's residual personality strengths. Whatever the reality limitations, striving for structure, familiarity, and predictable routine should be a cardinal principle in management of the demented.

Regular contact with a familiar and knowledgeable professional, such as the family physician, may be extremely helpful to both the patient and family. Supportive psychotherapy by such a person should be based upon careful psychological evaluation and knowledge of the patient's level of cognitive functioning, as assessed by serial mental status examinations. Therapy should be directed toward maximizing independent functioning within the patient's limitations. This requires helping the patient utilize preexisting personality strengths and adaptive mechanisms of defense to cope with diminished intellectual resources, e.g., intensification of obsessive-compulsive traits, such as keeping a detailed notebook as an aid to memory or enlisting the patient's participation in adhering to a daily schedule. On the other hand, accentuation of maladaptive defenses may impair coping skills, e.g., the patient prone to the use of projective mechanisms (blaming his failures on others) may become paranoid as dementia progresses. When based upon an established relationship of trust, the physician's sensitive exploration of such reactions may be used to suggest alternate, more realistic reactions to the patient, thus aiding him in reality testing and fostering more mature defenses.

Assisting the demented patient to accept realistic limitations depends upon the counselor's understanding of the processes of grief and mourning in response to loss. People who are experiencing a progressive decline in intellectual functions are suffering the loss of the very essence of their selfhood. The loss of memory, judgment, basic coping skills, higher integrative functions, and the uniquely personal aspects of personality strikes at the roots of self-identity and self-esteem. The concept of one's self as an autonomous, capable, independently functioning person is lost. Such a dissolution of the self almost invariably produces reactions of grief—which can become depression, and anger—which can become rage. Characteristic defense mechanisms are called upon to handle these affects, but their efficacy is frequently compromised by the dementing process which makes them necessary. In the late phase of Alzheimer's disease, the destruction of the cortical substrate of personality may strip the patient of all but the most primitive defense mechanisms, with profound regression as the consequence. The care required by such patients is similar to that of very young children.

Earlier in the dementing process, and with stable dementias, a supportive psychotherapeutic approach should address the grief process, aiding the patient in the work of mourning on the model of psychotherapy of reactive depression. Some patients are receptive to expressing their feelings about the losses they are experiencing, and are relieved to find a person who understands their anger and depression. Anger turned against the self in the form of guilt or unrealistic fantasies of self-blame for their plight can often be productively explored. Adaptive defenses should be encouraged, and those which are maladaptive subjected to reality testing.

Denial is a common defense. Some demented patients dwell upon the better-remembered, more pleasant historical past, thus avoiding the painful present with its recurrent reminders of impaired functioning. Such a defense may even be accompanied by an insistence that there is "nothing wrong." This may be alarming to relatives, as well as physicians, who tend to regard patients' denial as pathological. The patient who verbally "denies" being ill, yet behaves in a manner appropriate to his disability, obviously "knows" the truth at some level of consciousness; such a working defense should be respected. Defenses should, in general, be regarded as adaptive, unless they interfere significantly with appropriate medical treatment and management, or produce behaviors damaging to the patient and other persons.

Supportive psychotherapy of demented patients largely focuses on the "here and now," with emphasis on current affects and defensive patterns, rather than on the influence of antecedent childhood conflicts. The counselor should, however, be sensitive to cues from the patient about the usefulness of exploring the past. Some patients benefit greatly from a kind of life-review, deriving a sense of pride and accomplishment from a "job well done." Others are helped by relating anger and depression about cognitive loss to similar emotional reactions to past losses. This may aid the patient in integrating bewildering current feelings with those which were better understood in the past, and may even reveal remote determinants of present intense affects. The latter can sometimes be productively explored.

Areas of stress to which the patient is particularly vulnerable should be an ongoing focus in supportive psychotherapy, as these will change as dementia progresses. The therapist needs to know the demands and goals of the patient's activities in vocational, social, and self-care areas. Activities which tax coping resources are identified, and the patient is assisted in redirecting his efforts into more appropriate channels. This must be done with a sensitivity to the maintenance of a sense of dignity and self-esteem in patients who regard their diminishing functional capacities as evidence of failure.

The family also receives the most help from an ongoing relationship with the same person who works with the patient. He must be prepared to assist them with their own feelings of grief, helplessness, guilt, and anger—all of which are common responses to dementia in a loved one. They should be encouraged to express these feelings and regard them as expectable. Family members' reactions to their ambivalent feelings may range all the way from denial of the dementia to abandonment of the patient. Such extreme reactions, inimical to the patient's welfare, should be pointed out and the family helped to alter them.

Families also need to be educated about dementia and what they can do to help the patient—e.g., the nature of the cognitive defect; the patient's need for structure and predictable routine; the patient's level of functioning and the kind of care needed; his coping skills and stress points. Ultimately, the family may need help in arranging residential placement and working through their emotions about such an outcome. Group therapy experiences in which common concerns are shared with families of other demented patients may be extremely helpful.

Psychotropic drugs are sometimes useful in the management of dementia, but the usual guidelines for their usage must be modified. This is necessary because most demented patients are elderly and their pharmacokinetics differ from younger patients (7); demented, as well as elderly, individuals are also particularly prone to delirium-producing side effects of many psychotropics. Many of the commonly used tricyclic antidepressants (e.g., amitriptyline; imipramine) and the low-potency phenothiazines (e.g., chlorpromazine; thioridizine) have potent peripheral and central anticholinergic side effects. The central anticholinergic effects frequently cause delirium in the elderly and in the demented. If its source is not recognized, the delirium may be interpreted as a worsening of the dementia; the offending drug dosage may then be increased rather than reduced or removed. As a general rule, the psychotropics should be started in very low doses and increased very gradually, with close attention to possible adverse side effects. Often the required dosage is one-third or one-half of that used in younger patients.

Nighttime insomnia and daytime agitation are common problems in dementia. Sleepless nights may produce a delirious overlay to the dementia, with greater disorientation and memory loss, illusory and hallucinatory phenomena, and even delusional thinking occurring at night. Daytime functioning is, in turn, impaired by agitation and a carryover of psychotic symptoms. A vicious cycle may be established when daytime agitation further impairs sleep. An initial approach to this problem is the prescription of enough bedtime hypnotic to ensure a full night's sleep. Flurazepam or temazepam may be tried first; chloral hydrate is a rational second choice (7). Barbiturates should be avoided because of their propensity to produce paradoxical agitation and rebound insomnia. When insomnia is corrected, the patient's daytime cognitive functioning frequently improves. If agitation and psychotic-like symptoms still persist, a daytime neuroleptic may be useful, e.g., haloperidol or thioridizine, in divided daily dosages of 0.5-2 mgs and 20-75 mgs, respectively.

Persistent psychotic symptoms, such as hallucinations and paranoid delusions, secondary to a dementing process can be regarded as target symptoms, just as in the functional psychoses, and treated with a neuroleptic. Haloperidol, in a initial daily dosage of 0.5-2 mgs, with cautious increases as necessary, is a good choice. The goal should be to moderate psychotic symptoms to the extent that they impair the patient's functioning, not necessarily to abolish them completely. Paranoid ideation in particular may be extremely resistent to drug treatment; overly vigorous attempts to correct it with neuroleptics may product excessive sedation and severe extrapyramidal side effects.

Depression occurs frequently in demented patients. Many physicians regard it as an expectable concomitant of dementia and are nihilistic about treatment. In addition, depression may not be diagnosed if vegetative signs of depression, such as psychomotor retardation or agitation, inability to concentrate, insomnia, and anorexia, are erroneously attributed to the dementia. In general, patients with early or stable forms of dementia who meet the DSM-III criteria for major depression (2) should be treated in the same manner as younger patients with depression. Such patients frequently respond to somatic treatments with a gratifying improvement in their quality of life. Antidepressants with relatively lower anticholinergic potential are rational choices, e.g., desipramine or trazadone in initial daily dosages of 25–50 mgs and 50–100 mgs respectively. ECT may be used with patients who do not respond to antidepressants, or those with severe cardiac disease. Unilateral ECT may minimize post-ECT delirium, and patients often require fewer treatments than those who are younger and physically healthy. Less severe depressions in the demented patient should be treated with psychotherapy.

REFERENCES

1. Lipowski ZJ: A new look at organic brain syndromes. *Am J Psychiatry* 1980;137:674–678.
2. American Psychiatric Association Committee on Nomenclature and Statistics: *Diagnostic and Statistical Manual of Mental Disorders,* ed 3. Washington, DC, American Psychiatric Association, 1980.
3. Engel GL, Romano J: Delirium, a syndrome of cerebral insufficiency. *J Chronic Dis* 1959;9:260–277.
4. Lipowski ZJ: *Delirium*. Springfield, IL, Charles Thomas, 1980.
5. Wells CE: Chronic brain disease: An overview. *Am J Psychiatry* 1978;135:1–12.
6. Beck JC, moderator: Dementia in the elderly: the silent epidemic. *Ann Intern Med* 1982;97:231–241.
7. Thompson TL, Moran MG, Nies AS: Psychotropic drug use in the elderly. *N Engl J Med* 1983;308:134–138 and 194–199.

GENERAL REFERENCES

American Psychiatric Association Committee on Nomenclature and Statistics: *Diagnostic and Statistical Manual of Mental Disorders,* ed 3. Washington, DC, American Psychiatric Association, 1980.
Lipowski ZJ: *Delirium*. Springfield, IL, Charles Thomas, 1980.
Wells CE (ed): *Dementia*. Philadelphia, FA Davis Co, 1978.

Chapter 4

SCHIZOPHRENIA
AND THE PARANOID DISORDERS
HOWARD S. SUDAK, M.D.

DEFINITION

According to DSM-III (1), "The essential features of the Schizophrenic Disorders are: the presence of certain psychotic features during the active phase of the illness, characteristic symptoms involving multiple psychological processes, deterioration from a previous level of functioning, onset before age 45, and a duration of at least six months. At some phase of the illness, Schizophrenia always involves delusions, hallucinations, or certain disturbances in the form of thought. The essential features of the Paranoid Disorders are persistent persecutory delusions or delusional jealousy, not due to any other mental disorder such as Schizophrenia, Schizophreniform, Affective, or Organic Mental Disorder." Although rather severe, exaggerated pictures are presented in this chapter for the sake of clarity, milder variations are more common. It is worth stressing that the group of schizophrenias confronts the student with an extremely confusing body of observational and theoretical data.

HISTORY

Despite a number of previous more enlightened periods (2), the idea of psychoses being evidence of possession by the devil was not permanently abandoned until the 19th century. Morel (1860) was the first to describe schizophrenic reactions as "demence precoce." In 1871, Hecker described a case of "hebephreniz," a term which he borrowed from Kahlbaum. Three years later, Kahlbaum introduced the term "catatonia" or "tension insanity." Kraepelin (1896) advanced schizophrenia nosology by suggesting that catatonic, hebephrenic, simple, and paranoid psychoses all be diagnosed under the term "dementia praecox." He viewed these illnesses as "organic" in nature, and used prognosis in classification. In 1906, Adolf Meyer suggested that these conditions be termed "reactions" because they were due to adaptive difficulties, rather than organic causes (3,4). The current major classification system was formulated by Eugen Bleuler in 1911. His work, *Dementia Praecox or the Group of Schizophrenias,* unified the primary disturbances and classified them on a more phenomenological basis than did Kraepelin. Bleuler considered "dementia praecox" an unsuitable term because many cases did not eventuate in dementia, and the onset was frequently not during the adolescent period. He preferred the term, "schizophrenia," as it emphasized the "split" or coexistence of contradictory tendencies, thoughts, and affects.

INCIDENCE

The general incidence rate of schizophrenia is approximately 1% of the population over 15 years of age—accounting for approximately 100,000 new cases per year (5). Although schizophrenia patients only account for 15–25% of all first admissions to public mental hospitals, their chronicity causes them to ultimately comprise about 50% of all the patients in state hospitals. Approximately two-thirds of the annual admissions are readmissions. With the advent of phenothiazines our state hospital beds shrank from a total of approximately 560,000 in 1955 to less than 200,000 by 1975. Since the number of admissions per year more than doubled (from 150,000 to 375,000) in that same period, one can see that the average lengths of stay markedly diminished.

There are no significant international, racial, sexual, or cultural variations in incidence. There are, however, cultural variations in the form of schizophrenia. Prevalence and, possibly, incidence are somewhat higher in low socioeconomic urban areas, i.e., those with the densest populations, highest crime rates, etc. This correlation is only applicable to large cities; it did not hold up in Hagerstown, Maryland, or Nova Scotia. These data are influenced by factors such as more intact family support systems in middle and upper-class socioeconomic groups and the migratory drift of schizophrenic patients toward the central city as they lose the ability to support themselves (6).

The age of onset ranges from late childhood to late middle-age. The disease occurs frequently in adolescence or early adulthood, although paranoid schizophrenia and other paranoid disorders occur significantly later. Kraepelin noted that 50% of the cases showed clear symptoms prior to age 25; onset over 40 is rare. Childhood schizophrenia is never diagnosed before age 5, and rarely before age 10 (7)—in contrast to early infantile autism, in which symptoms usually occur in the first year and always before age 5.

PRECIPITATION

Schizophrenia often appears to be precipitated by psychological stresses. Severe blows to one's self-esteem (narcissistic injuries), increased sexual (libidinal) urges, or a feeling of decreased control over sexual or aggressive impulses (particularly homosexual impulses) are frequent antecedents of a psychotic break. Using retrospective analysis, however, one may incorrectly appraise the consequences of the earliest symptoms as precipitants, i.e., a sexual indiscretion may be the result of the early phase of the disease, rather than its precipitant.

Approximately half of the initial episodes have no discernible precipitating events—only an insidious transition from a schizotypal or schizoid personality to the manifest psychosis. Affect seems to slowly become more rigid. The patient turns his or her attention inward, progressively becoming more withdrawn from the outside world. The family doctor may detect bizarre, obsessional or hypochondriacal ideation.

Patients who are aware of the changes in their personalities may become panic-stricken and present an acute suicidal risk. As they grow accustomed to their delusions over weeks to months of hospitalization, one often sees a marked diminution of this anxiety ("I understand it all now"). This is termed "restitution," in contrast to the earlier "breakdown phase," and this is achieved by modifying the external world of reality (8–12).

PSYCHOPATHOLOGY AND DIAGNOSIS (MENTAL STATUS IN SCHIZOPHRENIA)

Introduction

Bleuler emphasized that the major disturbance was due to a split within the thinking processes, rather than between thinking and affect. Thus, he felt the "primary symptom" was the loosening of associations, and he grouped these with the "secondary symptoms" of affective disturbance, ambivalence, and autism. These "fundamental symptoms" were seen as caused by the all-important associational defect; hallucinations, delusions, illusions, somatic symptoms, etc., were only "accessory" symptoms. People frequently refer to the "four A's"—"association defect, affect disturbances, ambivalence, and autism." Except for the associational defect, which he considered organic, Bleuler felt that all secondary symptoms were colored by the patient's life (13). For the sake of convenience, we can classify the symptoms in the following groups:

Formal Thinking Disorder

This refers to the thinking *form and process,* rather than its *content* per se. Initially, the splitting and loosening of associations may merely lead to vagueness and tangentiality. As the loosening becomes more extreme, it results in alliterations, analogies, clangs, blocking, flight-of-ideas, and, ultimately, scattering, fragmentation, and incoherence. As we listen to someone, we are normally aware of the progression of thoughts or ideas. In a mild loosening of associations, we may only notice that we're having some difficulty following the patient's train of thought. As associations become more and more loosened, it becomes progressively more difficult to follow the logical sequence from "paragraph to paragraph" and "sentence to sentence." Finally, even the words within a sentence lose their logical, grammatical sequencing, resulting in a "word-salad." In contrast to loosened associations, in a flight-of-ideas one can follow the associative links, but the patient's thoughts are racing—one thought leads to two others which lead to four others, etc.—and cannot all be expressed. The concept of "loosened associations" as a diagnostic hallmark of schizophrenia has been challenged by Andreasen (14). Condensations of speech may be responsible for the creation of neologisms. Contradictions are frequent. Pseudo-puns result when the concrete meanings of words are incorrectly used because the patient has difficulty with abstract concepts. Speech is often pressured and perseverative. The patient may be evasive or verbigerous. The use of proverb interpretations as a test for concrete thinking can be misleading, however, since this symptom is often present in organic brain syndromes or any diffuse cortical disease. Manic patients are more likely than schizophrenics to have flights-of-ideas, and may also have loosened associations. The schizophrenic's proverb interpretations may be more bizarre and idiosyncratic than those of patients with organic brain syndromes (15,16).

Schizophrenics frequently indulge in "dereistic" thinking, i.e., pleasurable thinking which tends to falsify reality, disregard logic, and become autistic fantasy. "Primary process," or wish-fulfilling, thinking employs condensation, displacement, substitution, and symbolization. Young children often employ this process, which may be understood as relating to the "pleasure principle," and ignores causal or temporal relationships. "Primary" process thinking is clearly seen in dreams, and may also be relevant to schizophrenic thinking. Psychotic thinking has, in fact, often been compared to the manifest dream.

Disturbances of Emotions

Quantitative changes, i.e., flattening or blunting of affect, often occurs, particularly after the end of the acute phase. The blunting of more refined feelings, such as sympathy, occurs in the early stages; more gross feelings, such as rage or sexual excitement, are often preserved longer. *Qualitative changes,* i.e., emotional lability and/or affect inappropriate to the thought content, are common. Thus, the patient may laugh as he speaks of his mother's death or cry as he relates a presumably pleasant experience (inappropriate affect). The patient who seems fearful as he tells of delusions of persecution is not considered to have inappropriate affect. The patient's lack of warmth and ability to empathize with others, plus the observer's difficulty in empathizing with the patient, are sometimes helpful in diagnosing schizophrenia. These affective changes are discussed in Corradi's work on the assessment of affect in Schizophrenia (17), and recently clinically validated by Reid *et al.* (18). Similar affective disturbances can also be noted in organic brain syndromes.

Alterations in Behavior

These are often subsumed under other headings: mannerisms; stereotyped behavior; various rituals, e.g., counting, touching, hoarding, decorativeness, assaultiveness; self-destructive and mutilative behavior. Although patients may ignore personal hygiene, openly display sexual behavior, behave irresponsibly, etc., the majority of behavior remains normal.

Disturbances of Volition

Patients may be stubborn, persistent, negative, suggestible, apathetic, paralyzed by ambivalence, or extremely impulsive. This category also includes the motor symptoms which are so prominent in catatonic excitement or stupor.

Disturbances of Perception (other than hallucinations)

These include: inability to differentiate between two tactile points on the body; impaired ability to become oriented in an artificially disordered environment; difficulties in attending to various visual or auditory cues. Currently, there is considerable interest in attempting to analyze visual tracking disturbances in schizophrenic patients (19–23).

Delusions

Delusions are false beliefs which may be conceptualized as disturbances of symbolization, rather than perception, i.e., the patient recognizes a "radio," but errs in interpreting its significance. Delusions have a personal meaning for the patient that is not shared by the patient's immediate social or ethnic groups. Delusions can be described as systematic, subtle, organized, grotesque, bizarre, fragmented, sexual, grandiose, persecutory, self-accusatory, nihilistic, or somatic. Primary delusions enlarge into many secondary delusions. "Ideas of reference" are beliefs that certain external events have special, personal significance. The presentation of concrete evidence to the contrary will diminish more normal ideas of reference or influence; psychotic "delusions of reference" will not, of course, be dispelled by such evidence. Everyone has had occasional neurotic ideas of reference. For instance, you walk into a room and everyone bursts out laughing. You wonder if they're laughing at you—is your fly unzipped? . . . are you trailing a stream of toilet paper? Once you have been reassured that the laughter had nothing to do with you, you are able to give up such a neurotic referential idea. Psychotic delusions of reference are fixed. A particularly common theme among schizophrenic patients is that their thoughts are being broadcasted, influenced, or controlled.

Hallucinations

Hallucinations indicate a profound loss of reality testing, and are not limited to schizophrenia (e.g., visual hallucinations are frequently seen in acute brain syndromes). Schizophrenics are prone to auditory hallucinations of a persecutory, grandiose nature; tactile, visceral, and gustatory hallucinations are less frequent. Olfactory hallucinations may indicate possible temporal lobe pathology.

Hallucinations can be defined as perceptions that are not based on external stimuli. In contrast, illusory phenomena are based on misperceived external stimuli, e.g., a child's teddy bear becomes a scary intruder in the dark. Illusions may or may not be psychotic; hallucinations and delusions are psychotic by definition.

GENERAL DIAGNOSTIC POINTS

Bleuler felt that eliciting evidence of the associational defect was pathognomonic for schizophrenia, and many people feel this is a diagnostic sine qua non. For practical purposes, the diagnoses may be tentatively made on the basis of observed delusions and/or hallucinations, i.e., psychotic material *in the face of a clear sensorium.* The term "clear sensorium" means that the following functions are all intact: orientation for time, place, person; recent and remote memory; calculation ability; retention and recall. It must be recognized, however, that hallucinations and a clear sensorium may also be present in some affective disorders and amphetamine psychoses. The current DSM-III (1) diagnostic criteria for a Schizophrenic Disorder are:
A. At least one of the following during a phase of the illness:
    1. Bizarre delusions (content is patently absurd and has *no* possible basis in fact), such as delusions of being controlled, thought broadcasting, thought insertion, or thought withdrawal
    2. Somatic, grandiose, religious, nihilistic, or other delusions without persecutory or jealous content
    3. Delusions with persecutory or jealous content if accompanied by hallucinations of any type

4. Auditory hallucinations in which either a voice keeps up a running commentary on the individual's behavior or thoughts, or two or more voices converse with each other

5. Auditory hallucinations on several occasions with content of more than one or two words, having no apparent relation to depression or elation

6. Incoherence, marked loosening of associations, markedly illogical thinking, or marked poverty of content of speech if associated with at least one of the following:
   a. Blunted, flat, or inappropriate affect
   b. Delusions or hallucinations
   c. Catatonic or other grossly disorganized behavior

B. Deterioration from a previous level of functioning in such areas as work, social relations, and self-care.

C. Duration: Continuous signs of the illness for at least six months at some time during the person's life, with some signs of the illness at present. The six-month period must include an active phase during which there were symptoms from A, with or without a prodromal or residual phase, as defined below.

Prodromal phase: A clear deterioration in functioning before the active phase of the illness not due to a disturbance in mood or to a Substance Use Disorder and involving at least two of the symptoms noted below.

Residual phase: Persistence, following the active phase of the illness, of at least two of the symptoms noted below, not due to a disturbance in mood or to a Substance Use Disorder.

Prodromal or Residual Symptoms

1. Social isolation or withdrawal

2. Marked impairment in role functioning as wage-earner, student, or homemaker

3. Markedly peculiar behavior (e.g., collecting garbage, talking to self in public, or hoarding food)

4. Marked impairment in personal hygiene and grooming

5. Blunted, flat, or inappropriate affect

6. Digressive, vague, overelaborate, circumstantial, or metaphorical speech

7. Odd or bizarre ideation, or magical thinking, e.g., superstitiousness, clairvoyance, telepathy, "sixth-sense," "others can feel my feelings," overvalued ideas, ideas of reference

8. Unusual perceptual experiences, e.g., recurrent illusions, sensing the presence of a force or person not actually present.

Examples: Six months of prodromal symptoms with one week of symptoms from A; no prodromal symptoms with six months of symptoms from A; no prodromal symptoms with two weeks of symptoms from A and six months of residual symptoms; six months of symptoms from A, apparently followed by several years of complete remission, with one week of symptoms in A in current episode.

D. The full depressive or manic syndrome (criteria A and B of major depressive or manic episode), if present, developed after any psychotic symptoms, or was brief in duration relative to the duration of the psychotic symptoms in A.

E. Onset of prodromal or active phase of the illness before age 45.

F. Not due to any Organic Mental Disorder or Mental Retardation.

Psychological tests, such as the Minnesota Multiphasic Personality Inventory (MMPI), Rorschach Inkblot Test, and Wechsler Adult Intelligence Scale-Revised (WAIS–R) may be helpful in making the diagnosis of schizophrenia. On the MMPI, schizophrenia is typically diagnosed by elevations on scales 8 (schizophrenia); 6 (paranoia); 9 (mania); and F (a validity scale) (24,25). Similarly, schizophrenia is diagnosed on the Rorschach Inkblot Test by the presence of: 1. thought disorder; 2. impaired reality testing; 3. evidence of poor emotional controls; and 4. evidence of a limited or ineffective interpersonal life (26,27). On the WAIS–R, there is some scatter between and within subtests and difficulty with thought processes, abstract thinking, and conceptual thinking ability.

It should be noted that many other "diagnostic criteria" for schizophrenia are less stringent than those in DSM-III (e.g., Feighner criteria; RDC or Research Diagnostic Criteria; CATEGO criteria in order of most to least stringent). DSM-III criteria were purposely made narrow to compensate for the American tendency to "overdiagnose" schizophrenia and "underdiagnose" affective disorders (as compared to British psychiatrists) (28,29).

CLASSIFICATION (DSM-III) (1)

Disorganized Type

The essential features are marked incoherence and flat, incongrous, or silly affect. There are no systematized delusions although fragmentary delusions or hallucinations in which the content is not organized into a coherent theme are common. Associated features include grimaces, mannerisms, hypochondriacal complaints, extreme social withdrawal, and other oddities of behavior.

This clinical picture is usually associated with extreme social impairment, poor premorbid personality, an early and insidious onset, and a chronic course without significant remissions.

In other classifications this type is termed Hebephrenic and in this sub-type, the thinking disorder, per se, is the most prominent feature.

Catatonic Type

The essential feature is marked psychomotor disturbance, which may involve stupor, negativism, rigidity, excitement, or posturing. Sometimes there is rapid alternation between the extremes of excitement and stupor. Associated features include stereotypes, mannerisms, and waxy flexibility. Mutism is particularly common.

During catatonic stupor or excitement, the individual needs careful supervision to avoid hurting self or others, and medical care may be needed because of malnutrition, exhaustion, hyperpyrexia, or self-inflicted injury.

Paranoid Type

The essential features are prominent persecutory or grandiose delusions, or hallucinations with a persecutory or grandiose *content*. In addition, delusional jealousy may be present. Associated features include unfocused anxiety, anger, argumentativeness, and violence. In addition, there may be doubts about gender identity or fear of being thought of as a homosexual, or being approached by homosexuals.

The impairment in functioning may be minimal if the delusional material is not acted upon, since gross disorganization of behavior is relatively rare. Similarly, affective responsiveness may be preserved. Often a stilted, formal quality, or extreme intensity in interpersonal interactions is noted.

The onset tends to be later in life than the other subtypes, and the features are more stable over time. If a biologically related family member of an individual who has this subtype also has Schizophrenia, there is some evidence that the subtype of the relative will also be paranoid.

Undifferentiated Type

The essential features are prominent psychotic symptoms that cannot be classified in any category previously listed or that meet the criteria for more than one.

Residual Type

This category should be used when there has been at least one episode of Schizophrenia but the clinical picture that occasioned the evaluation or admission to clinical care is without prominent symptoms, though signs of the illness persist. Emotional blunting, social withdrawal, eccentric behavior, illogical thinking and loosening of associations are common. If delusions or hallucinations are present, they are not prominent and are not accompanied by strong affect.

PARANOID DISORDERS

The DSM-III (1) definition of Paranoid Disorders is as follows: The essential features are persecutory delusions or delusional jealousy, not due to any other mental disorder, such as Schizophrenia, Schizophreniform, Affective, or Organic Mental Disorder. The paranoid disorders include Paranoia, Shared Paranoid Disorder (e.g., Folie a deux) and Acute Paranoid Disorder.

The boundaries of this group of disorders and their differentiation from such other disorders as severe Paranoid Personality Disorder and Schizophrenia, Paranoid Type, are unclear.

The persecutory delusions may be simple or elaborate and usually involve a single theme or series of connected themes, such as being conspired against, cheated, spied upon, followed, poisoned or drugged, maliciously maligned, harassed or obstructed in the pursuit of long term goals. Small slights may be exaggerated and become the focus of a delusional system.

There may be only delusional jealousy ("conjugal paranoia"), in which an individual may become convinced without due cause, that his or her mate is unfaithful. Small bits of "evidence," such as disarrayed clothing or spots on the sheets, may be collected and used to justify the delusion.

Associated features. Common associated features include resentment and anger, which may lead to violence. Grandiosity and ideas or delusions of reference are common. Often there is social isolation, seclusiveness, or eccentricities of behavior. Suspiciousness, either generalized or focused on certain individuals, is common. Letter writing, complaining about various injustices, and instigation of legal action are frequent. These individuals rarely seek treatment, and often are brought for care by associates, relatives or governmental agencies as a result of the individual's angry or litigious activities.

Differential diagnosis. In organic Delusional Syndromes, particularly those induced by amphetamines, persecutory delusions are common. In Schizophrenia, Paranoid Type, or Schizophreniform Disorder, there are certain symptoms, such as incoherence, marked loosening of associations, prominent hallucinations, and bizarre delusions (e.g., delusions of control, thought broadcasting, withdrawal or insertion), that are not present in Paranoid Disorders. Although delusions that others are attempting to control the individual's behavior are common in both Paranoid and Schizophrenic Disorders, the experience of being controlled by alien forces suggests Schizophrenia or Schizophreniform Disorder. In addition, the delusions in Schizophrenia are more likely to be fragmented and multiple rather than systematized, as in Paranoid Disorder.

Diagnostic Criteria for Paranoid Disorder:
1. Persistent persecutory delusions or delusional jealousy.
2. Emotion and behavior appropriate to the content of the delusional system.
3. Duration of illness of at least one week.
4. None of the symptoms of criterion A of Schizophrenia such as bizarre delusions, incoherence, or marked loosening of associations.
5. No prominent hallucinations.
6. The full depressive or manic syndrome (criteria A and B of major depressive or manic episode) is either not present, developed after any psychotic symptoms, or was brief in duration relative to the duration of the psychotic symptoms.
7. Not due to an Organic Mental Disorder.

Thus, a) the remainder of the personality is more intact than in paranoid schizophrenia; b) even less evidence of a thought disorder than in paranoid schizophrenia; c) more believable delusions than in paranoid schizophrenia; d) rate of deterioration is less steep than in paranoid schizophrenia; e) evidence of psychotic thinking is present (in contrast to paranoid personality).

To call a condition Paranoia requires six months' duration of the above symptoms; if less than six months the condition is called "Acute Paranoid Disorder;" if the illness appears to develop as the result of a close relationship with another person who already has such a disorder it is termed "Shared Paranoid Disorder."

Etiology

These paranoid illnesses are traditionally (probably erroneously) considered "psychogenic." They may be viewed on a continuum ranging from the "normal" use of the defense mechanism of projection at one extreme, through paranoid personality, paranoia, and possibly paranoid schizophrenia at the other extreme.

The "normal" use of projection is familiar to everyone, i.e., attributing one's own unacceptable ideas or impulses to another person, thereby transforming a subjective concept into an apparent "objective reality." This, of course, often provides the basis for prejudice. Everyone occasionally blames others, feels suspicious, or has (neurotic) ideas of reference. These mechanisms are exaggerated in frequency and intensity in paranoid personalities; they only assume psychotic proportions in the paranoid disorders and paranoid schizophrenia. According to Freud, paranoia is a "defense psychosis," attributed to unacceptable (and, consequently, repressed) aggressive or erotic impulses. For instance, to ward off an unconscious homosexual feeling, the patient may use reaction formation to alter, "I love him," to, "I hate him." He may project this thought to the other person—"He hates me," and then elaborate this into, "He is persecuting me." Delusional paranoid jealousy can be similarly traced: "I don't love him at all, she does!" Paranoid erotic delusions: "I don't love him. I love her because she loves me." Erotomania involves the patient's insistence that someone of the opposite sex secretly loves him. The patient may even attempt to contact this "secret admirer," as perhaps occurred with John Hinckley regarding Jody Foster.

Further Differential Points

Paranoid patients may have exacerbations and remissions. Hallucinations are rare and not prominent. Paranoid personalities (without delusions) maintain a life-long character pattern without deterioration, unless they develop paranoid schizophrenia. The differentiation between paranoid disorders and paranoid schizophrenia depends upon the preservation of other personality functions—e.g., affects; general reality-testing; organization and credibility of the delusional system; presence or absence of hallucinations; etc. Note that paranoid personality disorder is classified under "Personality Disorders."

The onset of frank delusional symptoms is rarely seen in patients under 30; they may be more frequent in males, and are usually persecutory or grandiose. Such patients are frequently hostile, self-righteous, and litigious. Since they rarely consider their delusions alien to themselves, they rarely seek help voluntarily. Paranoid delusions are particularly believable and systematized, i.e., the patient logically rationalizes his delusions with the rest of his life. They usually contain a small element of truth, which often provokes a counter-attack by the accused person. The patient views this counter-attack as a confirmation of the other's aggression, thus reinforcing the delusion and driving the patient further into isolation. For some recent articles on this topic, see Kendler, 1981 (30), Oxman and Tucker (31), Lorenz (32). Kendler, in 1982 (33), indicates that the paranoid psychoses are similar and dissimilar to both schizophrenia and affective disorders, i.e., similar to affective disorders in that there is a preponderance of females; similar to schizophrenia in that there is a preponderance of lower socioeconomic classes; dissimilar to both in that there is an increased incidence in immigrants. He further speculates that these illnesses may be psychological rather than organic.

PSYCHOTIC DISORDERS NOT ELSEWHERE CLASSIFIED (DSM-III) (1)

Schizophreniform Disorder

This disorder is essentially the same as schizophrenia, but the duration (including prodromal, active, and residual phases) ranges from two weeks to six months. Schizophreniform Disorder is classified outside the category of Schizophrenic Disorders for several reasons: greater likelihood of emotional turmoil and confusion; tendency toward acute onset and resolution; greater likelihood of recovery to premorbid levels of functioning; no increased prevalence of schizophrenia among family members, as compared with the general population. Several studies indicate that the best way to differentiate between these two disorders is to maximize the differences in their external correlates—hence the six month criterion.

Brief Reactive Psychosis

Sudden onset of a psychotic disorder that persists for a maximum of two weeks, with eventual return to premorbid level of functioning. The psychotic symptoms appear immediately after exposure to a recognizable psychosocial stressor that would evoke significant symptoms of distress in almost anyone —e.g., loss of a loved one; psychological trauma of combat. The experience invariably involves emotional turmoil, manifested by rapid shifts from one dysphoric affect to another. This diagnosis should not be made if increasing psychopathology was apparent immediately before exposure to the psychosocial stressor.

Associated Features. Perplexity and confusion are frequently present. Bizarre behavior may include peculiar postures, outlandish dress, screaming, or muteness. Suicidal or aggressive behavior may also be present. Speech may include inarticulate gibberish or repetition of nonsensical phrases. Affect is often inappropriate and volatile. Transient hallucinations or delusions are common. Silly or obviously confabulated answers may be given to factual questions. Disorientation and impairment of recent memory may occur. The disorder usually appears in adolescence and early adulthood. The psychotic symptoms usually clear within one or two days. By definition, this diagnosis is not applicable to any psychotic symptoms that persist for more than two weeks. Transient secondary affects such as loss of self-esteem and mild depression, may persist beyond the two weeks, but the patient eventually returns to the premorbid level of functioning.

Schizoaffective Disorder

At the present time, there is no consensus on the definition of this category. It should be used if the clinician is unable to differentiate between Affective Disorder and Schizophreniform Disorder or Schizophrenia. Procci (34) reviewed the differential diagnoses regarding Schizoaffective disorders. Andreasen (35) defines "Schizoaffective Schizophrenia" as an episode of affective illness in which preoccupation with mood-incongruent delusions or hallucinations dominate the clinical picture when affective symptoms are no longer present.

Atypical Psychosis

This is a residual category for cases involving psychotic symptoms (delusions, hallucinations, incoherence, loosening of associations, markedly illogical thinking, or behavior that is grossly disorganized or catatonic) that do not meet the criteria for any specific mental disorder.

Childhood Schizophrenia (Dementia Precocissima)

The relationship between childhood and adult schizophrenias is not clear. Fish (36), among others (37), feels that the childhood syndrome is probably a more severe form of adult schizophrenia. Loretta Bender (38) and, more recently, William Goldfarb (39) stress the organic aspects of this disorder in children. Note: although DSM-III preserves the diagnosis of "Infantile Autism" (originally described by Leo Kanner [40]), the diagnosis of "Atypical-Development Disorders" and "Childhood Onset Developmental Disorder," (Margaret Mahler's "Symbiotic Psychoses") are not included (41). Schulsinger and Mednick's study of children of severely schizophrenic mothers showed that future schizophrenic spectrum individuals were passive babies with short attention spans (42). Cantor et al. feel that the disorder should be defined by its symptoms and signs, rather than the age of onset (43).

ETIOLOGY

Introduction

The etiology of schizophrenia is unknown. The two major theoretical formulations are the "organic" and the "functional," but most psychiatrists combine them. The resultant view is that these are a group of reactions, not necessarily homogeneous, with multiple determinants, ranging from primarily organic to primarily psychological. Thus, an individual with minimal organic predisposition requires more environmental stress to provoke overt schizophrenia than one with a greater predisposition. This speculative scheme does not disprove the theory to which many psychiatrists subscribe, i.e., that there are at least two major kinds of schizophrenia—one organic and one psychological. Some psychiatrists, however, prefer the Unitary theory, i.e., all mental illness can be viewed on a continuum from "normal" to a "not-normal but not functionally psychotic" which would include neuroses, character problems, psycho-physiological problems, etc.; and a "functional psychoses" group which would include schizophrenia and the affective psychoses. The Unitary theory implies that there are only quantitative differences among these illnesses in terms of the degree of psychopathology. This author and most psychiatrists feel that psychiatric illness should not be viewed on such a continuum. There seem to be clear qualitative and quantitative differences between functional psychoses and non-psychoses;

the qualitative difference is best exemplified by the breakdown of reality testing, the sine qua non of psychoses.

Evidence for Genetic Factors

Most of the following figures are based on Kallman's studies with siblings and 953 twin-pairs, 268 of whom were monozygotic (44). Kallman postulated a specific recessive factor which predisposed the affected individual to schizophrenia. His data showed a direct relationship between the degree of consanguinity with an index case and the incidence of schizophrenia. Consanguinity refers to the degree of genetic sharing between individuals—i.e., the greater the consanguinity, the greater the sharing. It is extremely difficult to separate the genetic and environmental similarities which result from close blood-ties. One solution is to compare the concordance rates for schizophrenia in monozygotic twins raised apart and M-Z twins raised together. Kallman found a concordance rate of 76% for M-Z twins who had been separated by age 4 or younger, and a rate of 91% for M-Z twins raised together. One of the major difficulties involved in such a study is the small number of M-Z twins who have been raised apart who are discordant for schizophrenia by the time they reach adulthood. Differentiating schizophrenia from borderline states presents another problem. There are only minor difficulties establishing true monozygosity, e.g., complete blood typing.

It is interesting that both the age of onset of clinical symptoms and the clinical picture vary in M-Z twins concordant for schizophrenia. Some of the newer Scandinavian studies do not replicate Kallman's figures, e.g., only two out of eight pairs of identical twins in Norway were concordant for schizophrenia. Tienari (45) found no concordance in sixteen pairs of identical twins in Finland; however, his studies contain only male index cases, which may partly bias the results. In another Norwegian study, Kringlin, cited by Rosenthal (46), found only 40% concordance. In a comparison of monozygotic and dizygotic concordance ratios (not rates), Pollin et al. (47) found a ratio of 3.3 for schizophrenia, in contrast to a ratio of 1.3 for neuroses. This evidence seemed to support the presence of some genetic factors.

Wender (48) studied the records of 39 children born of schizophrenic parents, who had been adopted by normal parents before the age of 1 year. He compared them with 47 children of normal parents who had been adopted by normal parents before the age of 1 year. Thirteen of the first 39 became schizophrenic or schizoid. Only 7 of the second 47 developed any sort of mental illness, and the illnesses were generally less severe than those of the other group. He also studied the natural and foster parents of schizophrenic children, and the foster parents of normal children. The largest incidence of symptoms of mental illness was found in the natural parents of schizophrenic children—10 couples in each group. In another study, Zahn

(49) found that the natural parents of schizophrenic children gave more deviant word associations than the adoptive parents. A fascinating study of quadruplets with schizophrenia was done by Rosenthal and Quinn (50). Stabenau (51) reviewed some of the nature/nurture problems in 1968, and these were also addressed by Heston (52) in 1977.

In general, increased consanguinity with an index case does seem to increase concordance. Tucker's review of the 11 best twin studies (7) demonstrated a higher concordance rate in monozygotic twins in all but one (means: 61% concordance in monozygotic, 12% in dizygotic twins). Seymour Kety has extensively reviewed and confirmed much of this genetic hypothesis literature and his studies are almost, but not entirely, universally accepted. A recent critique was done by Lorna S. Benjamin (53). Kety's rebuttal can be found in the same journal (54).

Other risk rates for incidence of schizophrenia among the relatives of schizophrenics have been reported: 16% risk for each child of a schizophrenic parent; 40–70% risk for each child if both parents are schizophrenic; 3% risk for nephews and nieces of a schizophrenic; 2% risk for first cousins. Others have calculated an 11% risk rate for nephews and nieces.

Kendler found a positive correlation between schizotypal personality disorder and schizophrenia. He determined there was no correlation between paranoid psychosis (delusional disorder) and the schizophrenic spectrum disorders (55,56).

Evidence for Biochemical Factors

The search for biochemical abnormalities in schizophrenics has a history of repeated false leads. Researchers often attempt to identify a biochemical alteration as the expression of an inherited genetic trait—e.g., using diseases such as PKU disorder (phenylketonuria) as prototypes. Unfortunately, methodologic problems (diagnostic difficulties, lack of a suitable control group) often preclude the validation of promising studies. Studies with control groups rarely take into account the secondary influences of chronic hospitalization with institutional fare. For example, Kety, Pollin et al. (57) found that large quantities of coffee accounted for the large hippuric acid spots noted in the urinary chromatograms of schizophrenics. McDonald (58) showed that the limited amounts of orange juice given to schizophrenic patients in state hospitals accounted for their high ceruloplasmin levels; this may also explain their high lactate/pyruvate levels, alpha-2 globulin abnormalities, "S" protein abnormalities, etc. (59–61). Stabenau (62) showed that consumption of tea in large quantities could account for abnormal DMPEA levels.

A number of other biochemical abnormalities have been reported in schizophrenics. For instance, Meltzer's (63) and others (64) work on CPK levels; Smithies and Osmond's adrenochrome study (65); transmethylation studies (66); 6-hydroxydopamine (67); etc. The adrenochrome theory postulated that, due to a genetic deficiency, some psychotomimetic, i.e., a chemical which causes a reaction mimicking a psychosis—builds up. Because dopamine so closely resembles mescaline, the thought was that possibly the block was in the metabolic pathway leading to norepinephrine (which would result in an excess of a dopamine-like compound). Methyl-donors were later postulated to make schizophrenics worse and methyl-acceptors to improve them. This approximates the view that dopamine and mescaline could be in some sort of dynamic equilibrium—pushed toward the latter by methyl donors and towards the former by acceptors.

Since almost all of the chemical agents successfully used to treat schizophrenia seem to have profound effects on extra-pyramidal systems, considerable interest has been focused on dopaminergic systems. Janice Stevens (68) analyzed clinical electroencephalographic and experimental data in relation to: the particular value of dopamine-blocking (DA) agents in the treatment of schizophrenia; the nearly unique distribution of dopamine axons to the neo-striatum and the limbic-striatum; the special anatomic relationship of the striatum to limbic structures. The lack of dopamine-hydroxylase in these pathways precludes the production of nor-epinephrine; the neurotransmitter must, therefore, be dopamine. Stevens suggests that the schizophrenic's characteristic fear, sense of unreality, or heightened or distorted sexual and sensory perceptions may be closely related to the limbic system's physiology and striatal filter. Hence, some of the extra-pyramidal effects of the major tranquilizers may be mediated by dopamine-blocking effects on the basal ganglia, whereas the anti-psychotic effects of these drugs may be mediated by the dopamine-blocking effects on the limbic system, cortex, and hypothalamus. In general, there is excellent point-to-point and proportionate correlation between an agent's effectiveness as a dopamine blocker and its potency as an anti-psychotic. Neuroleptics bind in a dose-dependent manner to post-synaptic DA receptors in striking parallel with clinical doses of the drug. So far, however, this has only been shown for extra-pyramidal DA receptors—not yet for limbic receptors. Dopamine agonists (e.g., L-Dopa, amphetamines) do seem to worsen schizophrenia.

Amphetamines are the best psychotomimetic agents for mimicking schizophrenia. However, apomorphine, a potent agonist, has no psychotomimetic effect, and Van Kammen et al. (69) recently showed that amphetamines can cause improvement in some schizophrenics. No one has convincingly demonstrated an increased turnover rate of dopamine, or abnormal resting or diurnal levels of prolactin or growth-hormone in schizophrenics—yet both of these are very sensitive to variations in dopamine levels. Also, no consistent increase in CSF HVA (the primary metabolite of DA) has been demonstrated in schizophrenics (even if probenecid is given first). Furthermore, methyl-tyrosine (AMPT), an effective blocker of DA synthesis, is only a mildly effective anti-psychotic. Paradoxically, clozapine, an anti-psychotic, has no DA effects. There is no correlation between the clinical potency of the butyrophenone group of tranquilizers and their ability to inhibit DA-sensitive adenine cyclase; it is, however, inhibited by phenothiazines. There are dozens of neurotransmitters besides DA (e.g., GABA, acetyl choline). Tranquilizers affect other systems too, however, clinical potency only correlates with affinity for DA receptors (labelled by H3-spiroperidol or H3-haloperidol). There is no correlation with alpha adrenergic, 5-HT, or histamine receptors (70–74).

Seeman, in 1977, demonstrated that double the number of DA receptors in the limbic system, caudate, and putamen are found in the brains of schizophrenics. Any counts must control for increased DA receptors caused by major tranquilizers. PET scans may enable us to count such receptors in vivo by tagging them with a radioactive neuroleptic (75). Seeman also believes the success of opiate blockers, such as naloxone, is an indication that endorphins may also play a role. Rotrosen (76), Snyder (77), Berger (78), Davis (79), and Manschreck (80) have all written review articles in this area. The variety of chemical theories range from Linus Pauling's "Orthomolecular Psychiatry" (81) (i.e., schizophrenics have vitamin deficiencies) to the beliefs of religious and lay groups that agitate for the widespread use of nicotinic acid dinucleotide (NAD) treatment. Theories that are not based on scientific foundations can do harm by arousing false or premature hopes in the families of schizophrenic patients (cf., Laetrile).

Miscellaneous Organic Factors

A focus on various endocrine systems stems from the increased incidence of schizophrenia at puberty and the knowledge that certain endocrinopathies can cause psychoses. No consistent evidence for endocrine or infectious causes of schizophrenia has ever been found. Much excitement was engendered by the "chemical psychoses" produced by psychotomimetic drugs such as mescaline and L.S.D.; however, these seem to be related more to acute brain syndromes than to schizophrenia. It is not clear whether the "stress psychoses" should be considered evidence for organic or environmental factors—e.g., severe sensory deprivation, concentration camp psychoses (82).

Many miscellaneous or "soft" neurological signs can be found in schizophrenic patients, e.g., finger agnosias, finger tip writing, tactile form recognition, tactile performance, object sorting, etc. Sixty percent of acute schizophrenics in Tucker's series showed these signs, as opposed to only 21% of acute non-schizophrenic psychiatric admissions. Tucker also reviewed a large number of studies showing various kinds of perceptual and sensory integration difficulties in schizophrenics. Although these signs may be "minor" in their manifestations, he feels they really represent major central nervous system dysfunction.

A number of investigators have cited CAT-scan changes in chronic schizophrenic patients—primarily in anterior aspects of the left hemisphere (83–89). Others have reported possible diminished regional cerebral blood flow in schizophrenics (90). Some histopathological evidence of low grade inflammatory changes have also been reported (91).

Evidence for an Environmental (Functional) Etiology

The inconclusiveness per se of all of the above studies may be indirect evidence in favor of a functional etiology; however, this could also have been said about any disease before its actual etiology was ascertained. Nonetheless, questions can be raised regarding the differences in concordance rates in M-Z twins, i.e., the fact that discordance increases when they are raised separately leaves room for at least some role for psychological factors.

The life-histories of various patients are often cited to illustrate the fact that schizophrenia's onset and clinical symptomatology—even the hallucinations and delusions—are unique in each case. Unfortunately it is difficult to be certain that a clinician's interpretations of past history are completely objective. Even the fact that a given patient's delusions are meaningful is no guarantee of a functional etiology; a paretic's delusions are also related to that individual's premorbid life. Nor is the fact that the patient accomplishes something by his illness direct evidence, since any illness involves at least some secondary gain.

The traditional psychoanalytic formulation (92,93) is that psychologic or organic factors arrest libido at an early stage of development (narcissistic level). When exposed to various stresses, libido may then become focused on the self. Some of the more current analytic thinking relates schizophrenia to adaptational failures in a defective ego.

It has become popular to study the interaction of schizophrenic patients with their families. Lidz (94) feels that the mother-child relationship is crucial, writing of the "schizophrenogenic mother." Wynne (95) classifies families' conceptual thinking patterns and notes the inconsistencies presented to the patient. After listening to separate tapes of family sessions when the patients were absent and tapes of patients without their families, trained personnel in Wynne's group were able to match the patients to their own families; they could also identify which families had schizophrenic members.

Jackson and Bateson write of the "double-bind" in which families place schizophrenic children (96). A classic example follows:

A young man in partial remission from his schizophrenia was visited in the hospital by his mother. When he impulsively put his arm around her, she stiffened. He withdrew his arm, and she said, "Don't you love me any more?" After he blushed, she said, "Son, you musn't be so embarrassed and afraid of your own feelings." The son thus received the message that preserving his ties with his mother required him to show and not show affection.

Certain extreme positions are primarily of heuristic interest here. Szasz (97), for example, states that "mental illness," as we define it, is a myth, and schizophrenia represents the patient's retreat from an unpleasant reality. Unfortunately, this rather glib theory has a certain appeal for many people who treat schizophrenic patients. A few years ago, Rosenhan (98) had subjects pose as schizophrenic patients to determine whether the staff of psychiatric hospitals would realize they were not sick. Kety (99) and Spitzer (100) published opposing viewpoints on the results of this experiment.

An existential view of schizophrenia has been expressed most articulately by R.D. Laing (101,102). Laing sees sanity and madness as "degrees of conjunction and disjunction between two persons where one is sane by common consent." Since the estranged "patient" can't see himself as real, he consequently invents a false self. By repressing both instincts and transcendence, our civilization creates a one-dimensional man. We call this madness "sanity," but all our frames of reference are ambiguous. For example, it's perfectly normal to say, "Men are machines;" but a man who says, "I am a machine," is deemed insane. Psychiatry is seen as a specialty that brainwashes, uses chemical straitjackets, etc. Although Laing does not deny the existence of psychosis, he states that there are lots of people at large who are more dangerous than psychotic patients, e.g., hydrogen-bomb manufacturers. He feels that psychotic behavior must be viewed in the context of interpersonal relationships, i.e., the psychiatrist's role, what the patient feels is expected of him, etc. Laing's views, which are somewhat reminiscent of Szasz's, are primarily of interest because they encourage thinking about schizophrenia in nontraditional ways. For a humorous refutation of Laing's theories, see Mark Vonnegut's commentary in *Harper's* (103), "Why I Want To Bite R.D. Laing."

Schizoid Personality (Constitutional Factors)

The etiological relationship between schizoid and/or schizotypal personalities and schizophrenia is unclear. There is a 34–63% premorbid incidence of such features in all patients with schizophrenia. This incidence is fifty times greater than that of schizophrenics' unaffected siblings, and two times greater than that of their parents. Schizophrenic patients with premorbid "schizoid" features have a worse prognosis than those who apparently had no previous abnormalities; the premorbidly "schizoid" are, however, less likely to undergo acute deterioration than the premorbidly normal. The schizoid state does not necessarily indicate latent or incipient schizophrenia, since many people with schizoid personalities never become overtly schizophrenic. Additional data regarding these disorders are included in the chapter on Personality Disorders.

COURSE AND PROGNOSIS

The schizophrenic illnesses are generally malignant, i.e., they progressively worsen, often in a stepwise fashion, with each remission becoming less complete; occasionally there is a sudden exacerbation which fails to remit. One can never be certain that the illness has come to a permanent standstill in any phase. It is difficult to disentangle the disease's effects on back ward patients from those of chronic institutionalization and aging per se. The pseudo-dementia seen in schizophrenia differs from organic dementia in that it results from their inability to utilize their intellect. The life expectancies of patients in such hospitals are only three-quarters as long as normal age-matched controls. The presence of tuberculosis and other organic diseases is easily masked by the patient's deterioration. Currently, patients are kept in smaller hospitals attached to general hospitals in their own communities; this is preferable to isolating them from their families by placing them in large psychiatric institutions away from their rural homes. Unfortunately, the apparently enlightened movement to provide "the least restrictive environment" for psychiatric patients has often had tragic results. Chronic schizophrenics are pushed into "single occupancy dwellings," where they are easy prey for unscrupulous landlords and thieves.

There are certain useful prognostic indicators. Prognosis improves in direct relationship to the acuteness of the onset and its relation to external reality (with the possible exception of postpartum schizophrenic episodes). A premorbid schizoid personality and an insidious onset carry a poor prognosis though an acute case is more likely to undergo rapid deterioration than an insidious case with premorbid schizoid features. Being married at the time of admission improves the prognosis. The prognosis worsens as hospitalization is lengthened, and improves as remissions lengthen. Patients may recover from two or three attacks, but are rarely able to do so after four or five. While older age of onset carries less chance for a total remission, the patient is less likely to undergo acute deterioration. Cyclothymic features improve the prognosis. General statistics on patients in their first year of hospitalization indicate that: one-third will regain function and return home; one-third will return home, function at a decreased level, and undergo intermittent hospitalization; one-third will remain hospitalized. The following figures are based on a 15-year follow-up study conducted by M. Bleuler (104): one-fourth of all cases lead to a "pseudo-dementia;" one-fourth to marked personality deterioration; one-fourth to a mild defect; one-fourth recover. At present, over half of all first admissions return home with few, if any, symptoms; after five years, only half of this group remains unhospitalized. Data indicating that somatic treatments have doubled the number of successfully treated patients must be viewed with some skepticism. All such data contain errors due to biased sources (e.g., state hospital data is loaded with "failures;" the length of time needed to follow the life-course of just one schizophrenic, etc.). The prognosis is probably better for milder types of schizophrenia, and apparently varies according to social class and family "support"—e.g., Hollingshead and Redlich (105) found that lower class patients remain sick longer.

A number of investigators consider chronic, process, nuclear, non-remitting, and simple schizophrenia as having a "poor prognosis." "Good prognosis" schizophrenias include schizophreniform, schizoaffective, acute, reactive, and remitting schizophrenias (106–108). Diagnostic criteria for these two kinds of schizophrenia include: intense affect and a family history of affective disorder in the good prognosis group; apathy and family histories of schizophrenia in the poor prognosis group. Eighty percent of patients who fulfill the criteria for the good prognosis type of schizophrenia ultimately have good prognoses. It is only possible to accurately predict the subsequent course for about 50% of the patients in the poor prognosis schizophrenia category. Andreasen (109,110) feels that dividing schizophrenic symptoms into "positive" and "negative" types helps to clarify prognosis. Shader (111) cites a number of other diagnostic criteria, e.g., little overt hostility in the poor prognosis schizophrenic; many persecutory delusions and paranoia in poor prognosis, as compared to preoccupation with guilt and death in the good prognosis schizophrenic. He also notes that a hebephrenic picture denotes a poor prognosis.

DIFFERENTIAL DIAGNOSIS

Organic Psychoses

These almost always manifest sensorial changes, as well as delusions and hallucinations. The hallucinations are generally visual and tactile, although they may be auditory. A lumbar puncture is sometimes necessary to rule out CNS infections. State hospitals often see adolescents who seem to have a mixture of character defects and schizophrenia; many turn out to have abnormal EEG's and respond to anticonvulsants, such as mysoline. Temporal lobe seizures can mimic acute schizophrenic symptoms. Patients with amphetamine psychoses or bromide intoxication may be oriented and appear "schizophrenic." Electrolyte imbalances, uremia, hepatic coma, porphyria, collagen diseases, syphilis, high doses of steroids, lead intoxication, and many other conditions can all cause psychoses which appear "schizophrenic." It is, therefore, absolutely necessary to include a thorough physical examination and laboratory studies in the work-up of a psychosis.

Affective Psychoses

True manic excitement is more sustained and infectious, and the patient is much more distractible than the more bizarre schizophrenic whose attacks tend to be paroxysmal. The schizophrenic's onset is usually more insidious; his delusions are more grotesque, yet the patient seems less disturbed by them. A flight-of-ideas is generally associated with mania, while defects in associations are more characteristic of schizophrenia. Clangs and puns can be seen in both schizophrenics and manics. Somatic or nihilistic delusions occur more often with affective psychoses. Note that if schizophrenic-like symptoms precede or follow a period of elated or depressed mood, one cannot diagnose an affective disorder, but must call the condition schizophrenia or schizoaffective disorder.

Neuroses

The presence of psychotic thinking rules out the neuroses, except for dissociative reactions (fugues, amnesias, "hysterial psychoses"). The onset, particularly for hysterical psychoses, is usually even more acute than that seen in schizophrenia. The premorbid personality is more theatrical and labile than it is schizoid. The relation to external events and the dynamics are clearer (i.e., primary and secondary gains) than in schizophrenia, and affect is more normal. The "psychosis" (really a pseudo-psychosis) is more paroxysmal, with normal and apparently "psychotic" periods interspersed (these periods exist side-by-side in schizophrenia). Differential diagnosis may not be possible until the course of the illness has been established. Hysterical psychoses usually clear spontaneously after a few weeks in the hospital, sometimes less. Hysterical psychoses may also be classed as Brief Reactive Psychoses.

Other

Sometimes schizophrenia has to be differentiated from acute alcoholic hallucinosis, an illness primarily seen in chronic alcoholics after they have temporarily stopped drinking. Differentiating factors include the alcoholism history, presence of persecutory auditory hallucinations in the face of a clear sensorium, and affect appropriate to the hallucinatory content, i.e., the patient is terrified. While this condition was once thought to be related to schizophrenia, most authorities now believe the two are quite separate. Endocrinopathies—particularly adrenal and thyroid disorders—sometimes present problems in differential diagnosis. Mental deficiency may need to be ruled out in other cases. Borderline and narcissistic personality disorders (112) are considered in the chapter on Personality Disorders.

TREATMENT

Introduction

Since the etiology of schizophrenia is unknown, all treatments are basically empirical. Adherents of almost all theoretical schools occasionally employ drugs. Many pure-psychotherapy advocates disdain the use of shock therapy. A fairly standard treatment plan for an acute case usually includes: immediate hospitalization; supportive psychotherapy; interviews to gather data about premorbid personality, precipitating events, family structure, etc.; four- to six-week trials of adequate doses of one or two phenothiazines (sequentially) or other major tranquilizers; if medication does not help, a course of ECT (electro-convulsive therapy) may be tried. If the patient is acutely suicidal or in a catatonic stupor, one may elect to use ECT before lengthy trials of tranquilizers. See chapter on Pharmacology for further details of the pharmacotherapy of schizophrenia.

Phillip May *et al.* (113) reviewed five different treatments for schizophrenia: 1. individual psychotherapy; 2. drugs; 3. individual psychotherapy plus drugs; 4. electro-convulsive therapy; 5. milieu. Milieu therapy had the lowest release and success rates; drugs and psychotherapy had the highest success rates. Hospitalized patients who were merely treated with psychotherapy tended to spend more time in subsequent hospitalizations than any of the other groups.

Prophylaxis

Ignorance of etiology precludes any definitive prophylaxis in this case (this is not always true, e.g., Snow prevented further cholera epidemics by closing off the Front Street pump, although he had not identified the specific causal agent). Optimal child-health raising practices might decrease the incidence of schizophrenia, but this theory is not supported by concrete evidence. It certainly makes sense to at least try to identify and help disturbed children and/or their parents as early as possible.

Psychotherapy

The specialized techniques of classical, formal analytic treatment are not readily adaptable to such patients. Frieda Fromm-Reichmann (114) was one of the pioneers in treating schizophrenics with modified psychoanalytic therapy. She emphasized the patient's fears of closeness and his own hostility, as well as the importance of the therapist's attitude toward the patient. However, analytic treatment of schizophrenic patients is extremely arduous, and there is no solid evidence that it leads to more complete or longer lasting remissions than those obtained by other means. Thus, most psychotherapy with schizophrenics (aside from analytic) is face-to-face, and limited in frequency and depth of probing. Hanna Green's novel, *I Never Promised You A Rose Garden* (115), touches on some issues involved in the "analytic" treatment (or its equivalent) of a schizophrenic girl. Many people assume that the character of Dr. Fried in this novel was based on Dr. Frieda Fromm-Reichmann. In any event, the main character, Debbie, is not a very typical schizophrenic since she makes rapid, dramatic changes from psychotic to non-psychotic states. Other forms of psychotherapy are occasionally employed, such as John Rosen's "direct analysis" (116). In this, the therapist directly interprets and interacts with the patient, sometimes encouraging the patient to regress ("anaclitic treatment") in order to help him "grow-up" again. Rosen's statements about this form of treatment being more effective than standard types were apparently not supported by followup studies of his patients. In general, it is not clear how the duration of inpatient care correlates with treatment outcome (117).

"Milieu therapy" can be considered a form of psychotherapy. Maxwell Jones (118) developed the "therapeutic community" in England, i.e., a hospital setting wherein all personnel endeavor to establish a maximally therapeutic atmosphere. Some clinicians believe milieu therapy may be too stimulating for some schizophrenic patients (119).

Meyerson described the "total-push" treatment for chronic, institutionalized patients (120). The degree of improvement seen in such patients is probably directly proportional to the amount of attention they receive. The underlying schizophrenic process is not likely to respond to any kind of social contact. However, some of the regressive, withdrawn, and deteriorative features can probably be prevented, or partially reversed, by not banishing patients to months of isolation without any external stimulation. The "success" of milieu or total push therapies is understandable if one is knowledgeable about some of the current treatment "techniques" for chronic schizophrenia. The degrading, dungeon-like atmosphere in many chronic state hospitals is medieval at best, and provides an appalling commentary on our "enlightened" modern civilization. Sociologist Erving Goffman (121), mercilessly exposes such hospitals in his book, *Asylums: Essays on the Social Situation of Mental Patients and Other Inmates.* Other problems involved in treating chronic cases were addressed by Leona Bachrach (122) and in Susan Sheehan's (123) excellent book, *Is There No Place on Earth for Me?*

Stanton and Schwartz (124) describe patients' responsiveness to the dynamics of the hospital milieu. They attributed much of the regressed patients' soiling, for example, to strategic, intra-staff conflicts and circumstances, rather than random occurrences. Sociologist William Caudill (125) studied the "internal aspects" of a mental hospital by posing as an inmate for a short period; his findings were similar to those of Stanton and Schwartz.

Much enthusiasm has been generated in recent years by the work of Wolpe (126) and others who utilize "Behavior Therapy" in treating various mental disorders. These conditioning techniques have also been used with schizophrenics. When regressed schizophrenic patients socialize properly or remain continent, for example, they may be rewarded with tokens which can be redeemed for cigarettes, candy, etc. To date, there is no objective evidence to prove the therapeutic superiority of such techniques. Many psychiatrists feel these techniques are dehumanizing and rob patients of their last shreds of dignity. Conversely, one can argue that any method aimed at encouraging schizophrenics to behave in a less bizarre manner, stop soiling, dress appropriately, etc., may be extremely helpful in liberating them from the back wards of hospitals. Most authorities feel that behavior therapy can help modify patients' symptomatology.

Pharmacotherapy and ECT

These techniques will be covered elsewhere. Salzman (127) recently reviewed the usefulness of ECT in schizophrenia. Tardive Dyskinesia problems were recently reviewed by Jeste and Wyatt (128).

Psychosurgery

The idea of severing the connection between the frontal lobes and the thalamus (mainly the dorso-medial thalamic nucleus) was introduced by Moniz in 1935. Freeman and Watts began to perform frontal lobotomies (or leucotomies) in this country in 1946. This drastic, irreversible surgery has almost been abandoned because of its unpredictable results. Post-surgical patients were frequently left with bizarre "frontal lobe symptoms," such as hyperactivity, jocularity, shallow affect, and lack of normal restraint. The operation ostensibly worked best for patients with chronic paranoia with relatively well-preserved personalities; however, the use of phenothiazines can often achieve the same results with far less morbidity and mortality.

REFERENCES

1. American Psychiatric Association Committee on Nomenclature and Statistics: *Diagnostic and Statistical Manual of Mental Disorders,* ed 3. Washington, DC, American Psychiatric Association, 1980.

2. Schoeneman TJ: Criticisms of the psychopathological interpretation of witch hunts: A review. *Am J Psychiatry* 1982;139:1028-1032.

3. Zilboorg G, Henry GW: *A History of Medical Psychology.* New York, WW Norton, 1941.

4. Schneck JM: *A History of Psychiatry.* Springfield, Ill, Charles Thomas, 1960.

5. Strauss JS, Carpenter WT: *Schizophrenia.* New York, Plenum Medical Book Co, 1981.

6. Faris REL, Dunham HW: *Mental Disorders in Urban Areas: An Ecological Study of Schizophrenia and Other Psychoses.* Chicago, University of Chicago Press, 1939.

7. Pincus JH, Tucker GJ: *Behavioral Neurology.* New York, Oxford University Press, 1974.

8. Arieti S (ed): *American Handbook of Psychiatry,* ed 2. New York, Basic Books, 1981.

9. Friedman AM, Kaplan HI, Sadock BJ: *Comprehensive Textbook of Psychiatry,* ed 3. Baltimore, Williams & Wilkins, 1980.

10. Mayer-Gross W, Slater E, Roth M: *Clinical Psychiatry,* ed 3. Baltimore, Williams & Wilkins, 1969.

11. Kolb LC, Keith H, Brodie H: *Modern Clinical Psychiatry,* ed 10. Philadelphia, WB Saunders, 1982.

12. Redlich FC, Freedman DX: *The Theory and Practice of Psychiatry.* New York, Basic Books, 1966.

13. Bleuler E: *Dementia Praecox or the Group of Schizophrenias,* Joseph Zinkin (Trans). New York, International Universities Press, 1950.

14. Andreasen NC: Thought, language, and communication disorders: I. Clinical assessment, definition of terms, and evaluation of their reliability; II. Diagnostic significance. *Arch Gen Psychiatry* 1979;36:1315-1330.

15. Arieti S: *Interpretation of Schizophrenia,* ed 2. New York, Basic Books, 1974.

16. Jackson DD (ed): *The Etiology of Schizophrenia.* New York, Basic Books, 1960.

17. Corradi RB: Clinical assessment of affect in schizophrenia. *J Clin Psychiatry* 1978;39:493-496.

18. Reid WH, Moore SL, Zimmer M: Assessment of affect in schizophrenia: Reliability data. *J Nerv Ment Dis* 1982;170:266-269.

19. Holzman PS, Levy DL, Proctor LR: Smooth pursuit eye movements, attention, and schizophrenia. *Arch Gen Psychiatry* 1976;33:1415-1420.

20. Holzman PS, Kringlin E, Levy DL, *et al.:* Abnormal pursuit eye movements in schizophrenia: Evidence for a genetic indicator. *Arch Gen Psychiatry* 1977; 34:802-805.

21. Holzman PS, Kringlen E, Levy DL, *et al.:* Deviant eye tracking in twins discordant for psychosis: A replication. *Arch Gen Psychiatry* 1980;37:627-631.

22. Latham C, Holzman PS, Manschreck TC, *et al.:* Optokinetic nystagmus and pursuit eye movements in schizophrenia. *Arch Gen Psychiatry* 1981;38:997-1003.

23. Levin S, Jones A, Stark L, *et al.:* Identification of abnormal patterns in eye movements of schizophrenic patients. *Arch Gen Psychiatry* 1981;39:1125-1130.

24. Lahar D: *The MMPI: Clinical Assessment and Automated Interpretation.* Los Angeles, Western Psychological Services, 1978.

25. Newmark CS, Gentry L, Simpson M, *et al.:* MMPI criteria for diagnosing schizophrenia. *J Pers Assess* 1978;42:366-373.

26. Exner JE Jr: *The Rorschach: A Comprehensive System.* New York, John Wiley & Sons, 1978, vol 2.

27. Weiner I: *Psychodiagnosis and Schizophrenia.* New York, John Wiley & Sons, 1966.

28. Skodol A: Schizophrenic and Other Psychotic Disorders, presentation at "Psychiatric Update: Beyond DSM-III," Oglebay Park, West Virginia, June 9-11, 1982.

29. Endicott J, Nee J, Fleiss J, et al.: Diagnostic criteria for schizophrenia: Reliabilities and agreement between systems. Arch Gen Psychiatry 1982;39:884–889.

30. Kendler KS, Hayes P: Paranoid psychosis (delusional disorder) and schizophrenia: A family history study. Arch Gen Psychiatry 1981;38:547–551.

31. Oxman TE, Rosenberg SD, Tucker GJ: The language of paranoia. Am J Psychiatry 1982;139:275–282.

32. Lorenz M: The language of paranoia—meeting place of mental events and verbal constructs. Am J Psychiatry 1982;139:319–320.

33. Kendler KS: Demography of paranoid psychosis (delusional disorder): A review and comparison with schizophrenia and affective illness. Arch Gen Psychiatry 1982;39: 890–902.

34. Procci WR: Schizo-affective psychosis: Fact or fiction? A surveyof the literature. Arch Gen Psychiatry 1976;33:1167–1178.

35. Andreasen N: Diagnostic Controversies, presentation at "Psychiatric Update: Beyond DSM-III," Oglebay Park, West Virginia, June 9–11, 1982.

36. Fish B: Neurobiologic antecedents of schizophrenia in children. Arch Gen Psychiatry 1977;34:1297–1313.

37. Ornitz EM, Ritvo ER: The syndrome of autism: A critical review. Am J Psychiatry 1976;133:609–621.

38. Bender L: Childhood schizophrenia: Clinical study of one hundred schizophrenic children. Am J Ortho-psychiatry 1947;17:40–56.

39. Goldfarb W: Emotional and intellectual consequences of psychologic deprivation in infancy: A revaluation, in Hoch PB, Zubin J (eds): Psychopathology in Childhood. New York, Grune & Stratton, 1955, pp 105–119.

40. Eisenberg L, Kanner L: Early infantile autism. Am J Orthopsychiatry 1956;26:556–566.

41. Mahler MS, Gosliner BJ: On symbiotic child psychosis: Genetic, dynamic and restitutive aspects. Psychoanal Study Child 1955;10:195–212.

42. Parnas J, Schulsinger F, Schulsinger H, et al.: Behavioral precursors of schizophrenia spectrum: A prospective study. Arch Gen Psychiatry 1982;39:658–664.

43. Cantor S, Evans J, Pearce J, et al.: Childhood schizophrenia: Present but not accounted for. Am J Psychiatry 1982;139:758–762.

44. Kallman FJ: Schizophrenia, in Heredity in Health and Mental Disorder. New York, WW Norton Co, 1953, pp 143–181.

45. Tienari P: Psychiatric illness in identical twins. Acta Psychiatr Scand, Supplement 171, Volume 39, 1963.

46. Rosenthal D (ed): The Genain Quadruplets. New York, Basic Books, 1963, pp 576.

47. Pollin W, Allen MG, Hoffer A, et al.: Psychopathology in 15,909 pairs of veteran twins: Evidence for a genetic factor in the pathogenesis of schizophrenia and its relative absence in psychoneurosis. Am J Psychiatry 1969;126:597–610.

48. Wender PH, Rosenthal D, Zahn TP, et al.: The psychiatric adjustment of the adopting parents of schizophrenics. Am J Psychiatry 1971;127:1013–1018.

49. Zahn TP: Word association in adoptive and biological parents of schizophrenics. Arch Gen Psychiatry 1968;19:501–503.

50. Rosenthal D (ed): The Genain Quadruplets. New York, Basic Books, 1963.

51. Stabenau J: Heredity and environment in schizophrenia: The contribution of twin studies. Arch Gen Psychiatry 1968;18:458–463.

52. Heston LL: Schizophrenia: Genetic factors. Hosp Pract 1977;12:43–49.

53. Benjamin LS: A reconsideration of the Kety and Associates study of genetic factors in the transmission of schizophrenia. Am J Psychiatry 1976;133:1129–1133.

54. Kety SS: Studies designed to disentangle genetic and environmental variables in schizophrenia: Some epistemological questions and answers. *Am J Psychiatry* 1976;133:1134-1137.

55. Kendler KS, Gruenberg AM, Strauss JS: An independent analysis of the Copenhagen sample of the Danish adoption study of schizophrenia. Part II The relationship between schizotypal personality disorder and schizophrenia. *Arch Gen Psychiatry* 1981;38:982-984.

56. Kendler KS, Gruenberg AM, Strauss JS: An independent analysis of the Copenhagen sample of the Danish adoption of schizophrenia. Part III The relationship between paranoid psychosis (delusional disorder) and the schizophrenia spectrum disorders. *Arch Gen Psychiatry* 1981;38:985-987.

57. Kety SS: Biochemical theories of schizophrenia. *Int J Psychiatry* 1965;1:409-446.

58. Kety SS: Progress toward an understanding of the biological substrates of schizophrenia, in Fieve RR, Rosenthal D, Brill H (eds): *Genetic Research in Psychiatry.* Baltimore, Johns Hopkins University Press, 1975.

59. Sardesai VM, Ward V, Provido H, *et al.:* The effect of schizophrenic factor on liver tryptophan oxygenase. *Commun Psychopharmacol* 1977;1:439-446.

60. Frohman CE, Arthur RE, Yoon HS, *et al.:* Distribution and mechanism of action of the anti-S protein in human brain. *Biol Psychiatry* 1973;7:53-61.

61. Frohman CE: Plasma proteins and schizophrenia, in Mendels J (ed): *Biological Psychiatry.* New York, John Wiley & Sons, 1973, pp 131-148.

62. Stabenau JR, Creveling CR, Daly J: The "pink spot," 3,4-DMPEA, common tea, and schizophrenia. *Am J Psychiatry* 1970;127:611-616.

63. Meltzer H: Muscle enzyme release in the acute psychoses. *Arch Gen Psychiatry* 1969;21:102-112.

64. Schweid DE, Steinberg JS, Sudak HS: Creatine phosphokinase and psychosis. *Arch Gen Psychiatry* 1972;26:263-265.

65. Hoffer A, Osmond H, Smythies J: Schizophrenia: A new approach. II. Result of a year's research. *J Ment Science* 1954;100:29-45.

66. Baldessarini RJ, Stramentinoli G, Lipinski JF: Methylation hypothesis. *Arch Gen Psychiatry* 1979;36:303-307.

67. Stein L, Wise CD: Possible etiology of schizophrenia: Progressive damage to the noradrenergic reward system by 6-hydroxydopamine. *Science* 1971;171:1032-1036.

68. Stevens JR: An anatomy of schizophrenia? *Arch Gen Psychiatry* 1973;29:177-189.

69. Van Kammen DP, Bunney WE Jr, Docherty JP, *et al.:* d-Amphetamine-induced heterogeneous changes in psychotic behavior in schizophrenia. *Am J Psychiatry* 1982;139:991-997.

70. Peroutka SJ, Snyder SH: Relationship of neuroleptic drug effects at brain dopamine, serotonin, a-adrenergic, and histamine receptors to clinical potency. *Am J Psychiatry* 1980;137:1519-1522.

71. Snyder SH: Biochemical factors in schizophrenia. *Hosp Pract* 1977;12:133-140.

72. Frederickson P, Richelson E: Dopamine and schizophrenia—A review. *J Clin Psychiatry* 1979;40:399-405.

73. Snyder SH: Antischizophrenic drugs and the dopamine receptor. *Drug Therapy (Hosp),* May 1978, pp 29-34.

74. Kleinman JE, Weinberger DR, Rogol AD, *et al.:* Plasma prolactin concentrations and psychopathology in chronic schizophrenia. *Arch Gen Psychiatry* 1982;39:655-657.

75. Roche Report: Searching for the biology of schizophrenia: The wilderness of neurological variables. *Frontiers of Psychiatry* 1980;10:1.

76. Rotrosen J, Miller AD, Mandio D, *et al.:* Prostaglandins, platelets, and schizophrenia. *Arch Gen Psychiatry* 1980;37:1047-1054.

77. Snyder SH: Dopamine receptors, neuroleptics, and schizophrenia. *Am J Psychiatry* 1981;138:460-464.
78. Berger PA, Watson SJ, Akil H, *et al.:* Beta-endorphin & schizophrenia. *Arch Gen Psychiatry* 1980;37:635-639.
79. Davis GC, Buchsbaum MS, Bunney WE Jr: Research in endorphins and schizophrenia. *Schizophr Bull* 1979;5:244-250.
80. Manschreck TC: Current concepts in psychiatry. Schizophrenic disorders. *N Engl J Med* 1981;305:1628-1632.
81. Pauling L: Orthomolecular psychiatry. *Science* 1968;160:265-271.
82. Bowers MP: Psychoses precipitated by psychotomimetic drugs: A follow-up study. *Arch Gen Psychiatry* 1977;34:832-835.
83. Golden CJ, Moses JA, Zelazowski R, *et al.:* Cerebral ventricular size and neuropsychological impairment in young chronic schizophrenics. *Arch Gen Psychiatry* 1980;37: 619-623.
84. Golden CJ, Graber B, Coffman J, *et al.:* Structural brain deficits in schizophrenia. *Arch Gen Psychiatry* 1981;38:1014-1017.
85. Jernigan TL, Zatz LM, Moses JA Jr, *et al.:* Computed tomography in schizophrenics and normal volunteers: I. Fluid Volume; II. Cranial asymmetry. *Arch Gen Psychiatry* 1982;39:765-773.
86. Nasrallah HA, Jacoby CG, McCalley-Whitters M, *et al.:* Cerebral ventricular enlargement in subtypes of chronic schizophrenia. *Arch Gen Psychiatry* 1982;39:774-777.
87. Weinberger DR, DeLisi LE, Perman GP, *et al.:* Computed tomography in schizophreniform disorder and other acute psychiatric disorders. *Arch Gen Psychiatry* 1982; 39:778-783.
88. Luchins DJ, Weinberger DR, Wyatt RJ: Schizophrenia and cerebral asymmetry detected by computed tomography. *Am J Psychiatry* 1982;139:753-757.
89. Andreasen NC, SMith MR, Jacoby CG, *et al.:* Ventricular enlargement in schizophrenia: Definition and prevalence. *Am J Psychiatry* 1982;139:292-302.
90. Mathew RJ, Duncan GC, Weinman ML, *et al.:* Regional CSF in schizophrenia. *Arch Gen Psychiatry* 1982;39:1121-1124.
91. Stevens JR: Neuropathology of schizophrenia. *Arch Gen Psychiatry* 1982;39:1131-1139.
92. Freud S: Psycho-analytic notes on an autobiographical account of a case of paranoia (dementia paranoides), in *The Complete Psychological Works of Sigmund Freud,* st'd ed. London, Hogarth Press, 1958, vol 12, pp 3-82.
93. Freud S: Some neurotic mechanisms in jealousy, paranoia, and homosexuality, in *The Complete Psychological Works of Sigmund Freud,* st'd ed. London, Hogarth Press, 1955, vol 18, pp 222-232.
94. Lidz T, Fleck S. Cornelison AR: *Schizophrenia and the Family.* New York, International Universities Press, 1965.
95. Wynne LC, Singer MT: Thought disorder and family relations of schizophrenics: I. A research strategy; II. A classification of forms of thinking. *Arch Gen Psychiatry* 1963;9:191-206.
96. Jackson DD (ed): *The Etiology of Schizophrenia.* New York, Basic Books, 1960.
97. Szasz TS: *The Myth of Mental Illness.* New York, Harper & Row, 1961.
98. Rosenhan DL: On being sane in insane places. *Science* 1973;179:250-258.
99. Kety SS: From rationalization to reason. *Am J Psychiatry* 1974;131:957-963.
100. Spitzer RL: More on pseudoscience in science and the case for psychiatric diagnosis. *Arch Gen Psychiatry* 1976;33:459-470.
101. Laing RD: *The Divided Self.* Pelican Paperback Edition, 1965.
102. Laing RD, Esterson A: *Sanity, Madness and the Family.* Pelican Paperback Edition, 1970.

103. Vonnegut M: Why I Want to Bite R.D. Laing. *Harpers,* April 1974.

104. Bleuler M: A 23-year long longitudinal study of 208 schizophrenics and impressions in regard to the nature of schizophrenia, in Rosenthal D, Kety SS (eds): *The Transmission of Schizophrenia.* London, Pergamon Press, 1968, pp 3-12.

105. Hollingshead AB, Redlich FC: *Social Class and Mental Illness: A Community Study.* New York, John Wiley & Sons, 1958.

106. Goodwin DW, Guze SB: *Psychiatric Diagnosis,* ed 2. New York, Oxford University Press, 1979, pp 28-50.

107. Bland RC, Parker JH, Orn H: Prognosis in schizophrenia: Prognistic predictors and outcome. *Arch Gen Psychiatry* 1978;35:72-77.

108. Hawk AB, Carpenter WT, Strauss JS: Diagnostic criteria and five-year outcome in schizophrenia. *Arch Gen Psychiatry* 1975;32:343-347.

109. Andreasen NC: Negative symptoms in schizophrenia. *Arch Gen Psychiatry* 1982;39: 784-788.

110. Andreasen NC, Olsen S. Negative v positive schizophrenia: Definition and validation. *Arch Gen Psychiatry* 1982;39:789-794.

111. Shader RI (ed): *Manual of Psychiatric Therapeutics.* Boston, Little Brown & Co, 1975, pp 63-100.

112. Spitzer RL, Endicott J, Gibbon M: Crossing the border into borderline personality and borderline schizophrenia: The development of criteria. *Arch Gen Psychiatry* 1979;36: 17-24.

113. May PRA, Tuma AH, Dixon WJ: Schizophrenia—A follow-up study of results of treatment: I. Design and other problems; II. Hospital stay over two to five years. *Arch Gen Psychiatry* 1976;33:474-486.

114. Fromm-Reichmann F: *Principles of Intensive Psychotherapy.* Chicago, University of Chicago Press, 1950.

115. Green H: *I Never Promised You a Rose Garden.* Signet Pocket Books, 1964.

116. Rosen JN: *Direct Analysis: Selected Papers.* New York, Grune & Stratton, 1953.

117. Caton CLM: Effect of length of inpatient treatment for chronic schizophrenia. *Am J Psychiatry* 1982;139:856-861.

118. Jones M: The concept of a therapeutic community. *Am J Psychiatry* 1956;112:647-650.

119. Van Putten T: Milieu therapy: Contraindications? *Arch Gen Psychiatry* 1973;29: 640-643.

120. Myerson A: Scrutiny, social anxiety, and inner turmoil in relationship to schizophrenia. *Am J Psychiatry* 1948;105:401-409.

121. Goffman E: *Asylums: Essays on the Social Situation of Mental Patients and Other Inmates.* Doubleday Anchor Paperback, 1961.

122. Bachrach LL: Overview: Model programs for chronic mental patients. *Am J Psychiatry* 1980; 137:1023-1031.

123. Sheehan S: *Is There No Place On Earth For Me?* Boston, Houghton-Mifflin Co, 1982.

124. Stanton AH, Schwartz MS: *The Mental Hospital.* New York, Basic Books, 1954.

125. Caudill W: *The Psychiatric Hospital as a Small Society.* Cambridge, Harvard University Press, 1958.

126. Wolpe J: *The Practice of Behavior Therapy,* ed 2. New York, Pergamon Press, 1973.

127. Salzman C: The use of ECT in the treatment of schizophrenia. *Am J Psychiatry* 1980; 137:1032-1041.

128. Jeste DV, Wyatt RJ: Therapeutic strategies against tardive dyskinesia. *Arch Gen Psychiatry* 1982; 39:803-816.

Chapter 5

AFFECTIVE DISORDERS
GLENN C. DAVIS, M.D.

> Sometimes he came to me in a very cheerful state of mind, when he
> used to say, "how happy he was, and that he could scarcely express the
> supreme felicity which he experienced." At other times, I found him
> plunged in the horrors of consternation and despair. Thus most acutely
> miserable, he frequently, and with great earnestness, intreated me to put
> an end to his sufferings.
>
> *Philippe Pinel (1)*

In the above passage, Pinel, a founder of moral psychiatry, described a
patient with manic depressive illness in terms which identify many major
features we recognize today. Elegant descriptions of depression and mania
may be found throughout recorded history. Nevertheless, the last several
decades of research into affective illnesses, and enormous advances in our
understanding of central nervous system function, have led to the construction of homogeneous depressive syndromes with characteristic patterns of
family history, course, and biological changes. The diagnosis of depression
has been refined to the point that the syndromes have predictable treatment
responses.

This chapter describes the signs and symptoms of affective disorders, as
well as their epidemiology, course, outcome, etiology, and treatment.

OFFICIAL DIAGNOSIS OF AFFECTIVE ILLNESS

Affective disorders are illnesses characterized by persistent alterations in
mood and the disruption of a number of central nervous system physiologies. DSM-III (2) contains six syndromes in the Affective Disorder Group
(Table I). Of these six syndromes, we will describe in detail the first four:
Bipolar Disorder; Major Depression; Cyclothymic Disorder; Dysthymic
Disorder. The Atypical Affective Disorders are a residual and poorly
described set of syndromes which we will not describe in detail, since little is
known about their diagnostic value.

```
+---------------------------------------------------+
|                                                   |
|                     TABLE I                       |
|           AFFECTIVE DISORDERS (DSM-III)           |
|                                                   |
|             Major Affective Disorders             |
|             1. Major Depressive Disorder          |
|             2. Bipolar Disorder                   |
|                                                   |
|          Other Specific Affective Disorders       |
|             3. Dysthymic Disorder                 |
|             4. Cyclothymic Disorder               |
|                                                   |
|             Atypical Affective Disorders          |
|             5. Atypical Depression                |
|             6. Atypical Bipolar Disorder          |
|                                                   |
+---------------------------------------------------+
```

MAJOR DEPRESSIVE EPISODE

Depressive Mood Versus Depressive Illnes

The cardinal feature of a major depressive episode is the presence of depressive mood. Nevertheless, the presence of unhappy, unpleasant, dysphoric feelings, even on a long-term basis, is not sufficient for a diagnosis of affective illness. Mood is altered, impaired, or influenced in MOST psychiatric disorders (Table II). Schizophrenia has characteristic abnormalities of affect as do the organic brain syndromes. Indeed, the frustrations, challenges, and surprises of daily living normally produce happiness, gloom, irritability, and a host of other mood states. Just as congestive heart failure may be the physiological expression of a number of cardiovascular diseases, depressive mood is a common outcome of a number of disorders. When is the presence of depressive affect a part of an affective disorder? Affective disorders are distinguished by *pervasive* and *persistent* disturbances of mood which are resistant to the reality of pleasurable experience (anhedonia), and are accompanied by characteristic alterations in drives. Affective disorders may be considered to be serious primary disturbances in the regulation of mood; other illnesses may produce alterations of mood as concomitant or secondary features.

Signs and Symptoms of Major Depressive Episodes

DSM-III criteria for major depressive episodes were selected on the basis of several decades of research. Taken together, DSM-III criteria for Major Depression and Bipolar Disorder produce reasonably reliable, valid, and

TABLE II
DISORDERS WITH AFFECTIVE FEATURES

Diagnosis	Affects
Schizophrenia	flat, fearful, paranoid
Schizoaffective	affect may be depressed or manic
Primary Dementia	labile, may mimic depressed mood
Substance Induced States	may produce any affect, commonly depressed mood
Abstinence Induced States	commonly anxious or depressed mood
Organic Affective Syndrome	labile, anxious, or depressed mood
Adjustment Disorder	anxious or depressed mood

homogeneous syndromes. Patients whose symptoms meet criteria for a major depressive episode have a predictable response rate to antidepressant treatment, as well as a predictable illness course. There are five categories of symptoms present in major depressive episodes: characteristic mood changes; neurovegetative symptoms; psychomotor alteration; cognitive disruption (which may include thought disordered psychotic features); and functional consequences. DSM-III extracts from these characteristic signs and symptoms those features which best differentiate depressive syndromes from other illnesses which produce depressive moods.

1. *Mood Changes:* Unhappiness, sadness, loneliness, agony, darkness, gloom, despair, apathy, sinfulness, deadness, pain, and hopelessness are common words used by depressed patients to describe their mood. Many depressed individuals seem more irritable than depressed. Many patients appear unable to identify internal mood states, and, additionally, have poorly developed mood language (a developmental problem called alexithymia) (3). Many patients with alexithymia express mood somatically, for example, using the language of pain.

2. *Neurovegetative Symptoms:* Neurovegetative symptoms (also called hypothalamic symptoms or biological concomitants of depression) include sexual drive (libido), impairment of peripheral sexual function, sleep abnormalities, and disruption of gastrointestinal function. Other symptoms, which may reflect impairment in drive functions, include decreased energy level, interest, motivation, and initiative. Certainly significant weight loss in any patient should suggest the possibility of a depressive process. Recent studies have demonstrated that peripheral sexual function (such as erection, ejaculation, or vaginal secretion), as

well as libido (sexual drive) are affected by depressive illness. Sleep abnormalities tend to be of three sorts: trouble falling asleep; disruption of sleep continuity (e.g., multiple awakenings); early morning insomnia. Early morning insomnia is the most characteristic feature of major depressive episodes. REM latency, the time from sleep onset to the beginning of rapid eye movement sleep (usually about 90 minutes), is often shortened in major depressive episodes (4). Spontaneous crying spells are common in depression, though not diagnostic.

Another interesting feature of depression is a disruption of the normal diurnal rhythm of mood (usually mood is better in the morning than the evening). Patients with major depressive disorders frequently feel the worst upon awakening. The disruption of diurnal mood rhythm is often associated with early morning awakening. Many of these symptoms, including decreased energy, interest, and motivation, may stem primarily from neurovegetative drive impairment; they may, however, be related more fundamentally to impairment in cognitive function.

3. *Cognitive Symptoms:* Attention, concentration, interest, and motivation are significantly impaired in affective disorders. In fact, depression appears to be associated with a generalized deficit in many aspects of information processing and learning. In addition to the impairment in the information processing aspects of cognition, depression is characterized by a disorder in the content of cognition. Self-reproach, guilt, worthlessness, wishes to be dead, suicidal feelings, and even hallucinations and delusions may be present. A formal thought disorder may also be present, particularly disruptions of language usage called fluent disorganization. Fluent disorganization refers to the fact that while language production may be smooth and grammatical, it is often tangential, circumstantial, and may lose its point.

Thus, there is *primary* cognitive impairment in depression—that is, the depressive illness disrupts cognitive information processing. There is also *secondary* cognitive impairment. "Secondary cognitive impairment" refers to impairment produced as a consequence of depressive illness and include a sense of aloneness, isolation, separateness, weakness, helplessness, inefficiency, and hopelessness. These symptoms often remain long after the primary recovery from the neurovegetative and mood aspects of the syndrome.

Psychotic features, such as hallucinations and delusions, may be present in major depressive episodes, as well as in schizophrenia and organic brain syndromes. Commonly, delusions of self-deprecation and self-accusation, ideas of reference, and paranoid ideas may be present. In general, delusions and hallucinations in affectively ill individuals tend to be mood congruent. Congruence is the judgment by the examiner that the content of the delusion or hallucination is consonant with depressive feelings. For example, the delusion of "having fallen from grace with the Lord" may arise from guilty ruminations about the past, in which a sense of failure and poor self-esteem, coupled with a religious upbringing, may steer thought content in this delusional direction. Mood incongruent delusions may also be present in depression. Bizarre delusions, seemingly unrelated to depressive content, are considered part of the depressive process if they disappear, along with other, more typical symptoms, during treatment. The notion of congruence is clinically meaningful, but subjective and often unreliable.

4. *Motor Symptoms of Depression:* Depression is often associated with psychomotor retardation. In recent years, this clinical wisdom has been confirmed with ambulatory activity monitoring devices. While there is a reduction in all body movements, the emphasis is on *psychomotor* retardation to highlight those movements most integrated into communicative aspects of mood, thought, and personal presentation of self. Thus, facial movements and gestures are particularly reduced. Depression may also be associated with increases in movements, i.e., often associated with pacing, wringing, and heavy utilization of facial and temporal musculature. Muscle tone may be increased throughout the body.

5. *Functional Consequences of Depression:* Depression is a disastrous disease with enormous morbidity. The impact of depression on the individual's sense of self, role in society, and job functioning may be overwhelming. Depressive illness causes social stigma and consequent demoralization. There is still a societal tendency to characterize the depressed patient as weak, flawed, and incapable, rather than ill. Often these antiquated beliefs are reinforced by stigmatizing behaviors of depressed patients, such as suicide attempts, self-injury, or financial misjudgments.

Epidemiology of Depression

In discussing epidemiologic features of Affective Disorders, it is useful to examine the epidemiology of depressive symptoms, as well as that of Major Depressive and Bipolar Depressive Disorders (see references 5–10 for details of epidemiology presented here).

Epidemiology of Depressive Feelings. The point prevalence of depressive symptoms ranges from 13–20% of the total population. Depressive symptoms are twice as prevalent in women as in men. There appears to be an inverse relationship between social class and rates of depressive symptoms. No racial differences in prevalence of depressive symptoms are seen when social class is taken into account (7). Married persons and those with intimate, nonmarital relationships are consistently found to have lower rates of depressive symptoms than unmarried persons.

Epidemiology of Patients with Major Depressive Disorder. Women have a twofold greater prevalence of major depression than men. The point prevalence appears to be 3.2% in adult men, and 4–9% in women. Studies report 82–201 new cases per 100,000 men, and 247–7800 new cases per 100,000 women. The age of onset of major depression ranges from the middle to late 30s—39 for females; 49 for males (6).

Epidemiology of Patients with Bipolar Depressive Episodes. The prevalence of bipolar depressive disorder is approximately equal in men and women. Bipolar illness has a lower point prevalence than major depression (0.6–0.8% with 9–15 new cases per 100,000 men; 7–32 per 100,000 women). Rates of bipolar depression are slightly higher in the higher social classes. No racial differences are found. There is no association between marital status and the rates of bipolar depression, although an excess of marital conflict (relative to normal persons) has been reported in the marriages of bipolar persons. The age of onset of bipolar depression is significantly younger than that of onset of major depression (usually late 20s).

MANIC EPISODES

Mania and the Affective Disorders

We have discussed the symptoms of depressive episodes without regard to the subtype of Major Affective Illness. The criteria for a depressive episode in Major Depressive Disorder are the same as those for Bipolar Disorder, depressed episode. What distinguishes Bipolar Disorder from Major Depressive Disorder? Clearly, it is the presence of a previous manic episode. If we examine a 20-year-old individual and find that his symptoms meet the criteria for major depressive episode, and he has no history of mania, the patient will be diagnosed as suffering from a Major Depressive Disorder. Possibly, within a year or two, or even ten years, such an individual may have a manic episode. When the manic episode occurs, it is possible to diagnose Bipolar Disorder. It is not possible to predict a person's vulnerability to mania on the basis of depressive symptoms. On the other hand, a family history of mania suggests possible vulnerability to bipolar illness. A family history of depression is not helpful; there is an equal likelihood of bipolar and unipolar (another name for major depressive disorder) relatives among bipolar patients. Patients with Major Depressive Disorder tend to have unipolar relatives. A patient with a major depressive episode before age 25 is more likely to be bipolar than one with a later age of onset.

Mood Elevation Versus Mania and Hypomania

Distinguishing between mood elevation associated with the everyday vicissitudes of life and that associated with manic illness is similar to the problem of distinguishing between depressive feelings and disorders. Mania, like depression, is a syndrome in which mood elevation is only one feature.

Signs and Symptoms of Manic Episodes

Symptoms of mania may be grouped into mood changes, motor changes, thought disorder, and disruption of judgment and impulse control.

Mood Changes. While manic individuals are commonly described as having an expansive or elated mood, other moods may predominate. Paranoid and hostile moods are almost as common as elation in mania. Paranoid and hostile manic patients are often misdiagnosed as paranoid schizophrenics. Irritable mood is also a frequent expression of mania. This is particularly confusing, since irritability may also be an expression of depression; thus, on the basis of mood alone, it is often difficult to determine whether a bipolar patient is experiencing a depressed or manic episode. Rapid mood changes are characteristic in mania; the patient may laugh one minute and cry the next. In contrast to other syndromes in which lability of mood is characteristic, the stimulus in the manic is often appropriate, though the magnitude of response is out of proportion to the stimulus.

Motor Aspects of Mania. There is an increase in *ALL* rate aspects of behavior in mania, e.g., increased motor activity, speech, thought and decreased sleep. A typical manic patient is quite active, gesticulates, is facially expressive, speaks quite rapidly, and may have flight of ideas. Indeed, the patient may report pressure of speech or thought, i.e., "can't keep up with my thoughts." In an inpatient ward, the manic patient is frequently found in the "catbird" seat—that location on the ward in which one can best observe everything that is going on, usually near the nursing station.

Thought Disorder in Mania. Formerly, thought disorder was thought to be associated with schizophrenia. Recent studies (11) have demonstrated thought disorder (disruption of language, thought, and communication) in manics. The thought disordered symptoms of mania, like those of depression, tend to be fluent, that is, thought and language are tangential, derailed, and may demonstrate loss of goal. Pressure of speech and flight of ideas are also present in mania. Content aspects of thought and speech, such as hallucinations and delusions, may also be present in mania, though much less commonly than in schizophrenia. The hallucinations and delusions tend to be mood congruent—that is, the content may be consistent with the patient's grandiosity or paranoid presentation.

Impairment of Judgment and Impulse Control. Perhaps the most stigmatizing aspect of mania is the impairment of judgment. This loss of judgment may be manifested in buying sprees, sexual indiscretions, foolish business investments, and reckless driving. Judgment impairment is often completely congruent with the patient's grandiosity. Thus, a patient who normally collects antiques may feel he is a world renowned judge of antiques in his manic state—and spend his life savings on junk believing it to be valuable. Patients in manic states may get in fights, drink excessively, and engage in socially unacceptable behaviors. Hospitalization for mania is often necessary, both to rapidly initiate therapy and protect the individual from the damaging consequences of his own acts.

Sleep in Mania. The decreased sleep in mania is often described as a decreased NEED FOR SLEEP. While he may only sleep for a few hours, the manic patient wakes up bright and refreshed. Bipolar patients often SWITCH into mania in the early morning (e.g., 4 A.M.). Much research has been done on the psychophysiology and psychopharmacology of sleep, in the hopes of discovering the underlying etiology of affective illnesses (4).

THE COURSE OF AFFECTIVE ILLNESS

Major Depressive Disorder (MDD)

We will discuss several of the more common courses for Major Depressive Disorder. Major Depressive Disorder (MDD) tends to begin in mid-life. It is common to find patients who are treated for a single episode, and never experience another; perhaps one-half of patients suffering from MDD have single episodes. Other patients may experience an initial episode at age 45 and have another in 5 years. It is much less common for an individual to experience several episodes a year for the remainder of life.

A major question for affective illness research has been the effect of antidepressant treatment on the subsequent course of the affective illness. Tricyclic antidepressants appear to treat a given episode of MDD and provide protection against subsequent episodes. Nevertheless, maintaining patients on prophylactic treatment is associated with risk; patients with a record of frequent recurrences are the best candidates for antidepressant maintenance therapy. It is important to remember that affective illnesses are disorders that will spontaneously remit; prior to the introduction of antidepressants the average duration of a depressive episode was between six months and a year.

Bipolar Disorder

Bipolar Disorder is a recurrent illness. The likelihood of a single depressive and manic episode is small. Since bipolar illness usually begins in the twenties, the patient is vulnerable over a long span of life. A depressive episode occurs slightly more often than a manic episode as the initial expression of bipolar illness. It is uncommon for the number of depressive episodes to equal the number of manic episodes; depression usually predominates. Individual patients tend to have a consistent temporal pattern of depression and mania or hypomania, e.g., a manic episode may terminate with several days of depression. For other bipolar patients, a depressed episode may suddenly terminate with the onset of mania.

OUTCOME

Major Depressive Disorder

The treatment of affective illness has several components; there are specific (for acute episodes) and prophylactic (to reduce the intensity and frequency of subsequent episodes) approaches. As with many chronic medical problems, we are unable to "cure" depression. Vulnerability to affective episodes may "break through" the treatment of even the most well managed and compliant patient.

Suicide is the major mortality risk in affective illness. Fifteen percent of patients with Major Affective Illness may ultimately die by suicide (12). Morbidity is also great. Recurrent affective episodes have significant secondary effects on self-esteem and outlook resulting from the severe demoralization and stigmatization which so frequently occurs. Many of the apparent characterological features of depressed patients represent the impact of chronic illness on personality style.

Major treatment goals include prompt identification of episodes by the patient or significant others, prompt treatment in an appropriate setting, and maintenance of the highest possible level of functioning. Strict attention to rapid return to social and vocational functioning is a major secondary treatment goal. In treating a first episode, the physician should continue to see the patient for a number of months after recovery and discontinuance of antidepressant therapy. If there is no immediate recurrence, the physician should instruct the patient to call the physician if symptoms recur.

Manic Depressive Disorder

The major difference between the outcomes of Major Depressive and Manic Depressive Disorders is the greater likelihood of recurrent illness. The psychiatrist may expect to see the manic patient intermittently over many years with a mixture of daily visits during hospitalization, weekly and monthly outpatient appointments. Both the physician and patient should understand the probabilities of recurrence. The psychiatrist is likely to follow the patient with Bipolar Disorder more frequently, because of differences in episode frequency and the fact that lithium maintenance requires monitoring of blood levels. The psychiatrist is often consulted by other physicians about drug interactions with lithium.

OTHER SPECIFIC AFFECTIVE DISORDERS

Dysthymic Disorder

Dysthymic Disorder is a diagnosis in transition. The DSM-III criteria for Dysthymic Disorder are merely attenuated criteria for Major Depressive Disorder. As such, patients who meet these criteria probably represent a variety of underlying disorders; "subaffective" or atypical expressions of Major Affective Illnesses or so called neurotic and characterologic depression (not DSM-III categories). Also, the criteria for Dysthymic Disorder may not be adequate to distinguish dysphoric reactions to adverse life circumstances from depressive syndromes. Nevertheless, the criteria should be carefully applied in order to develop the data base for the future diagnosis of more valid syndromes.

The diagnosis of Dysthymic Disorder is precluded by the presence of psychotic symptoms. Another major feature of Dysthymic Disorder is that it may be present continuously—a fact which leads to the inclusion of many conditions that are probably not related to an episode of major affective illnesses. As might be predicted for such a heterogeneous syndrome, antidepressants are not as effective as they are for the Major Affective Disorders.

Cyclothymic Disorder

Cyclothymic Disorder criteria are attenuated criteria for Manic Depressive Disorder. Like Dysthymic Disorder, the presence of psychotic symptoms precludes diagnosis. Many affective disease researchers believe that cyclothymia is present in individuals who carry the bipolar genotype.

It is important to learn the criteria for each of the Affective Illnesses (see DSM-III). The criteria for diagnosis are those symptoms which best discriminate among affective illnesses, schizophrenia, and other AXIS I diagnoses. These disorders have many common symptoms that are not considered as criteria for diagnosis, since they do not discriminate well (are not useful in differential diagnosis).

ADJUSTMENT DISORDER
WITH ANXIOUS OR DEPRESSED PATIENTS

Although adjustment disorders are not affective illnesses, they are commonly associated with affective symptoms. Several empirical and nosological features separate affective illnesses from adjustment disorders. The diagnosis of adjustment disorder emphasizes mood alterations produced by the interaction of psychosocial stressors and the individual's adaptive characteristics. Criteria for affective illnesses emphasize the autonomous nature and to some extent unavoidable aspects of the affective symptoms. Affective illnesses may represent disordered physiologies, while adjustment disorders may be the maladaptive recruitment of normal physiologies. The criteria for adjustment disorders require that symptoms remit after the stressor ceases. The definition of maladaptive is that the symptoms produce impairment in social or occupational functioning, or that the symptoms are in excess of a normal or expectable reaction to the stressor. This last feature differentiates adjustment reactions from uncomplicated bereavement.

ETIOLOGY

Most psychiatric investigators believe there is a genetic vulnerability to affective illnesses, at least for the Major Affective Illnesses. Mendelian genetic research—that is, the study of transmission of traits through examination of the pedigrees of affectively ill probands, supports the notion of genetic inheritance, without strict support of straight Mendelian inheritance, e.g., autosomal dominant or recessive patterns.

Genetic Issues

In a review of affective illness in 83 monozygotic twin pairs in six studies (13), 71% were concordant for major affective illness. Of the concordant pairs, 81% were concordant for subtype; 19% were not. The concordance rate for dizygotic twins was 13%. Thus, concordance rates support genetic factors in the vulnerability to affective illness.

The data from seven studies of bipolar, and three studies of unipolar, probands suggest a morbid risk of about 7% for first degree relatives of bipolar probands for bipolar illness, and 8% for unipolar illness (13). The first degree relatives of unipolar probands had only a .4% risk of bipolar illness and 6% risk of unipolar illness (13). Thus, family history studies suggest that patients with bipolar illness have family history links with unipolar illness, though unipolar patients do not appear to have family history ties to bipolar illness.

Biogenic Amine Hypotheses

Bunney and Davis (14) and Schildkraut (15) postulated that serious depressive disorders arose from a functional deficiency of norepinephrine (NE) within limbic areas of the brain. This hypothesis was based upon a dramatic increase during the 1960s in the understanding of the role of biogenic amines in the brain. More specifically, the putative neurochemical effects of a variety of drugs (antidepressants, stimulants, and drugs which affect biogenic amine synthesis or catabolism) suggested an imbalance in amine function in depression. It was postulated that depression is produced by drugs which deplete catecholamines and serotonin, such as reserpine and tetrabenzaine, and drugs which block synthesis, such as alpha-methyl tyrosine. In rats treated with reserpine, antidepressants reverse various behaviors that are thought to be related to the physiology of depression. Plasma and CSF studies of biogenic amine metabolites in depressed and manic patients have tended to support the hypothesis that affective illness is due to a disturbance in catecholamine function. Urinary levels of the major NE metabolite, 3-methoxy-4-hydroxy phenylglycol (MHPG), have been reported to be lower in depressive episodes than in manic states.

Alterations in serotonin metabolism have been found in the brains of depressed patients who have died by suicide. Other investigators (16,17) have implicated serotonin neurons in the pathophysiology of depression. Maas (18) proposed the existence of two types of depressive disorders: 1. a function of abnormal noradrenergic function (the low MHPG group); 2. a function of abnormal serotonergic function (the low 5-hydroxy-indolacetic acid [5HIAA] group). If this hypothesis were true, the NE-associated depressions should respond to desipramine (an antidepressant with predominantly NE effects), and the serotonergic depressions to amitriptyline (an antidepressant that raises both serotonin and NE).

The involvement of biogenic amines in the pathogenesis of depression is not supported by all studies. Stimulant drugs which increase both NE and serotonin are not effective antidepressants. Furthermore, the NE—increasing properties of antidepressants are immediate, while antidepressant effects require weeks. In addition, there are several clinically effective antidepressant drugs that do not raise NE or serotonin, either acutely or chronically.

The current version of the biogenic amine hypothesis for the etiology of affective illness focuses upon neurotransmitter receptor regulation. While the acute effects of antidepressants increase biogenic amines, the subacute and chronic effects appear to reduce receptor sensitivity.

BIOLOGICAL MARKERS AND AFFECTIVE ILLNESS

Biogenic Amine Markers

Although biogenic amine theories of affective illness remain unproven, the measurement of biogenic amines, their metabolites, catabolic enzymes, and receptors continues to be a useful strategy for investigating subtypes of affectively ill patients.

Sleep Research
Sleep architecture is disrupted in affectively ill patients (4). Patients with Major Affective Disorders tend to have "short REM latencies"—that is, the time from sleep onset to the first rapid eye movement period during sleep is shorter than comparable normal volunteers. In addition to giving researchers a potential marker of an affective episode, this finding suggests several neurochemical strategies for the investigation of the etiology of depression. It is interesting that cholinergic drugs administered during the night precipitate REM periods almost instantaneously. Some investigators have proposed a cholinergic hypotheses of depression (19).

Endocrine Abnormalities
Disruption of Hypothalamic-Pituitary-Adrenal Regulation: In the 1950s, adrenal steroids and their metabolites were studied in patients with affective illness, and found to be abnormal. By the 1970s, more sophisticated endocrine challenge tests became widely used since they have been found to be more sensitive indicators of abnormal endocrine physiology than basal hormone levels. The dexamethasone suppression (DST) test is one such challenge test.

DST. Dexamethasone is a synthetic corticosteroid which, when administered exogenously, suppresses ACTH secretion and its consequent influence on cortisol levels for 24–48 hours. In pituitary or adrenal tumors, the feedback system is not intact, and cortisol levels remain elevated. In Major Depressive Disorders, the pituitary does not suppress normally; plasma cortisol "breaks through" or "escapes" dexamethasone suppression. There has been a good deal of recent research on the specificity and sensitivity of the DST in affectively ill individuals. While this test should not be used routinely in clinical practice, it does appear to have good specificity (90%) but poor sensitivity (50%) for unipolar and bipolar depressions (20). The DST is the first laboratory test found to have some value in confirming a functional psychiatric diagnosis.

TRH-TSH. Prange *et al.* (21, 22) found that 40% of depressed patients had a blunted or absent TSH response to the administration of synthetic TRH. This procedure has also been proposed as a laboratory test for depression. The suggestion that the thyroid is involved in affective illness has a long history. Both hypothyroid and apathetic hyperthyroid states produce profound depressive symptoms that can only be reversed with electroconvulsive therapy. Prange (21) also found that antidepressant responses in depressed women could be speeded up by concomitant treatment with thyroid hormone. In spite of these early positive studies, confirmation has not been uniform.

TREATMENT OF AFFECTIVE DISORDERS

Introduction

The treatment of the major affective disorders includes the selection of one of a number of specific antidepressant medications, and a host of psychosocial and interpersonal therapies. A depressed patient may be hospitalized, either because of suicidal impulses or severe dysfunction in the home environment that is adversely influencing recovery. Initial treatment involves antidepressant therapy, as well as the development of adequate rapport and a working relationship with the patient. Depending upon the severity of the depression, interpersonal therapies are initiated when there has been sufficient recovery of affective and neurovegetative function. Interpersonal therapies focus upon aspects of the individual's character and environment that may interact with the depressive process, if not precipitate episodes. Interpersonal therapies also seek to bolster self-esteem, and provide a reality-test for the patient's concern about being morally or intellectually deficient. Social therapies target reintegration into family life and social and vocational environments.

Pharmacotherapy and ECT

The clinical pharmacology of antidepressants is described in the Psychopharmacology chapter of this book. Specific antidepressant therapies bring about recovery in 70–80% of DSM-III diagnosed major affective episodes. ECT is associated with an even higher recovery rate (90%) in well-selected depressive episodes.

Psychotherapy

Psychotherapy alone is not a specific treatment for affective episodes, but Klerman et al. (23) have demonstrated that the combination of antidepressants and psychotherapy is more effective than antidepressants alone. The combination of psychotherapy and pharmacotherapy or the use of antidepressants alone were found superior to psychotherapy alone. Considering the extensive secondary effects of depression on personality, it is not surprising that the combination of therapies was found more effective than just drug treatment. Insight-oriented psychotherapy focuses on developmental difficulties that are thought to be related to the etiology of disorders. There is no empirical evidence that affective illness is acquired, either through early life experience or developmental difficulties. Patients are helped by psychotherapies that: focus on adaptation and self-image; structure adaptive cognitions; provide a cognitive explanation for the experience of depression. While there is little evidence to support a psychological etiology for the major affective illnesses, dynamic psychiatry enables us to understand much of the content of the depressive process. Psychoanalytic theory provides a window on the individual's thought processing during the affective episode, thus highlighting the relationship of depressive thought to premorbid character style and conflict.

Freud, in *Mourning and Melancholia,* (24) highlighted the similarity of depression to grief for a lost loved one. The concept that the psychological consequences of object loss due to death might be similar to the experience of loss of an internalized object is still a major psychoanalytic concept. Abraham (25) also pointed to the similarity between depression and grief, and saw depression as an expression of infantile disappointment. Sandor Rado (26), a theorist who combined psychoanalytic thought with adaptation concepts of biology, saw depression as a response to the patient's perception of danger. Rado suggested that depression was produced by a loss which endangered the security of the individual. Fenichel (27) attributed depression to the loss of self-esteem, while Bibring (28) highlighted the experience of helplessness and powerlessness. Spitz (29), in his study on "anaclitic" depressions in infants, and Bowlby (30), in his studies of the loss of a parent in childhood, have emphasized the impact of real, rather than perceived loss, in examining the depressive process.

MAJOR PROBLEMS POSED BY AFFECTIVE DISORDERS

Early Identification by the Patient of an Episode

A patient is frequently referred for treatment months after the onset of an affective episode. During this period, the depressive process will have had significant impact on adaptation and character; this produces more morbidity and slows recovery.

Concomitant Illnesses or Character Features

Many patients have other mood symptoms, e.g., dysphoria, in addition to affective illness. The identification of affective disorder symptoms, and their separation from characterological moods and life's miseries, are essential to effective treatment. This is not always an easy task.

Refractory Illness

Twenty-five percent of affectively ill individuals may not respond adequately to antidepressant treatment. The identification and management of treatment-resistant affective disorders is a subspecialty within psychiatry. Psychiatrists working in this subspecialty attempt to identify pharmacokinetic, pharmacodynamic, and disease differences that may account for treatment resistance.

Pharmacotherapy Integration with Psychotherapy

The integration of somatic and interpersonal therapies requires training. Adequate management depends upon initiating various treatment modalities at the right times and the assessment of individual patient characteristics that bear on management.

Compliance

Compliance and non-compliance are major factors in treatment success and failure. Therapists are trained to identify compliance issues, and strengthen compliance through the relationships they develop with patients. The treatment of bipolar illness has special problems associated with the presence of mania. Depressed patients occasionally resist treatment actively; manic patients do so commonly. The manic patient's grandiose sense of self, and broad lack of insight into the problems he is experiencing, often make him an unwilling collaborator in therapy.

REFERENCES

1. Pinel P: *A Treatise on Insanity,* Facsimile of the London 1806 edition. New York, Hafner Publishing Inc, 1962, p 56.
2. American Psychiatric Association Committee for Nomenclature and Statistics: *Diagnostic and Statistical Manual of Mental Disorders,* ed 3. Washington, DC, American Psychiatric Association, 1980.
3. Nemiah JC: Alexithymia: Theoretical considerations. *Psychother Psychosom* 1977; 28:199–206.
4. Karacan I, Williams RL, Salis PJ: Sleep and sleep abnormalities in depression, in Fann WE, Pokorny AD, Williams RL: *Phenomenology and Treatment of Depression.* New York, Spectrum Publications, 1977, pp 167–186.
5. Boyd JH, Weissman MM: Epidemiology of affective disorders: A reexamination and future directions. *Arch Gen Psychiatry* 1981;38:1039–1046.
6. Perris C: A study of bipolar (manic-depressive) and unipolar recurrent depressive psychoses. *Acta Psychiatr Scand* 1966;42(suppl 194):1–89.
7. Hirschfeld RMA, Cross CK: Epidemiology of affective disorders: Psychosocial risk factors. *Arch Gen Psychiatry* 1982;39:35–46.
8. Weissman MM, Klerman GL: Sex differences in the epidemiology of depression. *Arch Gen Psychiatry* 1977;34:98–111.
9. Clayton PJ: Bipolar affective disorder—techniques and results of treatment. *Am J Psychother* 1978;32:81–92.
10. Weissman MM, Myers JK: Rates and risks of depressive symptoms in a United States urban community. *Acta Psychiatr Scand* 1978;57:219–231.
11. Andreasen NC: Thought, language, and communication disorders. *Arch Gen Psychiatry* 1979;36:1325–1331.
12. Goodwin DW, Guze SB: *Psychiatric Diagnosis.* New York, Oxford University Press, 1979.

13. Gershon ES: The search for genetic markers in affective disorders, in Lipton MA, DiMascio A, Killam KF (eds): *Psychopharmacology: A Generation of Progress*. New York, Raven Press, 1978, pp 1197–1212.

14. Bunney WE Jr, Davis JM: Norepinephrine in depressive reactions. *Arch Gen Psychiatry* 1965;13:483–494.

15. Schildkraut JJ: The catecholamine hypothesis of affective disorders: A review of supporting evidence. *Am J Psychiatry* 1965;122:509–522.

16. Asberg M, Thoren P, Traskman L, et al.: 'Serotonin depression': A biochemical subgroup within affective disorders? *Science* 1976;191:478–480.

17. van Praag HM, Korf J: A pilot study of some kinetic aspects of the metabolism of 5-hydroxytryptamine in depression. *Biol Psychiatry* 1971;3:105–112.

18. Maas JW: Biogenic amines and depression. *Arch Gen Psychiatry* 1976;34:1357–1361.

19. Janowsky DS, Davis JM: Cholinergic mechanisms in mania and depression: Questions of specificity, in Belmaker RH, van Praag HM (eds): *Mania: An Evolving Concept*. New York, Spectrum, 1980, pp 267–280.

20. Carroll BJ, Feinberg M, Greden JF, et al.: A specific laboratory test for the diagnosis of melancholia: standardization, validation, and clinical utility. *Arch Gen Psychiatry* 1981;38:15–22.

21. Prange AJ, Wilson IC, Lara PP, et al.: Effects of thyrotropin-releasing hormone in depression. *Lancet* 1972;2:999–1002.

22. Prange AJ Jr: Patterns of pituitary responses to thyrotropin-releasing hormone in depressed patients: A review, in Fann WE, Karacan I, Pokorny A, et al. (eds): *Phenomenology and Treatment of Depression*. New York, Spectrum, 1977.

23. Klerman GL, DiMascio A, Weissman MM, et al.: Treatment of depression by drugs and psychotherapy. *Am J Psychiatry* 1974;131:186–191.

24. Freud S: *Mourning and Melancholia,* Riviere J (trans). New York, Basic Books Inc, 1959.

25. Abraham K: A short study of the development of the libido, in *Selected Papers in Psychoanalysis*. New York, Basic Books, 1960, pp 418–501.

26. Rado S: Mood cyclic behavior, in *Adaptation dynamics*. New York, Science House, 1969, pp 238–250.

27. Fenichel O: *The Psychoanalytic Theory of Neurosis*. New York, WW Norton, 1945, pp 387–414.

28. Bibring E: The mechanism of depression, in Greenacre P (ed): *Affective Disorders*. New York, International Universities Press, 1953, pp 13–48.

29. Spitz R: Anaclitic depression. *Psychoanal Study Child* 1946;2:313–342.

30. Bowlby J: Loss, sadness, and depression, in *Attachment and Loss*. New York, Basic Books, 1980, vol 3.

SELECTED ADDITIONAL READING

Nemiah J: *Foundations of Psychopathology*. New York, Oxford Press, 1961, chapters 10,12,13.

Paykel ES (ed): *Handbook of Affective Disorders. New York, Guilford Press, 1982*.

Belmaker RH, van Praag HM (eds): *Mania an Evolving Concept*. New York, Spectrum Publishing, 1980.

Akiskal H (ed): *Psychiatric Clinics of North America*. New York, WB Saunders, 1979, vol 2.

Akiskal H, Webb N: *Psychiatric Diagnosis*. New York, Spectrum, 1978.

Chapter 6

THE CHILD PATIENT'S MIND

THEODORE R. WARM, M.D.

The following chapters on child development are not meant to be a course in child psychiatry which would place greater emphasis on pathological conditions and specialized treatment approaches. This section emphasizes the basic intellectual and emotional development of the child which any doctor or other health professional needs to know in order to encourage the patient's cooperation, reduce the stress of medical interventions, and guide parents through medical and other commonly occurring dilemmas.

Psychiatric conditions stem from two main causes: 1. interference with actual brain function, either at an anatomical or biochemical level; 2. patterns of psychological reaction which interfere with effective problem solving. The first category includes organic brain syndromes, some types of mental retardation, schizophrenic and paranoid disorders, and many of the major affective disorders. Since these conditions result from organic/biochemical brain dysfunction, the treatment is primarily organic. Other etiologic theories about the cause and treatment of these conditions focus on social and learned factors (1,2). It is exceedingly important to recognize and deal with the social and family aspects of these mental conditions, however, for the most part, they are either secondary to the original condition or serve to aggravate the underlying organic problem.

The second group includes conditions which are due to faulty or inefficient psychological patterns of adjustment such as disorders of anxiety, personality, and conduct. These disorders can be classified according to a variety of different psychological theories, none of which is "right" or "wrong." A theory is a means of organizing observable data in a form which is useful. One parameter for categorizing psychological theories is whether it focuses primarily on the present or whether it focuses on relationships between past and present. Psychological theories which focus on the present are referred to as "transactional" or "behavioral;" those which relate the past to the present are "dynamic" (or "psychodynamic"). Both orientations are used in these chapters. The dynamic theories are emphasized because they are especially relevant to prevention by demonstrating the relationship between adaptive and maladaptive reactions and the person's earlier life patterns.

If the health professional is interested in prevention of nonorganic psychological conditions by the use of dynamic theory, knowledge of child development is essential. Within child development there are various organizational theories. Freudian psychoanalytic theory (which should not be confused with Freudian psychoanalytic treatment) is one of the most useful (3). Modern adaptations of dynamic "psychoanalytic" theory, however, is greatly influenced by ego psychology (4,5), transactional analysis (6), family structural theory (7), learning theory (8), intellectual theory (9), existential theory (10), epigenetic theories (11), and object relations theory (12). Those aspects of theory and the child's emotional and intellectual life which are most likely to be misunderstood will be emphasized in this section. These aspects are influential in shaping the adult's style of reacting—and that is the essence of dynamic psychiatry.

Child development is commonly divided into stages. Again, there is no "right" way to do this but one way is to divide up the person's life according to emerging characteristics. From a dynamic point of view, these early characteristics are crucial, suggesting ways that a child can develop confidence that life is generally pleasant and satisfactory. They indicate characteristics which society or parents have determined are either undesirable or are valuable and are therefore to be encouraged. They also identify those influences in a child's life which establish patterns that are relatively unchangeable. Ethological studies indicate that animals go through critical periods of learning (13,14), and apparently this is relatively true also of the human infant (15-17). Certain personality characteristics become relatively fixed in infancy; others can be influenced as they develop if the adult understands the way the child's mind functions. The following chapters will highlight these issues, especially where they intersect with medical practice and treatment.

REFERENCES

1. Laing RD: *The Politics of Experience*. New York, Ballantine Books, 1967.
2. Szasz T: *The Myth of Mental Illness*. New York, Harper & Row, 1961.
3. Brenner C: *An Elementary Textbook of Psychoanalysis*. New York, International Universities Press, 1955.
4. Freud A: *The Ego and the Mechanisms of Defense*. New York, International Universities Press, 1946.
5. Hartman H: *Essays on Ego Psychology*. New York, International Universities Press, 1964.
6. Harris TA: *I'm OK—You're OK: A Practical Guide to Transactional Analysis*. New York, Harper & Row, 1969.

7. Minuchin S: *Families & Family Therapy.* Cambridge, MA, Harvard University Press, 1974.
8. Hilgard ER: *Theories of Learning.* New York, Appleton-Century-Crofts, 1956.
9. Piaget J: *The Construction of Reality in the Child.* New York, Basic Books, 1954.
10. Binswanger L: *Being-in-the World.* New York, Basic Books, 1963.
11. Erikson EH: *Identity and the Life Cycle:* New York, International Universities Press, 1959.
12. Mahler MS: On the first three subphases of the separation-individuation process. *Int J Psychoanal* 1972;53:333–338.
13. Hess EH: Imprinting—An effect of early experience. *Science* 1959;130:133–141.
14. Harlow HF, Harlow MK: Effects of various mother-infant relationships on rhesus monkey behavior, in Foss BM (ed): *Determinants of Infant Behavior.* London, Methuen, 1969, vol 4.
15. Spitz RA: Hospitalism: An inquiry into the genesis of psychiatric conditions in early childhood. *Psychoanal Study Child* 1945;1:53–74.
16. Provence S, Lipton RC: *Infants in Institutions: A Comparison of Their Development with Family-Reared Infants During the First Year of Life.* New York, International Universities Press, 1962.
17. Kennell J, Klaus M: *Parent-Infant Bonding.* St. Louis, Mosby, 1982.

Chapter 7

INFANCY

THEODORE R. WARM, M.D.

The first year of life is usually referred to as "Infancy," ending when the child escapes from its previous locomotive dependency by learning to walk. *Intellectually,* the baby is basically orienting himself to the world (1). He must learn to differentiate between himself and his environment (as represented by concepts of autism, symbiosis, and separation/individuation [2]), and learn to recognize specific individuals. Since his memory is only good enough to remember a few people, the child first recognizes the person most available to provide for his needs. As *motor* control over neck and trunk develops, the child can sit; hands become useful for clinging, exploring, and eating. Legs can be used for rolling and crawling, but are not yet strong enough to support the body in an erect position. The skin and mouth are centers of *sensory* responsivity. Holding, stroking, and cuddling produce dramatic responses which can be soothing or disquieting to the baby. The mouth is used for exploration, familiarization, and eating. Sucking becomes a means of feeding and emotional comfort. The baby is weaned in stepwise fashion near the end of this stage. The child's *emotional* development, an outgrowth of the above characteristics, is organized around the ability to relate to people (3). The experience of an early enjoyable interaction with another human requires the presence of a relatively constant parent or caretaker (because of the child's underdeveloped memory) and lays the groundwork for the development of the capacity to have future comfortable relationships (4). Children who are severely "deprived" during the first year of life do not later develop a natural, comfortable ability to relate to others; furthermore, their intellectual development is irrevocably stunted. These principles are derived from studies of extremely deprived children, and whether they are applicable to everyday life depends upon the principles of extrapolation, i.e., if severe deprivation causes severe problems, will moderate or mild deprivation cause moderate or mild problems (5,6)? This reasoning is not clearly established as applicable but is reasonable to assume for the time being.

The most common misunderstandings about infants are: 1. The baby is too young to care whether different people provide care. Actually, a baby needs constancy and familiarity because of his weak ability to remember and associate comfort with a person. 2. The baby must learn self-control and obedience is another common misunderstanding. Many parents believe that during the first year of life, the child should learn to not touch breakables, control excretory sphincters, and obey authority. The stress on learning self-control often stems from the parents misinterpreting the child's normal egocentrism as being meanness or selfishness.

These various views of babies are the logical extension of thinking that babies are miniature adults and represent misunderstandings of childhood characteristics. Actually the infant needs indulgence and personal attention to establish the very characteristics which will permit "maturation" and "civilizing." The infant needs to feel loved and enjoy pleasing his parent which then becomes the main source of parental influence, i.e., the child obeys because he wants the parents' approval. This is by far the most efficient and thorough way to teach a child. If this bond has not developed, the child can only be influenced by threats and punishment and this unfortunately becomes the core of the interaction between parent and child, establishing a negative tone. What is worse, the child only learns to behave in a civilized manner when there is threat of negative consequence and thus the early basis for development of a conscience will not be established.

The results are very different when the child is cared for by an adult who puts the welfare of the child above his or her own needs and ambitions, and who recognizes the child's characteristics and needs. The infant develops a pleasure in relating to others and a pleasure in mastering new skills, which expands enormously as his legs and speech begin to develop in the next stage of development.

REFERENCES

1. Heidelise A, Brazelton TB: A new model of assessing the behavioral organization in preterm and full term infants—two case studies. *J Am Acad Child Psychiatry* 1981; 20:239-263.

2. Mahler MS: On the first three subphases of the separation-individuation process. *Int J Psychoanal* 1972;53:333-338.

3. Kessler J: Reciprocal relationship of mental and emotional development in early childhood, in *Psychopathology of Childhood*. Englewood Cliffs, NJ, Prentice-Hall, 1966, pp 18-43.

4. Erickson EH: Eight stages of man, in *Childhood and Society,* ed 2. New York, WW Norton & Co, 1963.

5. Harlow HF, Harlow MK: Effects of various mother-infant relationships on rhesus monkey behavior, in Foss BM (ed): *Determinants of Infant Behavior.* London, Methuen, 1969.
6. Provence S, Lipton RC: *Infants in Institutions: A Comparison of their Development with Family-Reared Infants During the First Year of Life.* New York, International Universities Press, 1962.

Chapter 8

TODDLER STAGE
THEODORE R. WARM, M.D.

The toddler stage, ages 1–3 years, is characterized by the child's running, curiosity, independence, stubbornness, and speech development. In psychoanalytic terminology, this is referred to as the "anal stage" (1). Read this section slowly, using your imagination. Try to imagine what things look like from the children's point of view since this is crucial to understanding their thinking and feelings.

Just as an exercise in an imagination, think what you as an adult look like to a little two-year-old. If she looks straight ahead, what does she see? A crotch or knee. If she looks upward she sees belly or breast protuberances, and your face is mainly chin and nostrils. While this may have little psychological significance, it should remind you that things appear different when you're small. What does a table look like to a two-year-old? Can you remember lying on your back as a child, looking up at the bottom of the dining room table and chairs? There are unfinished boards, screw heads, labels. ("Do not remove this label under penalty of law"), and probably some crud around the edges. That is what a table looks like to a two-year-old. A dog looks as big as a horse does to you. How would you like to be running around the corner of the dining room doorway and have that stare you in the face? Almost nothing seems the same to the toddler as it does to you. To understand two-year-olds, you must constantly imagine the view from their stature and their immature minds. Adults watching two-year-olds are grinning and chuckling much of the time. What are they chuckling at? They are watching the child try to push a golf ball into the mouth of a pop bottle, or looking under the sink to see where the water goes as it disappears down the drain. The child does not have the intellectual capacity to understand about hollow pipes, etc.; things that can't be seen cannot be conceptualized (2). It's like the adult's attempts to conceptualize the fourth dimension. The child's inability to understand what happens to things when they are out of sight makes life full of incomprehensible disappearances. These disappearances don't seem to upset the child unless the item is greatly valued—a blanket, stuffed bear, or parent; the immature inability to conceptualize then causes the child to become very upset. Thus, the ability that has made the child appear so naively comical is the very characteristic which also makes her vulnerable to life's events and susceptible to anxiety.

By this age the child has developed a very good memory, and can clearly retain the visual image and loyalty of the caretaker (referred to as object constancy). The ability to conceptualize time and space is still immature, and so the child doesn't understand about hours, days, and weeks. If the parent has been around the child a lot, the child learns to believe that the parent will reappear—providing the parent doesn't stay away too long. One-year-olds can be left with a familiar person for several hours, three-year-olds can generally be left with a familiar person for a half to a full day.

During the toddler period, children sometimes cry when parents leave. There are two preferable ways to handle this: 1. Don't leave; 2. alert the child ahead of time, leave them with a familiar person, and let them cry. Later the parent assesses whether this experience was too upsetting to the child by determining how long the child wailed or whether there was a subsequent regression in other areas of functioning. The parent can also handle crying by sneaking away when the child is not looking. Although this method alleviates the parent's upset over the child's tears, you can easily see that it is not good for the child. Because there was no signal of the departure, the child constantly wonders when the next disappearance will occur and clings to the parent with even more persistence. The child may even begin having temper tantrums which the parents misunderstand so they may punish the child or perhaps sneak away in order to escape the aggravating behavior. Such attempts at dealing with the problem may actually make it worse.

If a child is put to bed before the sitter arrives and the parents leave and then the child awakens to find the parent gone and a stranger there, you can guess how the child will react. The child may then be afraid that the parents will again disappear if she goes to sleep. That night and subsequent nights there appears a "sleep disturbance;" it is really a "separation problem." This problem can be avoided by having the sitter arrive before the child goes to bed, even if the parents are not leaving for several hours. While it is expensive and inconvenient, this approach is not as troublesome as trying to undo the problem by having parents reassure a screaming child of their presence in the middle of the night or consulting with their physician.

There are similar risks in hospitalizing children. In order to minimize the stress of illness, medical procedures, and living in a strange environment, the parents should spend as much time with the child as possible, and leaving a familiar object such as a teddy bear when they need to be away. Many knowledgeable pediatricians permit parents to sleep in the child's room which provides the child with a maximum sense of security. While medical personnel may find this arrangement inconvenient, they need to be reminded of its importance to the child.

Toddlers do many other "humorous" things. They run stiff-legged, bobbing from side to side like a penguin, usually in a helter-skelter manner. While running into your knees is funny, running into the coffee table or outside into the street is not. Again, the characteristic makes her appear cute; also makes her vulnerable. The street looks like a sidewalk to a toddler. At best she can learn not to cross a certain line such as the curb or lawnstrip. At this age, the child is just not sophisticated enough to understand about such dangers and can't be trusted. The parent must know where the child is at all times; if there is a potential danger, the child should be in sight. While this may be a lot of trouble for the parent, it saves wear and tear on the child and the Emergency Room physician who has to suture the head that fell off the dining room table or pass a naso-gastric tube to pump out laundry soap, witch hazel, cigarettes, etc.

Some parents try yet another way to teach the child self-control. They beat her. Spanking appears to be a shortcut for teaching the child self-control. This method is used by some parents who do not have a close love relationship which they could use to influence the child or by parents who are impatient or who think that spanking a child is good for her—a common misconception. Although this approach occasionally works, it does so at the cost of the child becoming extremely inhibited and compliant about everything, and hardly able to stand up for her own rights. Fortunately, most parents don't have the stomach to punish the child enough for this to occur. If the parents primarily use hitting as a means of discipline, the child may learn to stop "the bad behavior," but unfortunately, she only stops when hit and she learns to hit others when she's angry or wants to make a point, just like the parent; these patterns then lead later to other problems such as fighting in the neighborhood or classroom (3).

A toddler should be disciplined by removing the child or object, sitting her on a chair (the parent may need to remain close enough to enforce this), scolding, supervision, and rewarding good behavior. This method does not provide immediate results but its effects, however, last longer, and the harmful effects of injurious, frightening discipline are avoided.

Since toddlers have an immature understanding of cause and effect, they are likely to think that events that follow one another necessarily have a cause and effect relationship. For example, a child may pull a tablecloth from the table and get hit on the head by a falling plate; the relationship between these two events is obvious and sensible. On the other hand, a child who develops appendicitis after sneaking an extra piece of candy may develop erroneous ideas about the causes of the illness. Some children think that medical personnel are punishing them for being bad because they have come to associate pain with punishment and associate both with having been bad. Medical personnel need to be alert to correct such misunderstandings.

The child's understanding of cause and effect is further complicated by his inability to distinguish between thought and action. A three-year-old who is having angry, resentful thoughts about a baby brother, and the brother actually begins to cry, thinks he has caused the crying. Could something terrible happen to a parent because the child is angry about being punished? The child might want to stay close to the parent to see that nothing bad happens. The child's clinging to the parent would have the outward appearance of a "separation problem." The fear and guilt associated with having angry thoughts may persist into adult life, causing great inhibition and suffering. Fortunately, the development of language at this toddler stage can be helpful in clarifying the misunderstandings if the adult is alert and understanding.

A little child learns to talk in a funny way—"ma ma," "da da," "wa wa," "ga ga" (crackers). It's no wonder that parents end up using words like "doo doo" and "pee pee." Although the language sounds silly, it is an outgrowth of the child's immature verbalization and conceptualization. The development of speech is particularly important because it provides a means of problem-solving without necessitating trial and error behavior. The child can think through a task without having to act on it immediately, e.g., ask for a toy on a high shelf, rather than climb up and be hurt by falling; call across the street to get mother's attention rather than run into the road. This greatly expands the child's capacities for learning self-control.

Parents commonly teach children certain words that are apparently important to our family and social structure, e.g., "red," "blue," "green," "ball," "milk," "bye bye," "nap," "no no," "one plus one is two." Other important words are often not specifically taught to little children; words expressing emotions, such as "happy," "scared," "mad," "sad," "sorry" (4). Knowledge and use of these words shows the child that such feelings are legitimate, acceptable, and permits a way of expressing the feelings through words rather than only through action.

Let's get back to the funny part of watching toddlers. They are really stubborn. They are recognizing that they can think and act as separate people (5), and they delight in practicing their independence. They love to say, "no"—which is, after all, the word they hear the most. In fact, adults sometimes enjoy tricking them into saying "no."

"Do you want a bath?"   "No"
"Clean up your toys."   "No"
"Do you want some ice cream?"   "No"

Being in control becomes a central issue for the toddler at about the same time the parents decide to teach the child to use the potty or toilet. Smart parents try not to make an issue out of "who is the boss." The real task is to get the child to want to perform the desired action. Toilet training should not be started until the child is: 1. aware of the sensation of imminent defecation; 2. able to signal the parent by word or action; 3. able to control the sphincter; 4. able to walk to the potty and probably pull her own pants down. This readiness may occur as early as 14 months, but 18 months is more common; if it isn't apparent by two years, the parents should probably go ahead and try anyway. The child should be shown the potty and taught the words to designate feces. The potty is used to avoid the child's occasional fear of falling into the toilet and being flushed away. Parents should encourage the child to use the potty by reflecting mild displeasure with continuing messes and very great pleasure with successes. Thus, the child is made to feel happy and proud about doing what the parents want rather than what comes natural, i.e., to let things fall where they will. It is true that the whole process sounds very manipulative and smacks of brainwashing. If you want a child to give up one side of her natural tendency, namely, to be mean, selfish, and dirty—you'll have to either beat it out of her or outfox her. This is a blunt, abbreviated way of stating the issues. A more professional statement of the issues is that the immature child is naturally egocentric, accepting of excretions, and has little control over hostility. While intimidation is an effective means of modifying these characteristics, a better method is to get the child to "want" to overcome these tendencies, through self-control and mastery. (In psychoanalytic theoretical terms, the mental capacity of mediating between the child's urges and the demands of the parents is referred to as the "ego.")

Actually, the process of civilizing isn't embarked upon in such a deliberate manner by most parents, but it amounts to the same thing. Usually the parent naturally shows pleasure and pride at the "right time" and the child learns by mimicking and by enjoying the parents' approval. But that is the real key. The child has to enjoy the parents' approval. That really becomes the potent influence over the child—a much more efficient influence than punishment! But that requires that the parents have spent a lot of time with the child so that an attachment can occur and it requires that a lot of that time was pleasant so that it becomes desirable for both the child and for the parent. The love relationship is not only great as a way of influencing the child, but it really is what makes having children be a nice experience; it makes parents smile out of inner pleasure rather than only out of amusement; and it establishes the child's ability to relate warmly, pleasantly, intimately, and securely to others.

REFERENCES

1. Freud S: The sexual life of human beings, in *The Complete Psychological Works of Sigmund Freud,* st'd ed, Strachy J (trans). London, Hogarth Press, 1963, vol 16, pp 303–319.
2. Piaget J: *The Construction of Reality in the Child.* New York, Basic Books, 1954.
3. Warm T: An approach to psychiatric school consultation: What's good about bad behavior. *J Am Acad Child Psychiatry* 1978;17:708–716.
4. Katan A: Some thoughts about the role of verbalization in early childhood. *Psychoanal Study Child* 1961;16:184–188.
5. Mahler, MS: On the first three subphases of the separation-individuation process. *Int J Psychoanal* 1972;53:333–338.

Chapter 9

PRESCHOOL STAGE
THEODORE R. WARM, M.D.

The period of a child's life beginning around age three and ending around six is referred to in this chapter as the preschool period of development. In the broadest terms, during this phase of development *a child learns he or she is a child.* The change is from the toddler's assumption that we are all equal in ability, regardless of size, to the view of the grade school child in which the differences in generations are clearly recognized. At that point children work in groups and begin to exclude adults. In between the toddler and the grade school periods is preschool during which the child is learning that he or she is a child. Children in this age group imagine taking on the roles of their parents or other heroes. They mimic and are highly competitive. Because of their grandiose view of their own abilities, they expect to win all the time and are poor losers. The child may imagine being married to one or another parent, but he gradually comes to grips with the fact that they are of a different generation. The acceptance of one's place in one's own generation is an important psychological and intellectual landmark that allows the child to more realistically compare himself with others. Failure to overcome this intellectual hurdle leaves the child comparing himself with people who are older, bigger, and more educated which constantly gives the child a feeling of inadequacy and contributes to chronic feelings of inferiority.

This preschool period of life might be referred to as the "age of measuring." Children love to use rulers to compare lengths and sizes. In the process of learning to categorize and compare, they finally accept the destiny of their own generation. The remainder of this chapter is organized into descriptive categories. Each category is followed by some common situations which a physician might encounter. Utilizing the concepts explained in the previous section, first imagine what kind of problems might develop from the situation. Then consider what you might say or do to prevent the problem.

112

Intellect

The child's understanding of cause and effect remains rather primitive. When two events happen in sequence, the child usually assumes that the first has caused the second. They still have significant remnants of "magical thinking," in which a child assumes that thinking or wishing about an event will make it actually occur (1). Wishes become somewhat more realistic. Instead of wishing for all the candy in the world, a child will wish that his father or mother were wealthy and would buy all the candy in the world. Children learn to classify objects by colors, shapes, and by whether objects are generally used by boys, girls, or grownups. They are extraordinarily curious and begin to ask many "why" and "how" questions. For example: "Why is the sky blue? Where did my brother come from? How did he get out? How did he get in?" Children are generally quite uninhibited in their questions. This naivete gives them an admirable aura of openness and the ability to ask penetrating questions. Their ability to understand the answers to such questions remains quite limited. As a child is able to increasingly think through his questions and problems, he is spared from needing to act upon every idea. He shows an increased ability to sit still, pay attention, and engage in fine motor activities, such as use of scissors and coloring inside the lines.

Situations
1. The doctor learns that his four-year-old patient had been sneaking candy just before he became sick with fever and vomiting. (This child could probably use some reassurance that the candy did not cause his sickness.)
2. The boy is admitted to the hospital and operated on for appendicitis. (The medical intervention, including removal from the home and having the body cut with a knife could be viewed by the child as punishment for his transgression by sneaking candy.)
3. In the hospital, the child is obviously staring at other patients who have eyes bandaged, I.V.'s running, limbs casted or missing, and other deformities. He does not ask questions about these children. (It is important to try to accurately prepare children for what they will experience at the hands of the medical profession. At times we do not consider what the child will observe in other patients. The child patient makes assumptions about what happened to the other children which are so scary that he asks no questions.)
4. Later that year, the boy's mother mentions that he leaves any play situation in order to carefully observe her changing the diaper of his baby sister but again makes no comments. (The child can have similar

misunderstandings at home as he did in the hospital and assume that parts of body can be removed and that this accounts for the difference between his genitalia and his sister's.

Play

Children continue to enjoy gross motor activities on tricycles, big wheels and climbing toys. They begin to develop fine motor coordination and can make representational drawings, such as persons, houses, or flowers. Their rhythmical abilities are poor as they struggle to learn to skip and to play the sticks, tambourine, or triangle in the rhythm band. Their language matures and they use better grammar. They are able to understand and relate fairly complicated stories which contain simple symbolic messages—for example, what happens to the person who is unwise enough to build a house of straw, rather than of brick. And they are particularly excited at the prospect in the story of outwitting and overcoming the big, mean, powerful figures (who often symbolically represent parents).

Children request increasingly realistic props to fulfill their strong urges for fantasy play in which they mimic adults, especially parents. Their fantasy life may become very real to them—especially when they take on the roles of adults or create imaginary companions, be they animals, children, or permissive parents. The children at times believe their own imagination and expect both their happiest wishes and worst fears to come true. The distinction between reality and fantasy becomes well separated only towards the end of the next stage of development, about age ten.

Situations

1. The doctor learns that the boy's father is becoming aggravated because his persistent efforts to teach his son basketball are not successful. (Neurological development at this stage has generally not progressed far enough for such coordinated rhythmical activities. The father needs to be reassured.)

2. The boy's mother is sympathetic to the father because she suffers similar frustration in trying to teach her four-year-old daughter to embroider. (Fine motor coordination has not progressed enough for most children to successfully engage in such meticulous handwork.)

3. The parents mention other ideas for toys—such as model cars to glue together or a play doctor kit. (Most model car projects require too much fine dexterity for children of this age. Toys that encourage the child to act out life situations which have been stressful can be very helpful.)

Peers
Play with other children shifts from being bossy and demanding towards being more cooperative and sharing roles and toys. The child is learning to understand what pleases others and how to alter his own behavior accordingly. This enormously important step in socialization makes the child quite appealing to the adult. At times this naturally leads the child to believe that anything can be obtained by just being cute and pleasing. Relationships are also influenced by a reversal in the child's pleasures. Whereas previously there was often pleasure in selfishness and cruelty, there is now a pleasure in sharing and helpfulness. While these nice, civilizing characteristics are emerging, the child remains quite competitive and poorly tolerates failure.

Situations
1. The doctor learns that the four-year-old has been left in charge of the two-year-old sister so the mother and older sister can keep the appointment. (At this stage, a child may show great interest and tenderness in caring for others, and may want to assume the adult role. On the other hand, the child's ability to persist in such supervision is quite variable and she lacks the proper judgement to supervise a younger child.)
2. The doctor is told that the four-year-old tries to play baseball with second graders. He ends up crying because he can't do as well as the older boys and they are disgusted with his disregard for the rules. (Most children in this stage of development cannot accept the rigid rules needed for such organized play and have not developed the capacity to be a "good sport.")
3. The doctor observes that the boy cries when he anticipates an injection. His embarrassed father thinks he is a sissy and shames him by comparing him to his brave eight-year-old sister. (Crying with pain is normal for children at any age. The capacity for bravery is usually not present until around eight or nine years of age. The father of this child needs to be reassured about that.)

School
By the end of this stage, most children attend some organized educational program, such as kindergarten and first grade while other children will have begun day care or nursery school earlier. The success of this experience depends in part upon the child's ability to tolerate separations; this, in turn, depends upon the previous separation experience, the child's preparation for the separation, and the parent's ability to transmit a sense of pleasure and security to the teacher. At first the teacher is viewed as a substitute for the

parents' protection and then later becomes a person to identify with and to mimic. Children often copy the teacher's role of being helpful to other children, perhaps instructing or chastising them. During this educational time, there is a gradual shift to pleasure in learning. At first the child enjoys learning those things which are personally interesting and appealing. By the end of the period, the child enjoys learning for the sake of mastery and accomplishment. If the adult's values are not adopted, the child only attempts to learn those things which are immediately interesting, pleasurable, and whose immediate relevance is obvious. That will cause difficulty in subsequent schooling.

Situations
1. The doctor is asked to treat a three-year-old girl for stomachaches which occur every morning before nursery school. He further learns that she plays cheerfully and without complaints after the bus leaves without her. (Stomachaches are one of the most common expressions of separation anxiety.)
2. Wanting to be thorough, the doctor debates in his mind about doing the medical work-up on an outpatient basis or hospitalizing the girl in order to do the evaluation more quickly and efficiently. (Hopefully the evaluation can be done as an outpatient. Hospitalizing a child for stomachaches which are actually due to separation anxiety will surely make both the symptom and the psychological situation worse.)

Emotions
The child's increased awareness of social interactions makes it easy for him to have hurt feelings. Temper continues to erupt, but not nearly as frequently or persistently as during the toddler stage of development. Conflict and fighting are focused on competition for friendships or roles in play, rather than only on possessions. Fears are prominent, especially at night, as the child's imagination seems very real. Night fears focus on kidnappers, attackers, monsters, and doctors' shots. Because of the child's fearful imagination, it is important to prepare him in advance for frightening or painful medical procedures. This preparation gives the child a proper signal as to when he should be afraid and when he can feel secure. Children who have experienced frightening medical or accidental traumas without preparation are often chronically anxious about the occurrence of the next frightening event. Some children will be more cooperative when they are well-prepared for medical procedures; some will be less cooperative. The primary purpose of advance preparation is to ensure mental health after the procedure, not to gain the child's immediate cooperation (2,3).

Situations

1. A mother tells the doctor that her four-year-old daughter has not liked nursery school since she broke a school paint jar and the teacher disciplined her by advising other children not to play with her. (Because of children's sensitivity to social interactions, such a discipline is much too severe. The mother should make some intervention.)

2. Another mother relates that her teenage son delights in playing monster, threatening to "get" the four-year-old if he doesn't behave. (The adolescent delight in exposing oneself to fearful fantasy situations is surely not shared by small children. It is an altogether unfair way of controlling or disciplining them.)

3. A mother uses the doctor's office as an opportunity to impress her four-year-old daughter with the importance of eating all of her vegetables so she won't get sick and have to come to the doctor for a shot. (While it is tempting for parents to use the fear and authority of the doctor to accomplish their own ends, enhancing the view of the doctor as punitive is certainly not helpful.)

4. The doctor is surprised and tempted to laugh at a boy's question as to whether the laceration on his head will get "stitches" and "sewn up" by a sewing machine. (This is an example of the myriad of misunderstandings which children have about medical procedures.)

Sexuality

From the beginning of this stage of development, most children discover their own genitals. If the opportunity presents itself, they will have a normal curiosity about comparing their own genitals with those of others. Since the boy's genital organ is more obvious externally, its presence is noticed by both girls and boys. The pleasurable sensation associated with pressure or rubbing of the penis or clitoris is discovered and this form of childhood masturbation is a common occurrence. Discovering pleasurable sensations in this part of the body is just another step in the sequence of bodily pleasures, e.g., the infant's oral pleasure from sucking and the pleasure of the skin from being stroked and held. Other bodily pleasures include sensations of muscular activity when the child is running, or anal sensations during defecation. These various bodily pleasures and their derivatives ultimately contribute to the bodily pleasures of adult sexuality (4).

The child's view of sexual pleasures remains immature, but gradually begins to incorporate concepts of the baby growing within the mother's uterus, concepts of birth, and beginning concepts and fantasies about impregnation by the oral or genital routes. The child's natural tendencies to compare himself with adults leads him to imagine being a parent. When children imagine being married and having children, it is natural for them to fantasize that they will marry someone who is familiar and caring. That person is often the child's own parent, usually but not necessarily of the opposite sex. The child views this rivalry for the other parent as quite realistic; the adult recognizes it as a fantasy. At times, the child feels angry with the parent for not fulfilling these wishes. He or she may assume that the parent feels as rivalrous, threatening, and angry as the child feels toward the parent. Imagined retribution and fearfulness may develop in the child. These concepts form the basis for the Freudian psychoanalytic theory of the "oedipus complex" (5). As the child gradually understands the generational differences, he gives up competing with the parent and accepts the destiny of relating to peers. Children may understand and attribute all manner of privileges and fears to the conflicts which occur in this interaction; these include fears that bodily injury might result from the parents' anger, or that various social or love advantages are attributed to the presence of obvious external genitalia (6). Psychiatrists who work with adult patients at times discover that remnants of these misunderstandings influence the sexual and family lives of adults.

Based upon the above description of children's thinking during this stage of development, some general guidelines for parents can be helpful. Parents should look for opportunities to answer their children's factual questions about the body, sex, and babies. Responding to the child's inquiry and curiosity is probably the best guideline as to when the child should learn the facts of life. On the other hand, children sometimes ask questions indirectly ("Why is Aunt Jane getting such a big tummy?"); these should be taken as an opportunity to educate the child. Body privacy should be encouraged, especially adult modesty in front of children. Exposure to adult genital nudity, as well as sleeping with children, generally heightens the above-described conflicts and may cause some greater difficulty in resolving them. Although these activities can also be expressions of openness and comforting, they carry risks of producing conflicts in the child which are usually not immediately evident. Because children take ideas very literally, they should not be threatened with injury to parts of their body. Physical discipline should be minimized as it is often interpreted as a threat to the body's integrity. Surgery and medical procedures may take on similar meanings, thus underlining the importance of realistic preparation of the child for medical intervention. Masturbation should be considered a normal but private matter. Children who do not respond to requests to honor the privacy of the body are probably using masturbatory pleasure to relieve other underlying tensions. Inquiry and searching to help relieve these tensions can be helpful to the child. Sex play and comparing genitals is normal among children. Children should generally be encouraged to learn about such matters by asking adults. In the same manner, explanations about adult sexual activities are preferable to the child's actually observing sexual intercourse; the child is likely to misinterpret the activity, and may even view it as a frightening struggle.

The effects of children's sexual fantasies and activities have been widely studied by psychiatrists in the process of doing therapy with adults. Most of this experience has been with Western European and American middle class society (7). It is difficult to separate exact scientific guidelines from social contexts on such matters. Certainly many societies use very different child-rearing practices relating to sexuality and intimacy (8). Also, they often value different adult personality characteristics which may be related to these early rearing principles. It is difficult to be persuasive and certain about the importance of the guidelines because while some persons exhibit obvious psychological difficulties that result from early childhood sexual misunderstandings, many other people are raised similarly and appear to be well-adjusted. No one knows why events, such as observation of sexual intercourse or nudity, have unfavorable influences on some people and not on others. Psychiatrists who recognize the difficulty of correcting adult problems with childhood origins tend to place great emphasis upon preventive measures and to offer conservative advice.

Whatever guidelines are given to parents, we should be very aware that children have a natural interest in sexuality and as with many other areas of interest, they develop misunderstandings. Clarifying those understandings through word and deed promotes mental health (9).

REFERENCES

1. Fraiberg S: *The Magic Years*. New York, Charles Scribner's Sons, 1959, pp 193–241.
2. Melamed BG, Siegel LJ: Reduction of anxiety in children facing hospitalization and surgery by use of filmed modeling. *J Consult Clin Psychol* 1975;43:511–521.
3. Mason EA: The hospitalized child—his emotional needs. *New Engl J Med* 1965; 272:406–414.
4. Freud S: Infantile sexuality, in *The Complete Psychological Works of Sigmund Freud*, st'd ed, Strachy J (trans). London, Hogarth Press, 1953, vol 7, pp 173–206.
5. Freud S: Infantile sexuality, in *The Complete Psychological Works of Sigmund Freud*, st'd ed, Strachy J (trans). London, Hogarth Press, 1953, vol 4, pp 261–267.
6. Thompson C: "Penis envy" in women, in *Psychoanalysis and Women*. New York, Brunner/Mazel, 1973, pp 52–57.
7. Parsons A: Is the oedipus complex universal? The Jones-Malinowski debate revisited and a south Italian nuclear complex. *The Psychoanalytic Study of Society*. New York, International Universities Press, 1964, pp 278–328.
8. Aries P: *Centuries of Childhood, A Social History of Family Life*. New York, Vintage Books, 1962, pp 15–32, 33–49, 241–268, 339–364, 365–404.
9. Rothchild E: Emotional aspects of sexual development. *Pediatr Clin North Am* 1969; 16:415–428.

Chapter 10

CONSCIENCE FORMATION
THEODORE R. WARM, M.D.

The conscience is that part of a person's thought process and emotional life that provides guidelines, goals, morals, and restraints, even when not required by the immediate consequences. The conscience functions automatically, and, for the most part, without much self-questioning or awareness.

By adult standards, the young child of two is selfish and egocentric. It is, of course, natural that he wants his own way and is unmindful of how he imposes on others. The parent attempts to teach the child self-control and consideration of others' rights, property, and feelings by providing consequences, such as praise or punishment. Gradually the child learns that certain actions result in unpleasant reactions from the parents and good things happen if he conforms to the parents' wishes.

The psychoanalytic term for those functions of the mind which size up reality consequences and exert self-control is the "ego" (1,2). Some people's behavior is always governed by a basic philosophy, i.e., you only get what you earn and you only impose upon yourself because of immediate consequences. At this level of development, stealing is quite acceptable, if there is little or no danger of getting caught; similarly, consideration for others is only practiced when there is a tangible payoff. Most civilized societies, however, value more altruistic attitudes and behaviors, in which the individual suppresses or delays personal urges in order to benefit others. Such values are embodied in laws, family life, religion, or nationalism; the counterpart in the individual is the conscience or "superego."

The development of altruistic attitudes and self-restraint begins early in childhood. Parents pressure children to forego some of their natural pleasures in order to be clean, neat, orderly, kindly, helpful. The child is taught that such behavior is not based just on the immediate consequences but that benefitting others should provide inner satisfaction and pleasure. This reversal of the natural feelings helps to establish the automatic aspects of the superego. While such values are admirable, it is easy to see that they can also be overdone. An individual should not be so giving that his own "rights" are lost. He should be aggressive enough to protest injustice to himself. The struggle over drawing the line between realistic self-interest (ego) and dedication to fairness and the interests of others (superego) continues throughout most people's lives.

Superego formation is not solely a process of reversing natural tendencies, it is also a process of learning and "internalizing" attitudes and behaviors. If the young child is loved by an adult, and if he is capable of experiencing love, he comes to value the adult's loving approval. The child tries to think and act in ways that will please the adult who will then show affection. The child of two or three learns that the adult values him more highly when he is more "altruistic," kind, sharing, helpful, or hardworking. Internalization occurs when the child evaluates himself according to the learned standards. When the child does not live up to the set standards, he experiences a devalued, self-punishing feeling which we call "guilt." Guilt is the feeling which prompts the person to not be self-serving, even if he could "get away with it." The conscience which is beginning at age three or four becomes harsh and rigid by age six when children view rules of conduct or games as irrevocable and expect severe consequences for any infraction (3). This results in their tattling on peers and refusal to play a game unless it is played "right." They are equally severe with themselves such that they often deny their guilt or blame others in order to avoid their own intolerable self-criticism. By age eight or nine, the conscience begins to soften as the children recognize that rules are made to serve a purpose and can be altered. They see variations in the standards of the other families as their horizons extend beyond their own parents.

On the positive side, the superego provides a set of goals to be reached. The satisfaction of striving for and reaching such goals is referred to as the "ego ideal." Although the conscience or superego can overburden the person with feelings of guilt and inadequacy, it can also provide the loftiest goals and greatest satisfactions. It is both the bane of the civilized person and yet the embodiment of civilization itself.

A simplified variation of psychoanalytic structural theory may help to illustrate the possible clinical variations that can be illustrated by diagramming the balance between the various types of mental functioning. When the baby is first born, it has various neurological reflexes (e.g., sucking response) and urges (e.g., cry, eat). These unfocused drives are referred to as the "Id."

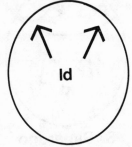

Later in life these urges for pleasure and satisfaction are expressed by sexual and aggressive behavior.

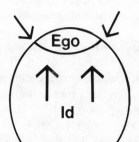

In addition to these basic drives, the baby's brain has programmed, organized capacities to respond to the environment, e.g., mirroring the caretaker's rhythm and movement; recognizing the "mother" by being more responsive to her face and presence. This beginning capacity to recognize reality and distinguish inner (fantasy) perceptions from external reality is referred to as the "Ego."

The child's experience and memory in the first year of life permits increasing recognition of the external world's demands. The ego's ability to recognize is joined by an increased capacity for control over the individual urges—especially in the second and third years of life. The child increasingly learns how to deal with external forces (i.e., the demands of the parents), while still achieving adequate satisfaction of personal urges. Referred to as growth of the ego, this stage can be diagrammed by an increasing size of the ego as it more frequently interposes itself between the persistent urges of the id and the expectations of the environment; for example, the child is expected to control urges to defecate rather than allowing immediate bowel evacuation.

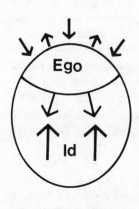

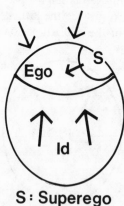

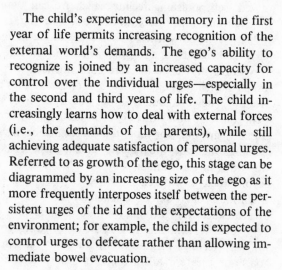

The final complication occurs when the external judgment of the loved and admired parents becomes internalized. Now the ego responds to internal pressures, even when the external world does not provide immediate approval or punishment. This aspect of the mind known as the conscience or "Superego" can be diagrammed as "large" or "small," according to how strongly it recognizes and exerts moral standards in controll-

S ꞉ Superego

ing the ego. There is, of course, not really an id, ego, or superego. They are not actually located anywhere in the brain; they are only a shorthand way of categorizing mental activity. Some variations may illustrate the clinical usefulness of this concept.

What would a person with a well-developed ego and a very small superego be like? We would expect him to have a keen sense of reality and good control over impulses, but little restraint from moral values. He would be clever and calculating, but would use his talents for his own selfish purposes. The person would be cleverly sneaky as a child, and con others successfully as an adult. While these characteristics might bring personal gain in business or politics, they would ultimately generate a lack of trust from others in relationships.

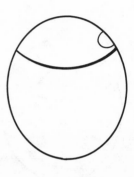

The ego could be well-developed and the super-ego deficits could be focal or partial. A person can be quite restrained and moral in many ways, but retain limited areas of inconsiderate, immoral, or illegal attitudes and behavior. These holes or "lacunae" (4) in the superego may also be unwittingly transmitted by the parents if they are punitive but simultaneoulsy reveal an admiration for the child's cleverness.

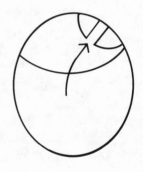

A small ego and a small superego would cause a person to be impulsive, aggressive and demanding, but capable of pleasurable, excited behavior. The person would have little self-control, and little awareness of others' reactions and expectations. The person would suffer little remorse or guilt, but would experience unhappiness over conflicts with others who would be viewed as unduly rejecting and restrictive.

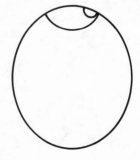

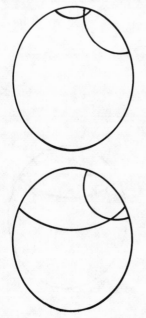

A rather pitiful variation can be seen where there is a small ego but a large superego. Such a person has high ideals, but is too impulsive to follow their own personal standards. The result is a constant feeling of remorse and guilt. The person repeatedly and sincerely promises to improve—only to be overcome by the next strong impulse.

Finally, we come to the "All American ideal" with a large ego and a very large superego. Such people are bright, alert, well-controlled, trustworthy, loyal, helpful, friendly, courteous, kind, obedient, cheerful, thrifty, brave, clean, and reverent. They are successful in middle class educational systems, but are frustrated by unreachable goals and worry about their relationships with others.

Although alterations of configurations of the ego and superego are most dramatically accomplished prior to school age, they can occur throughout adolescence and adult life. Ego changes are based on learning from experience. Educational discipline and consequences are important childhood influences and continue on into later life (5). The superego, however, is only altered by loving, admiring relationships, accompanied by a wish to emulate the admired person.

The concept of conscience is relevant for doctors and other health professionals who are sometimes consulted about conditions which reflect the vagaries of conscience activity, e.g., behavior disorders; learning disorders; delinquency; depression; hypochondriasis; suicide risks; and uncooperative patients.

REFERENCES

1. Freud S: The ego and the id, the ego and the superego, in *The Complete Psychological Works of Sigmund Freud,* st'd ed, Strachy J (trans). London, Hogarth Press, 1961, vol 19, pp 19–27.
2. Freud S: The ego and the superego, in *The Complete Psychological Works of Sigmund Freud,* st'd ed, Strachy J (trans). London, Hogarth Press, 1961, vol 19, pp 28–39.
3. Flavell JH: *The Developmental Psychology of Jean Piaget.* Princeton NJ, Van Nostrand, 1963, pp 290–297.
4. Johnson A: The genesis of antisocial acting out in children and adults. *Psychoanal Q* 1952;21:323–343.
5. Fraiberg S: Education of conscience, in *The Magic Years.* New York, Charles Scribner's & Sons, 1959, pp 242–282.

Chapter 11

GRADE SCHOOL STAGE
THEODORE R. WARM, M.D.

The grade school period of a child's life (age 6–12) is referred to in psychoanalytic theory as the latency period. This latter name refers to relative quiescence of sexual issues and family fantasied relationships, both of which were important in the preschool period and are again enlivened in adolescence. Many of us can remember this part of our life quite well and our memories are often nostalgic and pleasant.

The child makes great *intellectual* strides during this period of life. He begins to conceptualize the existence of things that he cannot see, e.g., organs and blood vessels within the body. (Schools often use giant plastic replicas of the eye and ear.) The child is now able to respond to doctors' explanations about sickness and treatment, and to participate more fully in his own care. Improved organization of ideas and perceptions enables the child to recognize right and left directionality and to categorize symbols—abilities which are prerequisites for reading. Delays in recognition of directionality or difficulty in translating shapes into sounds and meanings, will delay the child's ability to read and will be diagnosed as a learning disability (1).

Children of this age learn to categorize various items on the basis of common traits. This ability to generalize, along with the universal wish to make life more predictable, leads children to characterize various groups, e.g., teachers; policemen; thus begins the development of prejudices. A prejudice differs from a generalization in that the prejudiced believer only processes information which supports the generalization and rejects any contradictory information.

Considerable alterations in *relationships* occur during the grade school period. The child develops admiration and attachments to adults other than his parents, e.g., teachers; coaches; group leaders. These new attachments and admirations allow for some alterations of the superego by altering behavioral standards and ideals. Comparing the parent with other adults makes the child become increasingly aware of the parents' shortcomings.

126

This increasing disenchantment coupled with a more realistic view of sexual and family life, almost always raises in the child's mind the idea that they may be adopted. This universal fantasy accounts for the popularity of various folk tales based on the theme of "family romance." These tales involve children who were born to different parents; and in adulthood, they discover their real parentage and claim their rightful places in life.

Family patterns are increasingly evidenced during this period. Patterns emanating from unacknowledged marital conflict between the parents may cause problems in the children. In order to spare themselves from painfully recognizing their own difficulties, the parents focus upon a child as the source of the family unhappiness. Children who are scapegoated in this manner become programmed for continual adjustment problems. Delinquency in children also results from parents who obtain vicarious pleasure from the children's acting out, but chastise and punish them when they embarrass the family by getting caught.

The preschool age has ended when the child learns that he is a child—thus causing a considerable change in *peer relations*. Realizing that he cannot compete with adults, the child tends to segregate himself somewhat with same sex children of his own age. Great pleasure results from the sense of belonging to such groups, and excluding others from them. Informal neighborhood clubs begin to appear; each club has a leader, excludes someone from the membership, and keeps a secret, usually from adults. In the process of playing together, children pass on the rules of various games (e.g., jump rope, hide and seek), share secrets, tell "dirty stories," and educate each other about swear words both by conversation and by reading the inside walls of the public rest rooms.

Children of this age have lively *imaginations*. They enjoy reading and watching television movies about their heroes which over the years have changed from the Lone Ranger to Batman to Kung Fu to the Incredible Hulk and onward. Although children love to imagine themselves as heroes, exhibiting power and brilliance, they have developed the important ability to recognize the difference between fantasy and reality.

Children develop characteristic *habits* and *thoughts*. They enjoy repetition of sounds and things they are learning about. They jump rope endlessly, count the number of times they can bounce a ball off the garage door, and learn to count to a thousand. Their compulsive tendencies are revealed in organized collections of baseball cards, stamps, coins, and plastic models. Unorganized collections can be found on the floors of their bedroom closets; mementos of the past, such as a plastic cup with dried cocoa in it, feather from an Indian headdress, a flattened rubber ball, a kindergarten paper with a gold star on it, and a flashlight with corroded batteries. These collections bring them into conflict with their parents, who constantly claim the children are sloppy and irresponsible.

The *sexual* interests of children are more secret than absent. Children are regularly involved in swearing, sharing sexual information, and peeking at explicit magazines. Masturbation is common, and some mutual sex play between children of the same sex is not unusual; peeking in order to see some private aspect of the opposite sex is a regular pastime. These interests are generally kept fairly quiet and secret from adults.

The child gains considerable control over the expression of emotions during this period. At its end, the *difference between fantasy and reality* has been mastered; the child proves this to himself through constant exposure to fantasized dangerous situations. This "counter-phobic" interest in proving mastery over fearfulness is exemplified by children's enjoyment of supernatural and violent movies as well as exposing themselves to presumed dangers such as the roller coaster and fun house at amusement parks.

It is fairly common for children to develop *fears* about going to school. These fears are commonly manifested as headaches or stomachaches which are relieved by staying home instead of attending school. Such children usually feel unsafe in unfamiliar surroundings. Their parents commonly share similar anxieties about life's dangers and are unable to transmit a sense of confidence. Pent-up hostility is a common finding and needs a chance for ventilation. It is important for the child to re-establish regular school attendance immediately. The longer the child remains at home, the harder it becomes to re-enter the school system. Since such children frequently present with a variety of somatic complaints, the doctor has ample opportunity to help the child and provide the parents with some insight into the problem.

Doctors are frequently consulted about children who are overactive and have difficulty concentrating. These symptoms may reflect an attention deficit disorder but also may be a cover-up for a child's depressed moods (2). During the latency period, children can suffer from depressions similar to those found in adolescents and adults. Treatment includes an effort to identify the psychological stress that is causing the depression; but there is also an increasing interest in the treatment of such children by antidepressant medications (3).

The *implication for physicians* of the above characteristics is that the child is able to help in understanding and participating in medical treatment. The latency patient can use the intellect to help cope with the situation and understand sophisticated explanations. The child can conceptualize body parts and be helped by drawings and the physician's explanations. The child can learn about the body with a sense of pleasure and mastery, thus reducing fears of being an ignorant victim of illness and treatment. The child's compulsive tendencies may coincide with the need for regularity in treatments. He can help by getting pills, disposing of syringes, and planning diets; the child cannot be expected to take primary responsibility for participating in these regimens. Although the child can intellectually understand the reasons for most medical treatments and restrictions, he lacks the self-control necessary to apply the understanding without adult supervision.

By age 8, it is all right for the doctor to begin to encourage bravery. Prior to this age, gentle coercion against crying or protest only succeeds if the need of the child to show his feelings is strongly suppressed. The child should learn that complaining is legitimate and acceptable, but can be delayed. Bravery can be encouraged, but the doctor should acknowledge the underlying suppressed affect, and permit its expression later.

Children can generally tolerate elective surgery better as they become older. The emergence of speech as an effective reciprocal means of communication (2–3 years), is the first developmental landmark of the child's increased ability to tolerate procedures. The next landmark is better understanding of cause and effect, which occurs at age 5–6. The abilities to understand treatment intellectually and not take it personally are characteristics of the latency period which indicate the greatest tolerance for elective procedure. Most treatment cannot reasonably wait for a psychologically opportune time; when possible, however, surgery should be delayed until the middle of grade school period of development.

Once the child is in the hospital and not suffering acutely, an interest in actively helping others should be encouraged, e.g., cheering up or reading to smaller children. The satisfaction of actively helping another child gives the child experience in being active and helps alleviate the suffering of only being on the receiving end of getting help and treatment.

Some hospitals have scheduled meetings with child patients to discuss hospital experiences. These meetings can be used as a source of information and emotional support, as well as a way of helping others. The idea appeals to the latency child's appreciation of group peer experiences. While younger children primarily need the support of an adult, the grade school child can get considerable support from relating to other children. The stress of hospitalization, illness, and treatment, may, however, cause temporary regression to the need for comfort and nurturance from adults. The professional should honor the child's temporary need for indulgence. The restitution of maturation should be gradually and gently encouraged as the child's condition improves.

Finally, the physician should not be surprised if a child of this age does not always pour out his or her heart and reveal the innermost worries. While many are good at communicating with adults, quite a number of these children shun such intimate conversations. Their reluctance to elaborate on their inner thoughts and feelings is quite natural for their age. They should not be threatened or browbeaten into talking. The best approach is to re-explain why the information is needed, and anticipate and sympathize with the fears which might be interfering. If all efforts fail, adults should recognize the importance of the child's having at least one way of proving that he or she doesn't have to passively submit to every aspect of the whole intimidating medical experience.

REFERENCES

1. Kessler J: Learning disorders in school age children, in *Psychopathology of Childhood*. Englewood Cliffs, NJ, Prentice-Hall, 1966, pp 199–226.
2. Warm TR: An approach to psychiatric school consultation: What's good about bad behavior. *J Am Acad Child Psychiatry* 1978;17:708–716.
3. Cytryn L, McKnew DH Jr: Proposed classification of childhood depresson. *Am J Psychiatry* 1972;129:149–155.

Chapter 12

ADOLESCENCE
ELLEN ROTHCHILD, M.D.

"I see no hope for the future of our people if they are dependent on the frivolous youth of today, for certainly all youth are reckless beyond words . . . When I was a boy, we were taught to be discreet and respectful of our elders, but the present youth are exceedingly wise and impatient of restraint."

Hesiod, 8th Century B.C.

Before the last two or three decades, little medical attention was paid to adolescents. Since they seemed relatively healthy, pediatricians tended to ignore them and concentrate instead on combatting infant mortality and childhood infectious diseases. Once they reached puberty, adolescents were traditionally discharged from the pediatrician's practice. Earlier in this century, there were fewer adolescents. The socially defined duration of adolescence was also shorter because most people were expected to go to work and marry after high school. Adolescents have lately become far more conspicuous—both as a consumer group and a population with its own special needs and problems. As they have tried to meet these needs, physicians have been faced with several challenges: 1. How to determine "normal" situations that should be left alone; 2. how to identify situations that require intervention; 3. how to respond to medical situations in a manner which will support, or at least not hinder, psychologic growth.

"NORMAL" ADOLESCENCE

How Does Psychologic Change Occur?

The Latin term "adolescere," meaning "to become," implies some unfolding or metamorphosis. Experience, existing psychic structure, and innate maturational factors unique to this period are combined to facilitate this "becoming."

The biologic changes of puberty create new personal capabilities and possibilities for experience, as well as new adaptational demands. Intellect takes a maturational leap enabling abstract reasoning with several simultaneous variables (Piaget's "Stage of Abstract Operations"). The person learns to reason from hypotheses and mentally rehearse different choices of action. Adolescent behaviors represent an evolving mix of adaptations to, and outcomes of, maturation and current experience. This is a time when new impulses, feelings, and capacities must become integrated into a sense of the self as a person—hopefully a person who can reach his or her potential, has definite values and goals, and can act responsibly.

Anna Freud (1) tried to identify some average expectable components of this developmental phase:

> "I take it that it is normal for an adolescent to behave for a considerable length of time in an inconsistent and unpredictable manner; to fight his impulses and to accept them; to ward them off successfully and to be overrun by them; to love his parents and to hate them; to revolt against them and to be dependent on them; to be deeply ashamed to acknowledge his mother before others and, unexpectedly, to desire heart-to-heart talks with her; to thrive on imitation of and identification with others while searching unceasingly for his own identity; to be more idealistic, artistic, generous, and unselfish than he will ever be again, but also the opposite: self-centered, egotistic, calculating. Such fluctuations between extreme opposites would be deemed highly abnormal at any other time of life. At this time they may signify no more than that an adult structure of personality takes a long time to emerge, that the ego of the individual in question does not cease to experiment and is in no hurry to close down on possibilities. If the temporary solutions seem abnormal to the onlooker, they are less so, nevertheless, than the hasty decisions made in other cases for one-sided suppression, or revolt, or flight, or withdrawal, or regression, or asceticism, which are responsible for the truly pathological developments.
>
> While an adolescent remains inconsistent and unpredictable in his behavior, he may suffer, but he does not seem to me to be in need of treatment. I think that he should be given time and scope to work out his own solution. Rather, it may be his parents who need help and guidance so as to be able to bear with him. There are few situations in life which are more difficult to cope with than an adolescent son or daughter during the attempt to liberate themselves."

Echoing these sentiments, Kenneth Kenniston (2) writes:

> ". . . while we can outline provisionally the hallmark of a 'successfully-completed adolescence,' we cannot provide criteria for 'mental health' during adolescence itself. The concept of 'mental health,' slippery and elusive during all other stages of life, is almost useless during adolescence,

except perhaps as it describes the over-all direction of development. The adolescent routinely exhibits 'symptoms' that only reflect the routine trials of growing up, but which—were they to occur in later adulthood—would rightly be deemed ominous. Violent swings of mood and behavior, feelings of depersonalization and estrangement, hypomanic flights of ideas and frightening feelings of inner breakdown can all be merely the signs of routine inner turmoil, and need not bode ill for the adolescent's future."

Not everyone agrees that upheaval is characteristic. In a classic study of 73 nondeviant, "normal" white middle class boys, for example, Offer (3) found that a fourth of the group progressed smoothly toward a meaningful adulthood (and developed values similar to those of their parents) without showing much internal or external turmoil. On the other hand, many professionals (e.g., Blos [4]) view behavioral upheaval as the external reflection of certain internal psychologic tasks that must be accomplished in the passage from childhood to adulthood. These tasks are necessary to growth because they give the personality a "second chance" to experiment with new solutions to old conflicts, thus undoing earlier fixations and acquiring new adaptive possibilities.

The clinical distinction between "normal" upheaval (or its absence) and more ominous developments is not always easy. The "task" concept is one way to assess a given individual's standing, i.e., whether his behavior reflects the routine turbulence of forward movement or the agitation of truly blocked development.

The "Tasks" of Adolescence

There are essentially three tasks that tend to peak at sequential, though overlapping, stages of adolescence:

1. Adaptation to puberty (Early Adolescence);
2. Emancipation: resolving old dependent, parental attachments and forming new love ties to persons of the same generation (Mid-Adolescence);
3. Establishing an "identity": defining oneself and one's values in terms of gender, occupational commitments, standards, and beliefs (Late Adolescence).

The developmental characteristics that are expected during a given phase provide a rough framework for assessing normality. For example, one might expect that a modal 15-year-old (mid-adolescent) girl is: 1. responsibly caring for most of her body needs (not inviting mother to wash "hair that's too long for me to do myself"); 2. spending less time at home and more with friends, sometimes being argumentative at home but still inviting closeness with parents; 3. questioning, but still quite influenced by parental, societal, and peer beliefs; considering future life goals but not yet strongly committed. There are, of course, wide variations—depending upon socioeconomic circumstances, time in history, family attitudes, biological factors, and so on. The concept of a psychologic "growth curve" does, however, offer a rough framework for assessment.

Adaptation to Puberty. Puberty demands learning about the maturing body: how it responds sexually; how to care for it (i.e., whether to smoke, drink, pierce ears, become a vegetarian, use birth control, etc.); how to feel good about it and assume "ownership." Active exploration of the body helps define the self, e.g., using a mirror to see where the Tampax goes; determining where the good feelings that accompany masturbation are generated. Learning words that differentiate specific genital parts, such as vulva and clitoris, is a further cognitive aid. Ideally, becoming sexually active includes learning to share one's body without fearing loss of "ownership." The timing of puberty can affect adaptive capacities. For instance, a very early onset (e.g., at age 10) may prematurely challenge ego resources.

Many pediatricians routinely discuss sexual development with early adolescents. While youngsters avoid such discussions, the offer at least indicates the MD's willingness and availability to give information. Birth control information is probably the most common request. Concerns about bodily normality are also prevalent, especially if a physical examination is involved; reassurance to that effect may be appropriate. Concerns about sexual behavior and feelings are more likely to be discussed in group settings, such as school hygiene classes. Typical questions include: "Which way should your penis curve?"; "How can you tell a queer?"; "Why do they say masturbation doesn't hurt you, but tell you not to do it anyhow?" Some boys confuse wet dreams with bedwetting. Anxious parents may ask the physician to judge the adequacy of an embarrassed boy's genital development ("Doesn't he need hormone shots?"). Unless there is good medical reason for concern, such parents are best advised to let pubertal growth take its course. (Why they should be so concerned is, of course, another question.) Alarm over transient gynecomastia secondary to endogenous hormonal changes should be dealt with in the same manner.

Masturbation is an almost universal way of dealing with sexual thoughts and feelings. At this phase of development, genital masturbation helps to discharge tension and orient earlier pregenital (oral, anal) elements toward their eventual roles in sexual pleasure. Adolescents generally alternate between controlling and giving in to impulses; they are often ashamed of the inability to maintain control. The struggle for control is sometimes displaced onto other activities: repeated, unsuccessful attempts to diet; elaborate bedtime rituals; attempts at self-distraction through excessive busyness and exercise. Some youngsters quickly turn to intercourse as being "more normal." Exaggerated health worries and anxious scrutiny for minor bodily defects (like pimples) often reflect fears about having harmed the body. If a patient asks about masturbation, the physician can correct misconceptions about going crazy or loss of potency. It is less wise to say, "Don't do it," or "Go right ahead, it never hurts anyone;" neither of these polarities considers the individual's own struggle to mediate and control impulses. It is better to respect the person's desire for control and attempted solutions.

Emancipation. Infants gain a degree of autonomy by internalizing mental images of the parents which can temporarily assuage discomfort or guide action. The adolescent, however, must do the reverse, i.e., assure separateness by partially disengaging these object representations from mental representations of the self. Infantile perceptions of the parents as perfect or all-powerful must be modified, allowing the parents to assume human proportions. The intensity of old love ties to the parents becomes attenuated as emotional investment shifts to the self, contemporaries, and other significant adults. While not unique to this phase, this sorting out of self- and object-representations allows the adolescent to further determine identity differences from the parents, individual capacities and limitations, talents and interests. Clarity of self-representation fosters the ego's autonomy in choosing and directing action. Conflict between the adolescent and parents, perhaps most evident during mid-adolescence, is a major vehicle for disengagement. Besides fostering separation, it provides the individual with a means for distinguishing his/her own qualities and capacities from those of the parents.

Such conflicts may be expressions of old oedipal feelings, as well as adolescent and parental needs to interpose some safe distance. Sexual maturation implies that the youngster is becoming bigger, stronger, and sexually attractive enough to really compete with the parent. Primitive cultures dealt with this "threat" by sending the adolescent off to another village or imposing severe puberty rites; a possible counterpart in our culture is sending the young off to war. Some youngsters do separate from home geographically by boarding with relatives, attending boarding schools, or running away; they achieve physical, though not always emotional, distance. Many adult tasks and responsibilities, which ordinarily aid emancipation, are unavailable to the young. The job market is virtually closed to youth, and we prolong the period of dependency by encouraging longer schooling. Many American teenagers attempt to resolve the problem of declaring independence in the home while still clinging to childhood ties. They may alternate between contemptuous arrogance and superiority towards the parents, provocative baiting, moodiness, and episodic withdrawal to the basement or a friend's house, coupled with wishes to remain under parental protection and avoid venturing out into new experiences.

The following illustrates the bipolar conflict between dependence-independence, love and hate. A 14-year-old girl eagerly greeted her father when he returned home each evening; although she found every opportunity to sit close to and touch him, she complained angrily, "My father's always coming around and *bothering* me." Resolution of oedipal conflict is generally easier when the parents' interest in each other obviates the need to enter into covert (generally unconscious) flirtations with an attractive son or daughter. A classic example of the latter is the MD father who still doctors his teenage daughter (listening to the chest, poking the abdomen), ostensibly to avoid bothering his colleagues with trivial family illnesses he can handle himself; the daughter usually considers these actions seductive. Another potentially explosive variant involves a fatherless teenage boy whose mother has no other source of male companionship.

Emotional separation from the parents entails defining one's own ethics, beliefs, and interests. Previously unquestioned childhood assumptions about family standards and values must be examined at some point. During the emancipation effort, such assumptions may simply be rejected without much critical scrutiny. For example, youngsters who scorn their parents' values may deliberately fail in areas of parental success, and vice versa—a pseudoemancipation. In psychological terms, the need to repudiate old beliefs may temporarily weaken the superego; this accounts for some of the rashness, impulsiveness, and "delinquency" of this period. Physical and emotional separation from the parents—i.e., disavowing their mental representations in ego identification and superego components—also accounts for some of the loneliness, depression, and proneness to feeling unreal or depersonalized ("I'm the only real, living person walking through these school corridors and these others walking about are only imaginary."). Youngsters who are frightened by their feelings may never try to make the break from home and family. They remain like "good" latency children— conforming, compliant, troubling no one; unfortunately, their problems are less likely to be identified because they seem so easy to live with.

This period—roughly occupying the middle teens—is usually the most trying to parents. Apparently the situation has not changed greatly since Hesiod's day. Parents who can avoid being overly permissive in the face of arguing, sulkiness, and provocation can generally be more helpful; by setting reasonable limits, they give the youth a chance to test himself on something concrete and worthwhile. Both teenagers and parents are relieved when some of the intensity of old relationships is shifted onto new ones outside the family—e.g., hero worship; crushes; friendships; falling in love. These newer objects also provide new models for identification and elaboration of new interests and ideas.

Identity. Later adolescence focuses on consolidation of identity, i.e., individual beliefs; ideals; interests; capabilities; aspirations. Such activities are not, however, limited to this time period. The ability to think in abstract terms, while keeping several relative values in mind, enables definition of personal moral-ethical values. Emancipation is also a prerequisite for commitment to these values and standards.

The capacity for intimacy (including sexual intimacy) probably has a close relation to this task. Erik Erikson (5), known especially for his investigations into identity formation, notes that intimacy poses the threat of engulfing and being engulfed, if the boundaries of the self have not been delineated. Thus, mature love relationships (hard to define!) generally occur subsequent to finding the self. By later adolescence an individual should be familiar with his assets and liabilities, willing to be himself (not a carbon copy of what he thinks others want him to be), and sure that this self is a worthwhile person. Ideally he should feel ready to begin striving for competence in a chosen field, mutuality and reciprocity in relations with important others, and concern for the welfare of the wider community.

Summary

The use of age-appropriate activity and behavior norms can be useful in determining which behaviors are problematic. However, not everyone accomplishes all tasks at the same rate or level of completeness; much depends upon individual endowment, experience, and environment. The infinite number of possible variations among these factors also makes it impossible to define one "norm."

"Typical" Adolescent Conflicts and Defenses

Using psychoanalytic terms, puberty entails biologic and social pressures that heighten sexual and aggressive impulses, at a time when the ego and superego are relatively weak. In other words, the ineffectiveness of previous coping maneuvers increases the adolescent's fear of losing control over impulses. Old defenses still exist—e.g., the girl's *projection* that her father was always bothering her; *regressions* to more infantile behavior; *displacement* of old ties to new relationships; *subliminations* via creativity. New defenses that are fairly typical of this phase include:

1. *"Asceticism"*—the repudiation of pleasure or gratification in an attempt to combat "bad," or overpowering, instinctual urges. For example, the adolescent tries to forego eating or sleeping, determine how few clothes he can wear in winter, "swear-off" TV or sex. He may observe elaborate religious rituals—interspersed with breakthroughs of hedonistic indulgence.

2. *"Intellectualization"*—the exaggerated use of thought processes to control, rather then experience, feelings and impulses. Extreme intellectualization may be manifested in lengthy discourses on the virtues of communal living or legalizing pot (although the individual may not have tried either one), armchair theorizing instead of action, and unproductive ruminating over a "philosophy of life."

3. *Conformity to the peer group*—slavish imitation of the unique slang, special costumes, customs, and dance rituals which act as the peer group's barriers against the demands and pressures of the adult world. Conflict can be avoided by forfeiting individuality.

When not carried to extremes, these defenses can enrich the person's adaptive repertoire.

PARENTS AND ADOLESCENTS

Rearing an adolescent ushers in a new phase in parental development. The youngster may be an object of envy ("menopause-menarche syndrome"), someone to be put down; on the other hand, as the repository of the adult's unfulfilled ambitions, the child requires support (6). The parent's own adolescent feelings are apt to be revived, seeming to offer the parent a "second chance" to rework experience through the youngster. In a pathological form (a "superego lacuna"), parents vicariously enjoy, and unconsciously promote, delinquent or out-of-control sexual behavior in their young, simultaneously expressing disapproval and indignation (7). Teenagers respond to such ascribed "roles" in a variety of ways. Some comply, in effect "rescuing" the parent by becoming the externalized target of their problems. Some resist by either disavowing all family precepts or refusing to be controlled in a highly circumscribed area, such as eating. Some respond to the "double bind" with inhibition, confusion, and psychotic symptoms. Under healthier circumstances, children are the sources of the parents' further growth and posterity. The treatment of younger, more emotionally dependent adolescents is often aided by exploring the family situation—which isn't always easy.

MEDICAL CARE

J. Roswell Gallagher, a pediatrician, pioneered the establishment of "adolescent clinics." These clinics are staffed by specialists in disorders common to adolescents, e.g., dermatology (acne); gynecology (menstrual complaints, contraceptive information); orthopaedics (athletic injuries); psychiatry (emotional problems); dietetics (obesity); social service; educational psychology (school learning problems). Planning such a practice should include: 1. after-school clinic hours; 2. geographic separation from areas in which babies or elderly patients are seen; 3. private examining and consulting rooms. MDs in private practice sometimes accomplish these goals by reserving a special waiting room or day of the week for teenagers.

Some Emotional Aspects of Illness in Adolescence

The biologic and emotional disequilibrium may affect the course of some chronic illnesses, e.g., previously well-controlled epileptic seizures may become more frequent, only to stabilize again in later adolescence. As conformity to the peer group becomes more important, youngsters with long-standing physical handicaps (such as mild cerebral palsy) are likely to become more self-conscious and socially disadvantaged. Physical blemishes of any sort (pimples, crooked teeth) are harder to tolerate. The need to feel in control of body processes can result in unsafe, risk-taking behavior, e.g., a hemophiliac boy joins a motorcycle gang; a diabetic tries to stop taking insulin.

Emotionally-engendered complaints are common. Vague aches, pains, weakness, and fatigue may represent somaticized worries about harming the self through masturbation or other sexual activity; the youngster both fears and hopes that the MD will discover some real abnormality. Sleep disturbances may result from efforts to ward off masturbatory temptations; cancerophobia among adolescent girls commonly disguises conscious or unconscious fears about another kind of tumor, i.e., pregnancy. Anorexia nervosa (deliberate, severe starvation that obscures signs of sexual maturation) is a classic adolescent disorder. Pediatricians get many requests for gym excuses because this age group wants to avoid undressing in public.

Since youngsters in this age group can assume greater responsibility for their medical needs, they experience a greater sense of control over illness. For example, diabetics can be taught to give their own insulin, and cystic fibrotics to do much of their own chestclapping routines. Most youngsters can also administer their own medications.

Some Do's and Don'ts About Talking With Adolescents

Empathize, but don't identify, with them. Sympathy for their feelings is appreciated; indiscriminately siding with them against parental or societal precepts seldom helps. It's one thing for the teenager himself to criticize his parents; if you do so too, you'll be attacking some of his deepest attachments. Don't side with a weakened superego or appear corruptible. If he casually mentions forging a school pass to come for an appointment at a time convenient for you, consider choosing another time; question the need for illegal means. You can be a role model, but don't moralize; you're likely to end up sounding phony and pompous. Do not, however, side with denial of risky or dangerous behavior, such as drug or alcohol abuse.

Respect privacy. Don't be pushy or prying if he's reluctant to discuss something. While it's easy to force confessions and make an adolescent lose control of private thoughts, more trust is generated by letting him control the conversation. Let him be vague and guarded if he must. You *can* comment on how hard it seems for him to sort things out, and indicate your desire to understand the situation. He may feel more comfortable about talking at a return visit if he knows he won't be pressured.

Try approaching him as a therapeutic ally or cotherapist, e.g., solicit his ideas about working out a therapeutic plan, or his observations about how such a plan is actually working out. This allows him to assume responsibility for himself, and removes you from the impossible role of being omniscient.

It's often helpful to talk with a teenager both alone and with the parent. Don't exclude the parents totally. They too have feelings and you may well need their alliance. Seeing both together can also give you insight into family dynamics. If in doubt about the youngster's safety and good judgment, err on the side of caution and heed the parents' limits on his freedom. They've known him longer than you have, and their controls are apt to be better than his.

THE ADOLESCENT IN EMOTIONAL TROUBLE

There is a vast range of presenting symptoms. Psychiatrists may see: depressions, e.g., apathy, social withdrawal, declining school performance, misuse of drugs, somatic complaints; suicidal behavior or equivalents, such as exaggerated risk-taking and multiple "accidents;" psychotic behaviors, e.g., schizophrenic or manic-depressive illnesses, which may first appear during the teenage years; delirium secondary to substance abuse or systemic illness; anorexia nervosa and other somatopsychic disorders; antisocial behavior; chronic truancy and running away; school learning problems and phobias; sexual problems; intra-family conflicts; transient panic situations in which the individual's defenses are temporarily overwhelmed; etc. To determine the seriousness of a situation, ask yourself the following:

1. Is the behavior age-expectable, given the individual's particular environment and probable physical, intellectual, or emotional potential? This implies some knowledge of previous development and functioning.

2. Is the behavior transient, or has it persisted for too long? (1–2 weeks of misery is not uncommon, but several months of significant interferences with school, friends, or family is too long to ignore.) Phrased another way, is the individual "stuck" in working out a solution?

3. How hurtful is the behavior? Is there time to watch and wait, or is the individual at high risk for hurting himself or others?

4. Is it really the patient's problem—or someone else's? Is he a "calling card" for a parent or the family?

You may need more information than the adolescent can offer—from family, school, other agencies, or MDs. Some physicians in private practice share office space with a social worker or nurse clinician who can share in this job, make home visits, and offer counseling. Don't be afraid to ask for psychiatric consultation, or to suggest that the teenager discuss his concerns with a doctor who specializes in such problems. Know your community resources, such as programs for the retarded, handicapped, and teenage mothers; family counseling agencies; hotlines, rap centers, crash pads, group homes, and residential treatment centers; vocational guidance agencies; school social workers; juvenile court. Also consider using the homes of relatives as short-term cooling off places during family crises in lieu of a hospital.

Confidentiality and the rights of minors remain thorny treatment issues. Our social institutions have attempted to protect the young by selecting certain arbitrary chronologic cut-off points, such as age 18. Below these points, responsibility rests with parents; above them, the individual is deemed mature enough to be responsible for his actions. Until recently, it was illegal in Ohio to medically treat a person under 18 without parental knowledge and consent. The age was recently lowered to 16 for treatment of VD and drug-related problems, in the belief that maintaining confidentiality would encourage youngsters to seek help. In 1976, it became possible for a minor to obtain an abortion without parental involvement, though this law is again in question. A minor can no longer be held in a psychiatric hospital solely on parental instruction; he has the same right to a hearing as an adult. There will undoubtedly be further modifications of the legal age of responsibility; meanwhile, it's wise to know the law in your practice area.

Apart from the legal and social ethical dilemmas, one must determine how best to support individual growth. Is it proper, for instance, to arrange an abortion for a 14-year-old who comes in with a friend, without at least encouraging her to discuss the decision with her family? Should you respect a minor's request for confidentiality in a situation where the youngster is clearly endangering himself? Many would argue that parents need to know what's happening with their children if they are to care responsibly for them. Confidentiality is, therefore, a privilege—not a right—based upon the ability to assume adequate responsibility for the self.

It is fun and gratifying to work with this age group. One can often see much change within a short time. However, not everyone can tolerate the feelings adolescents arouse. If you feel uncomfortable with adolescents, acquire some referral resources.

REFERENCES

1. Freud A: Adolescence. *Psychoanal Study Child* 1958;13:255-278.
2. Kenniston K: *The Tasks of Adolescence.* Draft report submitted to Task Force III of the Joint Commission on the Mental Health of Children.
3. Offer D: *The Psychological World of the Teenager.* New York, Basic Books, 1969.
4. Blos P: *On Adolescence.* New York, Free Press of Glencoe, 1962.
5. Erikson E: *Youth and Crisis.* New York, WW Norton & Co, 1968.
6. Anthony EJ: The reactions of parents to adolescents and to their behavior, in Anthony EJ, Benedek T (eds): *Parenthood.* Boston, Little Brown & Co, 1962, pp 309-324.
7. Johnson A: Sanctions for superego lacunae of adolescents, in Eissler K (ed): *Searchlights on Delinquency.* New York, International Universities Press, 1945, pp 225-245.

Chapter 13

BEHAVIORAL, AFFECTIVE, AND PSYCHOPHYSIOLOGIC DISORDERS IN CHILDHOOD AND ADOLESCENCE

JUDITH W. DOGIN, M.D.

INTRODUCTION

The psychiatric disorders outlined in the DSM-III (1) can be grouped to include:

1. Mental retardation
2. Behavioral disorders (attention deficit and conduct disorders)
3. Emotional disorders (which impair a child's ability to relate or communicate)
4. Physical disorders (eating, stereotyped movement and others with physical manifestations)
5. Developmental disorders (pervasive and specific developmental disorders)
6. A variety of disorders common to childhood, adolescence and adulthood (organic mental disorders, substance abuse, affective and schizophrenic disorders, psychosexual and adjustment disorders).

MENTAL RETARDATION

Case I.

Jim was the 6 lb. product of a welcomed, uncomplicated pregnancy, labor, and delivery. His parents, concerned that he spoke only several words by age 2½, noted that he had generally developed more slowly than his siblings (crawling at 7 months, walking at 18 months). A full medical and neurologic evaluation at age 7 revealed that he was moderately retarded, with an I.Q. of 45. He was enrolled in a school for the moderately retarded, where he learned to care for his basic needs, read, and add and subtract. He completed the program, and obtained a high school diploma. He went on to work in a sheltered workshop while living in a group home in his community.

Mental retardation is defined as the sub-average general intellectual functioning of an individual whose tested I.Q. is less than or equal to 70; it is associated with deficits or impairment of adaptive functioning, and occurs before age 18. Individuals who are mildly retarded (I.Q.s in the range of 50-70), or "educable," comprise 80% of the mentally retarded. By age 5, they are usually able to communicate and function adequately socially. While academic achievement usually remains at the sixth grade level, by adulthood most individuals are able to be self-supporting. "Trainable" individuals with moderate mental retardation, in the range of 35-49 I.Q., comprise 12% of the retarded population. These individuals are able to talk and communicate, have basic daily living and social skills, and achieve second grade level academically; they usually require a sheltered setting through adulthood. The severely mentally retarded, 20-34 I.Q., comprise 7% of the retarded population. They have poor motor control, speech, and social development, and are often unable to communicate. They may be able to take care of elementary hygiene needs. The profoundly retarded, with I.Q.s of less than 20, comprise less than 1% of the retarded population. They display little development in all areas (almost like babies), and require much supervision.

The majority of the mentally retarded have ideopathic mental retardation. Twenty-five to 30% have a recognizable organic etiology, such as Down's Syndrome, P.K.U., fetal alcohol syndrome, congenital infection, congenital syndromes, or genetic illness, such as Tay-Sachs (2).

BEHAVIORAL DISORDERS

Case II.

"It's like a cyclone hit the house. He's into more drawers, cupboards, games, and rooms than I can count, and all in 20 minutes." This is how Mr. M. described his 7-year-old son Tim, who was interested in a great number of things but never seemed able to sit still or concentrate long enough to get anything done. Frustrated, he would quickly "pick a fight" with his sister or mother. Predictably, a loud argument would follow, with everyone going to separate corners of the house "to cool off." Similarly, in school, Tim would continually get out of his seat to sharpen his pencil, or offer to help others with their work. He rarely finished an assignment.

Attention deficit disorder with hyperactivity. The child exhibits inappropriate inattention, impulsivity, and hyperactivity relative to his chronologic and mental ages. These problems are reported by adults, including parents and teachers. Symptoms may be most prominent when a child is faced with a new situation or a task that requires attention. The peak incidence of this disorder occurs between the ages of 8 to 10. The inattentive child fails to complete tasks, doesn't listen, and is easily distracted; he has difficulty concentrating or sustaining attention, and difficulty engaging in play. Although there is no cognitive impairment, the impulsive child will act prior to thinking, shift from one activity to the next, and have difficulty organizing work. He or she will require a great deal of supervision, call out in class, and have difficulty waiting his turn in a group. The hyperactive child will run and climb excessively, have difficulty sitting still, and seem to always be on the go. He will fidget excessively when sitting, and may even move excessively while sleeping. These symptoms must occur before age 7, must be of greater than 6 months' duration, and not the result of schizophrenia, affective illness, or mental retardation.

Attention deficit disorder has previously been called minimal brain dysfunction or hyperkinetic syndrome. While the recognized onset is typically around age 3, diagnosis is usually made when a child enters school. It affects 3% of the population, runs in families, and occurs 10 times more frequently in boys than girls. There are three prognostic patterns: symptoms persist throughout childhood to adulthood; symptoms subside at puberty; hyperactivity decreases at puberty, but the inattention and impulsivity persist— leading to impairment in academic or social functioning. The attention deficit syndrome can be associated with negativism; temperamentally, a typical child has a tendency to bully others, is quick to anger, lacks discipline, and lacks self-esteem. Five percent of children also exhibit "soft" motor perceptual problems or mild EEG abnormalities. This syndrome is felt to be an organically-based disorder. Treatment can include special classroom settings, the use of stimulant medication, such as dexedrine methylphenildate or pemoline, and diets restricting sugars and food additives (2).

CONDUCT DISORDERS

Case III.

Beth, a 14-year-old, was noted to be somewhat shy, but courteous, at school. An average student, she was friendly with a group of girls described as "preppy." Her extracurricular activities included piano lessons and horseback riding. Her parents reported that she had "never lied, cheated, or broken a rule." They were at their wits' end, however, because she repetitively punched holes in the bedroom wall when angry. When enraged, she'd broken several lamps, and ruined a toaster "when it burned the toast." (Socialized, aggressive subtype)

Case IV.

Bill, a 15-year-old, was frequently absent from school. His teachers, feeling that "they hardly knew him," remarked that he associated with different acquaintances from week to week. Placed on probation for truancy, his parole officer discovered Bill shoplifting, fencing stolen goods, and using and selling marijuana to elementary school children. (Undersocialized, non-aggressive subtype)

Conduct disorders, characterized by the repetitive, persistent violation of either the basic rights of others or major, age-appropriate societal norms or rules, include: under-socialized aggressive; under-socialized non-aggressive; socialized aggressive; socialized non-aggressive. "Under-socialized" is defined as the inability to form a normal degree of affection or empathy, or bond with others. The under-socialized child has either few or superficial relationships which serve his advantage, and exhibits little guilt or remorse over violating basic rights or norms. The socialized child or adolescent shows some evidence of attachment, but may be callous or manipulative with those to whom he is not attached. The aggressive child or adolescent manifests violent behavior toward others, including raping, mugging, or committing homicide. The non-aggressive child or adolescent will come into conflict with norms by running away, engaging in substance abuse, lying, or stealing, without being physically violent toward persons or property. The problems of children with conduct disorders are typically complex. They may have poor self-esteem, as well as academic, social, and familial difficulties. These disorders occur five times more frequently in boys than girls. Treatment for conduct disorders ranges from firm limit-setting at home to placement out of the home in therapeutic settings or legal institutions (3–5).

EMOTIONAL DISORDERS

The *anxiety disorders* include separation anxiety disorder, avoidant disorder, and over-anxious disorder.

Case V.

John, a 10-year-old, had "absolutely refused" to go to school in the mornings since he began nursery school. His mother, insistent that he go, would drive him to school and walk him into the classroom daily. He had never had a babysitter because "the ruckus wasn't worth it. They would call us to come home anyway." Furthermore, John stated firmly that he would "never ever" sleep overnight at a friend's home. "They'll just have to stay over here."

The child with *separation anxiety disorder* exhibits excessive anxiety upon separation from loved ones, home, or familiar surroundings. Clinically, the child will refuse to sleep or visit at a friend's house, and will cling to parents at home when visitors arrive; he is unable to spend time alone, and may suffer from headaches, stomachaches, or vomiting due to anticipated separation. Often the child will exhibit fears of death, illness, wild animals, and muggers, which make it difficult for him to fall asleep at night. This anxiety often results in school phobia or avoidance.

The child with an *avoidant disorder* exhibits excessive avoidance of social contact with strangers, to the degree that it interferes with social functioning with peers. This child is usually very close to family members, and may be very unassertive and unconfident. Symptoms often develop around age 2, and the course may be quite variable.

The child with an *over-anxious disorder* exhibits excessive worry and fearful behavior, without a specific precipitant or stressor. The child may ruminate about the future, past, competence, or somatic problems, and may need constant reassurance; obsessional habits, used as attempts to master anxiety, are often prominent. This disorder is rather uncommon, and more marked in boys than girls. Treatment of these disorders often requires parental guidance, manipulation of home and school environments, and individual treatment for the child.

Other emotional disorders include reactive attachment disorder of infancy, schizoid disorder, elective mutism, oppositional disorder, and identity disorder.

The infant with a *reactive attachment disorder* exhibits impairment of social responsiveness and physical development. These infants, usually under 8 months, lack a social smile, fail to track a moving person, and do not play or babble with adults. They typically have poor muscle tone, weak cry and suck; motor development is delayed, and they may sleep for long periods of time. The etiology of this failure to thrive is felt to be either organic or interactional.

The *schizoid disorder* is marked by a defective capacity to form social relationships in children over 8 months old. It is marked by an inability to form or derive pleasure from close peer relationships, and avoidance of non-familiar social contacts. Symptoms must be present for more than three months. This entity is rare, and occurs more often in boys than in girls.

Case VI.

Mary, a 12-year-old, had been an excellent student in elementary school. In seventh grade, her grades plummetted. She withdrew from Girl Scouts and choir, and suddenly stopped talking. She was occasionally noted to ask her mother to get something for her, but was otherwise mute. During the previous year, Mary's grandmother had been very depressed over her husband's lingering death from cancer. Mary's mother, overwhelmed herself by the loss of her father, spent great periods of time with her mother. This drastically altered Mary's relationship with her mother, and the family's life in general.

Elective mutism is defined as the refusal to speak in all social situations, despite the ability to speak normally. While there may be some history of language delay and some mild articulation abnormality, the child basically has the ability to use language. This behavior has been observed in the overprotected child who is mentally retarded or has a mild speech disorder, or history of trauma. It is also rare, and occurs more often in girls than boys.

Oppositional disorder is marked by a pattern of disobedient, negativistic, and provocative opposition to authority which lasts for at least a six-month period in children aged 3–18. This opposition occurs in response to parents or teachers, even at times when it would be in the child's best interest to cooperate. School failure is common, as are violations of minor rules, tantrums, or argumentativeness.

Case VII.

Jane, a 16-year-old, found herself "unable to make any decisions— even deciding what to have for lunch is a major crisis." She spent several hours a day working for a national political movement, but, ironically, was "immobilized" when she faced decisions about academic schedules, seeing friends, and deciding what to do with friends. She found herself in several groups at school—the popular, fashionable, troubled—and was unhappy and uncertain about her role in each of them. Terribly uncomfortable about her sense of "being so unsettled," she sought counseling.

Identity disorder occurs most often in late adolescence, when one is faced with decisions about long-term goals, career choice, friendship patterns, sexual orientation behavior, religious identification, moral values, and group loyalty. The disorder is marked by severe subjective stress about one's identity.

Treatment for this disorder ranges from parent guidance to individual therapy. The etiology of the emotional disorders can be multi-faceted, ranging from an organic impairment of ego functioning and coping style to the intrinsic temperament reinforced or exacerbated by family interactions (3–5).

PHYSICAL DISORDERS

The *eating disorders* include anorexia nervosa, bulimia, pica, and rumination disorder of infancy.

Case VIII.

Hanna first became interested in gymnastics when she was 7. Her parents eagerly encouraged her interest. By age 10, she was very skilled, and competing locally; she was doing well socially and academically. At 13, she said, "Everything changed. I was growing, getting too big really. I wanted to be the smallest and the best." This 5′3″ girl found herself driven to exercise and practice. She was obsessed with dieting and maintaining her caloric intake at 600 calories per day, to keep her weight at 85 pounds. Her previously "perfect" relationship with her parents was marked by continual struggles over meals and food choices.

Anorexia nervosa, a disorder very common in adolescents and young adults, is marked by an intense fear of becoming obese, weight loss greater than or equal to 25% of the ideal weight, and marked disturbance of body image—which causes a feeling that one is fat, despite cachexia. This refusal to maintain a normal weight occurs without physical or mental illness. *Bulimia* is marked by recurrent episodes of binge eating of high caloric food, followed by repeated dieting, vomiting, and use of diuretics or cathartics. Despite an awareness of this pattern, the person seems incapable or afraid of stopping this behavior voluntarily. Binges are followed by a marked sense of disgust and self-deprecation. Etiological theories interpret anorexic and bulimic symptoms as ways of dealing with the struggles of adolescence and sexual development. Broader family theories interpret the individual's symptoms as expressions of family struggles and issues.

Pica, the persistent eating of non-nutritive substances, without an aversion to other foods, occurs in children between 12 and 24 months of age. This is usually a transient symptom associated with mental retardation, mineral deficiency, or, at times, poor supervision.

Rumination disorder of infancy is marked by repeated regurgitation, without nausea or gastroenterologic illness, for a one-month period; it occurs in 3- to 12-month-old children and is accompanied by weight loss or failure to gain weight. There is often a marked sense of satisfaction associated with regurgitation. This disorder is felt to be a result of an interactional problem between infant and caretaker. Treatment of the eating disorders includes parental guidance, and family and individual treatment. In cases of severe anorexia/bulimia, hospitalization may be required. Behavior modification has been helpful with anorexia and bulimia.

The *stereotyped movement disorders* are marked by involuntary, rapid movements of skeletal muscles or the involuntary production of noises or words. In the *transient tic disorder,* a voluntarily suppressed tic—usually of the facial muscles—varies in intensity, and occurs at least once a month for less than a year. The tic is noted to increase with stress or anticipation of stress, and to decrease when the child is absorbed in an activity or sleeping. It occurs in 12–24% of the population, and the prevalence in boys is three times that in girls. This disorder is felt to be primarily emotionally-based; the chronic tic disorder and Tourette syndrome are felt to have organic etiologies. *Chronic tic disorder* involves the involuntary, invariable movement of more than three muscle groups; this movement cannot be voluntarily suppressed, and must be present for more than one year.

> Case IX.
>
> Jason, a 9-year-old, explained that he was "tired of being teased all the time." Since he was a toddler, he would grimace or raise his eyebrow and blink uncontrollably. In elementary school, he began to grunt or make a barking noise when nervous. His father had a similar problem which was responsive to low doses of haloperidol.

Tourette's syndrome includes tics involving multiple muscle groups and vocal tics. The tics cannot be suppressed voluntarily, vary widely in intensity, and must be present for more than one year. The tics usually involve the head, torso, and upper limbs. The vocal tics can include clicking, grunting, barking, sniffing, coughing, or obscene words. The tics increase with stress and decrease when the person is sleeping. They can be associated with echokinesis (the repetition of another's actions), palilia (the repetition of one's own last words or phrases), mental coprolalia (the use of derogatory words or swearing), or obsessive doubting and compulsive actions. This disorder occurs most often in boys. Low doses of haloperidol have been found helpful in controlling the chronic tic and Tourette's syndrome.

Other disorders with physical manifestations. This series of disorders includes stuttering, functional enuresis, functional encopresis, sleep disorder and sleep-walking disorder. *Stuttering* is defined as the repetition, with increasing frequency, of the initial consonant or first syllable of a word, first word of a phrase, or the most important word of a phrase. The onset is usually before age 12, with peak incidence at 3½ to 5 years of age. Initially, a child has no awareness of the stuttering, which will spontaneously cease in 50–80% of cases. Treatment for stuttering includes speech therapy, individual therapy, and behavior modification.

Functional enuresis is repeated, involuntary urination that occurs after a child has been successfully toilet trained and dry for one year. It may be caused by the immaturity of the neuromuscular system, stress, or familial tendency to be enuretic. Treatment includes individual psychotherapy, behavior modification, and may employ low doses of imipramine.

Sleep-walking disorder. A sleep-walking child will repeatedly arise from bed during sleep, usually at least 30 minutes after initially falling asleep, and wander around the home with a blank stare. There is seemingly no response to the environment or other people, and the child can be awakened only with great difficulty. The next morning, the child has no memory of sleep-walking. The incidence increases with fatigue, stress, or sedatives. Seizure disorder or CNS disease may pre-dispose the development of sleep walking, which occurs most often in six to twelve-year-old children.

Case X.

Brian, a 10-year-old, has been hospitalized for three months following surgical resection of a bowel obstruction. Eager to "eat again and never need hyperalimentation again," he looked forward to returning home. For six weeks following his discharge, Brian would cry out in his sleep, sit up with a panicked expression, and sob. After being comforted by his parents, he would again fall asleep. He would wake up the next morning with no knowledge of what had happened. "My parents are nervous as all get out in the morning, and I don't remember a thing."

Sleep terror disorder. Children with sleep terror or pavor nocturnus, awake abruptly from deep sleep with intense anxiety and physiologic signs of sympathetic over-activity (increased heart and respiratory rates, dilated pupils, sweating, piloerection). As in the sleep-walking state, the child is unresponsive to comforting, and appears confused and disoriented, and may have perseverative motor activity. Thought by some to be an organically-based problem, it can occur at times of stress. Individual psychotherapy, as well as tricyclic antidepressants, have proved helpful (2,5).

PERVASIVE DEVELOPMENTAL DISORDERS

The pervasive developmental disorders include infantile autism, childhood onset pervasive developmental disorder, and the specific developmental disorders—including disorders of reading, arithmetic, language, and articulation.

Infantile autism, a very rare entity, is marked by a pervasive lack of responsiveness to others in a child less than 30 months of age. The lack of responsiveness is marked by inattention to people, failure to cuddle, lack of eye contact, and social unresponsiveness. Later in childhood, there is a lack of cooperative play and peer interaction. Deficits in language development are marked by a total lack of language, as well as echolalia. The disorder occurs most commonly in boys, and has been associated with congenital rubella, phenylketonuria, encephalitis, and meningitis, as well as other congenital CNS syndromes; most often, however, there is no diagnosable organic disorder. Therapy includes extensive parental guidance, and specialized educational settings, and, at times, psychotropic medication.

Case XI.

Stuart, a 4-year-old, was "driving his mother crazy." She reported that her son, terrified by loud noises such as vacuum cleaners, thunder, and car or smoke alarms, would either cling to her all day or rock on his rocking horse. He avoided contact with other children in nursery school, he became loud and disruptive when in a group. He would often repeat verbatim questions asked of him, and would approach strangers, to ask if they "had machines at home." At age 3 he could read a newspaper but could not identify odors. As an infant, his motor milestones were normal. He was slow to nurse and seemed to be an uncuddly baby.

Childhood onset pervasive developmental disorder is marked by gross, sustained impairment in social relationships, such as the lack of appropriate affective responsibility, inappropriate clinging, asociality, and lack of empathy. Onset occurs after 30 months of age and before 12 years, and is accompanied by three of the following symptoms: sudden excessive anxiety such as severe, free-floating anxiety, or catastrophic reactions to everyday occurrences; constricted or inappropriate affect; marked resistance to change in the environment; oddities of movement—such as peculiar posturing or walking on tiptoe; abnormalities of speech—such as question-like melody or monotonous voice; hyper- or hyposensitivity to the environment; and self-mutilation. There is a marked absence of delusions, hallucinations, incoherence, or excessive marked loosening of associations. Treatment is the same as for infantile autism.

The *specific developmental disorders* are marked by impairment in the age-appropriate development of reading, arithmetic, language or articulation skills, as judged by I.Q. testing or language evaluation. The reading disorder, often referred to as dyslexia, is manifested by omissions, additions, or distortions of words when reading aloud, reduced comprehension, and the inability to copy the written word correctly. Expressive or receptive language disorders, are marked by the failure to develop adequate vocal expression or comprehension. Treatment of each of these disorders usually involves a specific understanding of the deficit, followed by tutoring and/or psychotherapy.

Children and adolescents may also develop organic mental disorders and substance abuse problems. The schizophrenic illnesses can occur initially in adolescence. Affective illness can manifest in children with symptoms similar to those of adults; a careful evaluation is often required to document the required symptoms. A child with all of the entities listed above will present with academic, social difficulties, and difficulties functioning at home (6–9).

REFERENCES

1. American Psychiatric Association Committee on Nomenclature and Statistics: *Diagnostic and Statistical Manual of Mental Disorders,* ed 3. Washington DC, American Psychiatric Association, 1980.

2. Herskowitz J, Rosman N: *Pediatrics, Neurology and Psychiatry—Common Ground.* New York, MacMillan, 1982.
3. Chess S, Thomas A: *Temperament and Development.* New York, Brunner/Mazel, 1977.
4. Sahler OH: *The Child from Three to Eighteen.* St. Louis, Mosby, 1981.
5. Lewis M: *Clinical Aspects of Child Development.* Philadelphia, Lea & Febiger, 1982.
6. French A, Berlin I: *Depression in Children and Adolescents.* New York, Human Sciences Press, 1979.
7. Kandel D: Epidemiological and psychosocial perspectives on adolescent drug use. *J Am Acad Child Psychiatry* 1982;21:328-347.
8. Puig-Antich J: The use of research-diagnostic criteria for major depressive disorder in children and adolescents. *J Am Acad Child Psychiatry* 1982;21:291-293.
9. Easson W: The early manifestations of adolescent thought disorder. *J Clin Psychiatry* 1979;40:469-475.

Chapter 14

MENTAL RETARDATION
DONALD K. FREEDHEIM, Ph.D.

Mental retardation poses one of the unmet challenges to the behavioral sciences. World attention has only recently focused on the enormity of the problems presented by the demands of the retarded for public health, social welfare, and educational services. In diagnosing and treating the mentally handicapped, we need to take into consideration the realities that have often been neglected or overshadowed by the many myths associated with retardation.

Because retardation has been largely ignored by scientists and the helping professions, it is sometimes surprising to discover the scope of the problem. Estimates of prevalence vary between two and three percent, depending upon the criteria used to define the condition (1). At three percent, the number of Americans in the United States who are mentally retarded reaches over six million. But those affected by the condition far exceed the actual number of handicapped persons. Each retarded individual has two parents, probably one sibling, and at least one or more other close relatives. Using a conservative estimate for family members, a country of 230 million includes 34½ million people who are closely affected by retardation—well over 10 percent of the population.

DEFINITION AND CLASSIFICATION

The most current and widely accepted definition of mental retardation is as follows:

> Mental retardation refers to significantly subaverage general intellectual functioning existing concurrently with deficits in adaptive behavior, and manifested during the developmental period (2).

The above definition makes no reference to etiology, e.g., retardation associated with psychosocial or polygenic influences, or with a biological deficit. "Mental retardation" is a descriptive term for current behavior, and does not imply prognosis.

"Significantly subaverage intellectual functioning" refers to an individual I.Q. test performance which is more than two standard deviations below the mean—that is, I.Q. below 70. The upper age limit of the developmental period is 18 years.

Since mental retardation encompasses such a broad range of intellectual functioning, it is classified into categories according to degree of handicap. The standardized intelligence test is generally used to distinguish among categories, which have traditionally been associated with various labels. A current breakdown of subdivisions is presented in Table I, including general I.Q. boundaries plus educational and DSM-III (3) categories.

Although the "borderline" classification has been included in Table I, it should be noted that a "borderline" child may be termed retarded only if a sufficiently poor quality of adaptive behavior is present. Deficits in adaptive behavior vary according to age. During infancy and early childhood, the affected areas include: sensory-motor skills; communication skills; self-help skills; socialization. During childhood and early adolescence, affected areas include: basic academic skills; application of appropriate reasoning and judgment in mastery of the environment; social skills. In late adolescence and adult life, affected areas include vocational and social responsibilities and performances (4).

TABLE I
CLASSIFICATION OF MENTAL RETARDATION

Category	I.Q. Range	Educational Term	DSM-III
NON-MENTALLY RETARDED			
Borderline	69–80	Slow Learner	V62.89
MENTALLY RETARDED			
Mild	52–68	Educable	317.0
Moderate	36–51	Trainable	318.0
Severe	20–35	Trainable	318.1
Profound	< 19	Custodial	318.2

I.Q. ranges vary slightly according to the particular tests used. For example, the WISC-R test yields slightly higher I.Q.s than the Stanford-Binet (L-M). Classification should be made according to the test score received, and psychologists must be aware of the distinctions among the tests.

INCIDENCE

It is important to note the differential incidence among the categories of the retarded. With the exception of the "borderline" classification, as the incidence in this category can vary greatly, depending upon educational remediation and emotional functioning, the incidence of retardation decreases dramatically as I.Q.s lower. The vast majority (90%) of the retarded fall into the "mild" category. Approximately 6% comprise the "moderately" retarded, 3.5% the severely retarded, and 1%, the "profoundly handicapped."

There is some controversy over the total incidence of retardation in the population (1); most researchers agree that at least 2% of the population suffers from mental retardation. Obviously, the inclusion or exclusion of the "borderline" category can radically change the incidence figures in any population.

HISTORICAL CARE OF THE RETARDED

Despite the fact that a problem of this scope has always been present, the history of special care for the retarded goes back barely 100 years. In mid-nineteenth century Europe, humanitarian concerns, as well as medical and educational studies, marked the beginning of the separation of the retarded from those with other chronic conditions.

The first special institutes began in the mid-1800s. At first, progress was slow in developing methods for treating and training the mentally handicapped. There were many false claims of cures, which soon disillusioned both the public and the professionals. However, the work of Itard, Sequin, and others demonstrated that the retarded could be educated, and that many insights to medical and educational practices could be gained from working with these children (5).

Soon the small, well-tended facilities grew into large, over-crowded institutions. For the most part, they were built far from urban centers and completely isolated from the rest of the population. The mentally retarded of all types and degrees were literally herded together away from their families and neighbors. The existence of mental retardation remained an unbearable stigma. Its presence in families was hidden and looked upon with great shame.

At a time when public educational opportunities were expanding rapidly, the retarded were excluded from regular schooling. In the United States, this situation began to change very slowly. There were no significant changes until the early 1960s when President Kennedy's interest in the problem led to national action on behalf of the retarded (6).

Among the early suggestions for improved care for the retarded, was that the focus of service should shift from large, distant institutions to community-based centers. It has taken several years to adjust professional thinking toward this goal, and a great deal of educational work must be done before the community will accept this concept. Experience and demonstration are beginning to demonstrate the benefits of community programming for both the retarded and the public-at-large.

Just from an economic aspect, studies in the U.S. have shown that communities can save tens of thousands of dollars per child (!) by training and employing the retarded, rather than warehousing them. It costs a community far less to provide a moderately retarded individual with a sheltered workshop job, including home care and transportation, than to have him languish in an institution.

The trend toward community care is beginning to spread to other countries. In 1974, the World Health Organization considered community care one of its primary goals. The achievement of this goal will depend upon increased numbers of professional personnel trained to deal with the special needs of the retarded.

THE CHALLENGE OF MENTAL RETARDATION

Maturation is a slow and at times a difficult process for all children, involving the mastery of many tasks. When a child suffers from mental retardation, the growing process becomes more complex and more difficult. In addition to all the normal developmental tasks, retardation presents a whole set of new problems. These problems involve not only the child and the family, but, eventually, the community and society-at-large.

Mental retardation has just begun to interest scientists and those in the helping professions. The field of psychology, in particular, has only recently turned any significant attention to the area. Scientists are now beginning to recognize the potential wealth of information about human functioning which can be derived from the study of retardation. A single child offers the chance to study the interaction of normal and abnormal growth rates, involvement with parents and society, and the resulting developmental and adjustment problems.

The field of mental retardation also offers a great deal of opportunity for interdisciplinary work and cooperation. One piece of legislation for new facilities requires representation of no fewer than 14 disciplines. Clearly few institutions could meet this requirement.

Different disciplines have various roles in working with the retarded. At different ages, crucial decisions involve different areas of understanding, so no one discipline can claim exclusive responsibility. Early diagnosis may depend upon medical knowledge, school planning requires psychological and educational assessments, etc. To help families and children through any step of the process, cooperation and coordination among the various disciplines is necessary.

Every parent instinctually wishes for a physically perfect, intellectually normal child. To have less can only lead to disappointment and rejection. Society has recognized and accepted this rejection by providing hospitals and institutions for the retarded. The parents' feelings can be reinforced by an authority's advice to institutionalize the child. Not all parents can, however, tolerate their feelings of rejection, even if they are "legally" sanctioned. They become overcome with guilt which may not be manifested until many years after the placement (7).

A not unusual case in point is a family who had placed their Down's Syndrome child in an institution immediately following his birth. They had no other children and five years later finally brought themselves to visit their only child. They expected to find a bed-ridden, helpless infant; instead, they found a happy, playful boy functioning around the two-and-a-half year level. They came to the clinic to express their shock and disappointment over being deprived of the child's upbringing. The earlier guilt was now heightened by their anger at the physicians who had advised placement at so early an age.

If the parents elect to keep the child—sometimes over professional objections—the guilt may manifest as overprotection and overindulgence of the handicapped child. As the child grows, the parents may be afraid to let go; to do so would reveal their underlying wishes to reject the child completely. The situation is particularly difficult with retarded children, as their slower development tends to reinforce dependency. It is important to give the retarded every opportunity for independence, rather than sustain them in the dependent role. Finding appropriate opportunities is difficult enough, without contending with guilty parents afraid to show any pleasure at the child's growing freedom from the family.

The professional specialist's own attitude toward the retarded may greatly influence the parents' behavior toward, and future relationship with the child. Hasty decisions at the time of birth may be regretted years later. Although there may be a temptation to support immediate rejection wishes and place the child, recent experience has shown that it is often better to wait until both parents can discuss the meaning and implications of placement. Of course, this means that skilled counselors must be available to help the parents, even if such counseling requires several months of work.

In the majority of cases, the retardation is not discovered immediately. Parents who have come to expect normal development from their child must be reoriented. Although most professionals stress the importance of early diagnosis and intervention, actual identification of retardation may sometimes be forestalled for years. Most mothers are very sensitive to their own child's development, and will have early suspicions of retardation if the child is not progressing normally. When she confronts the doctor with her suspicion, more often than not, he will reassure her that the child will "grow out of" his slowness. Even if mental retardation is suspected, an evaluation may be delayed. The rationale is that a diagnosis of retardation would be detrimental to the parent-child relationship; thus, it is better to preserve some expectation of normality as long as possible. However, this reasoning overlooks two factors: 1. The mother's doubts and anxiety about her child may be more damaging than actual knowledge of a problem. 2. The parent-child relationship might benefit from professional help on the parenting of a handicapped child.

Since the first evaluation of a possibly retarded child is tentative at best, parents may have to contend with partial answers. Early identification of retardation is only beneficial to the child and parent if appropriate services and facilities are available to the family during the diagnostic period. In addition to counseling, services should include observation nurseries where preschool children can be observed by child development specialists.

DIAGNOSIS AND TREATMENT

The diagnostic process involves the determination of etiology, functional evaluation, and an estimate of prognosis. Although there have been many recent advances in the discovery of genetic, metabolic, and other causes of retardation, we cannot give a definitive cause of the problem in the majority of cases. Added to the burdens of parents are the questions as to reasons for the handicap. Lacking knowledge about the reasons for the handicap, parents substitute self-blame, mythical or magical causes, and project blame to the other parent.

The major medical categories of causes are:
1. Following infection or intoxication (such as rubella, toxoplasmosis);
2. Following trauma or physical agent;
3. Following disorders of metabolism or nutrition (such as PKU);
4. Associated with gross brain disease (e.g., neurofibromatosis, tuberous sclerosis);
5. Associated with diseases and conditions due to unknown prenatal influence (primary microcephaly; hydrocephalus, etc.);
6. Associated with chromosomal abnormality (Down's Syndrome); gestational disorders (prematurity).

Differential diagnosis is not an uncommon task in dealing with the retarded, especially since many children have associated problems—such as cerebral palsy, autism, or emotional disturbance. The likelihood of added problems increases in the retarded population, although not necessarily with the degree of handicap. In fact, the susceptibility to affective disorders may be negatively correlated with the degree of retardation. In any event, the confounding factors of associated sensory, motor, and emotional disabilities increase the difficulties of evaluation. It is important to treat any associated conditions, as such therapy may well result in improved intellectual functioning.

I.Q. is a necessary, although not sufficient, measure in the diagnosis of retardation. The most reliable instrument for assessing intellectual functioning is the intelligence test.

Recently in the United States there has been a growing controversy over the use of psychological tests to evaluate individuals (8). Tests of I.Q. have generated particular concern. It is argued that the limited information derived from I.Q. measures may do more harm than good because it is misinterpreted by both professionals and the public. Probably the most unfortunate use of such tests is for exclusion purposes. When educational tracking depends entirely upon intelligence tests, many children on the borderlines suffer from inappropriate placement. It is not unusual for a child's entire educational future to be decided on the basis of one I.Q. test, given during a single interview.

Only recently, and at great expense, have we begun to modify the laws. By placing less emphasis on I.Q. alone, we enable more children to benefit from educational and training programs.

The relative importance of I.Q. in the diagnosis of mental retardation is underscored by the revised definitions issued by the World Health Organization and American Association on Mental Deficiency. Diagnosis of the syndrome is now based on both behavioral criteria and intellectual assessment (2,9).

While we recognize the limitations of the I.Q. as an absolute criterion, it is important not to disregard its usefulness. New instruments are being developed to supplement the I.Q. in assessing children's learning skills. These tests attempt to evaluate the processes involved in learning, not just the end product.

Observation over time is an important part of the evaluation process. Ideally, opinions on the child's development might be obtained from a variety of specialists, including speech, neurological, and psychiatric personnel; the reality of having all the appropriate manpower available is, of course, difficult.

Depending upon the degree of the handicap and its complications, it is often best to wait for a period of perhaps six months before making precise statements about the child's eventual progress. Early information is most definitive for severely handicapped, older children. However, retesting is unually important, particularly when the child is on the borderline of retardation categories. Planning for the child's habilitation usually proceeds during the diagnostic process.

There is no known treatment for mental retardation per se. Since the major treatment mode is educational, decisions about schooling are critical. Collateral therapies, such as speech work or physical therapy, may proceed in conjunction with educational planning.

EDUCATIONAL IMPLICATIONS

Whether handicapped children should be integrated into a regular school or segregated into special classes is a central issue for all special educators. For other types of handicaps, the decision is made on the basis of the appropriate teaching situation. Blind children are usually integrated into regular classes from the earliest grades. Hard-of-hearing and deaf children, on the other hand, are usually educated in separate groups until they are able to receive information from regular teachers. There is no question that the severely mentally retarded child requires special classes and a curriculum geared to an appropriate level of development. There is no reason, however, why these classes cannot be held in close proximity to regular schools. The author once held a special class for moderately and severely retarded children in a church next to a public school. One of the classes from the public school met in the church, across the hall from the special group. As the year progressed, regular meetings were held to help the average school children understand the "special" children who were learning across the hall. The fantasies which the children had about the retarded group were striking. One child thought they had no mothers, because their behavior was so different. After a year of being near the special class, the average children had a much better understanding of the handicapped children.

The question of integrated education for the mildly retarded or borderline children is more controversial. Retarded children who are integrated into average classes generally perform better academically than their segregated counterparts. However, the special class child seems to have better social development.

The most significant legislative development in recent years has been the passage of Public Law 94-142, The Education for All Handicapped Children Act of 1975. Despite some current legal threats, this law clearly states that mentally retarded children be placed in the "least restrictive, appropriate setting." Criteria for placement include adequate evaluation and planning, with participation by approved professional disciplines and parents (10).

Despite the strong social and parental pressures toward mainstreaming mentally retarded children into regular educational channels, progress has been slow and at times painful (11). Advocates for mainstreaming tend to overlook the distinct advantages of special education for special children. The advantage of integration can be lost if the retarded child is not given adequate attention and time to complete assignments or understand concepts. Mainstreaming is only advantageous if the educational needs of the child are not neglected. The care needed to plan for the mentally handicapped often requires greater efforts than for average children. The physician's role in the planning is crucial to the assessment of the child's capabilities, parent and teacher education, and appropriate referrals for consultation.

In America, as elsewhere, we have the unfortunate phenomenon of the "six-hour retarded child"—i.e., the child who is identified as mentally handicapped during school hours, but who functions adequately away from this setting. We must learn to recognize the strengths and weaknesses of each individual child and avoid generalizations which stigmatize special groups.

As the retarded grow into adulthood, decisions must be made about their eventual vocational and living arrangements. Sheltered workshops and group homes can provide appropriate environments for those who cannot live independently. Since every human has an emotional need for companionship, social activities must also be arranged (12).

SOME PERSISTENT MYTHS

There are many professional workers in the sciences, including the social and behavioral fields, who have misconceptions about the mentally retarded; these myths prevent us from dealing realistically with the retarded. It is the responsibility of those in the field to inform their fellow workers, as well as the public, about the handicapped (13).

Because the retarded learn at a slower rate and remain longer on simple material, one myth is that they are easier to care for and understand than average children. Retarded children are, in fact, more complex—and consequently more difficult to deal with—than children of average intelligence. In the school system in my community, it used to be common practice to put the older, nearly retired teachers with the special classes. The rationale was that the retarded demanded less and, therefore, required less astute and perhaps less skilled teaching personnel. Many schools are now beginning to realize that the retarded demand more patience, understanding, and specialized teaching techniques than average children. The introduction of structured learning environments, behavior modification systems, and specialized materials is changing the traditional picture of sad-looking special classrooms. In some public schools, the personnel teaching the special classes have higher degrees than those teaching the regular classes.

It should be pointed out, however, that these changes are just beginning to emerge in a few school systems in the United States. For most retarded children, the educational program is still confined to watered-down versions of regular classes, occasional excursions to demonstrate practical life skills, and generally monotonous routines.

Another myth that still pervades professional circles is that the retarded are insensitive, or less sensitive to their handicap than the average person might be. Again, those who live or work with the retarded become aware of just how sensitive they are and how they have learned to cover up their feelings. There are very few reports in the literature on how the retarded view themselves. Unfortunately, retardation limits self-expression. Also, retarded children are unconsciously trained to be insensitive to themselves. The training begins with workers who may talk about the child in front of him. The parents pick up this behavior and also believe that the child does not know when people are talking about him. We forget our own awareness of being the subject of conversation—an awareness shared by very young children. It is not difficult to imagine how we might react if we were spoken of as objects that had no understanding of what was being said. We would come to believe that we had no feelings or sensitivity toward ourselves. Thus, the handicapped child is actually trained to "tune himself out" and become insensitive to his own reactions.

Parents also attempt to hide their own feelings toward their handicapped child, particularly when these feelings are sad or negative. While such actions are appropriate, they do limit the child's knowledge of feelings.

Parents also attempt to protect their children from knowledge of their disability. There are parents who have actually done their children's school work for them, in order to keep them enrolled in regular classes and not identified as retarded.

The attempt to keep one's children ignorant of their condition was brought sharply to my attention during a counseling session with the parents of a six-year-old. When I mentioned that their son would be much better off knowing that he was retarded, the mother immediately burst into tears. I tried to point out that his self-awareness would be a real asset in his social development, and give him some chance for independent living. She could not be convinced, however, that he would be better off if he had a realistic awareness of his retardation.

In working with the mildly retarded, especially as they move into adolescence, it is important to help them understand the areas and degree of their handicap. Admittedly, it is not an easy or pleasant task to tell a teenager that he cannot drive a car or anticipate marriage. Many of the mildly retarded have the same ambitions as average children. They know about the world around them. They watch television and, perhaps aided by their parents, try to convince themselves that they are no different from anyone else. If a mentally handicapped person is to function in the community, however, his best asset is the knowledge of his own limitations—which should give him the foresight to ask for help in situations in which it is needed. How often do people mess up the plumbing because they are reluctant to call an expert? Being aware of one's limitations can, hopefully, prevent them from causing problems. In order to help the retarded and their parents cope with the inevitable feelings of hurt that accompany such self-knowledge, professional workers must be sensitive to the psychological adjustment necessary to deal with such information.

A third myth is that the retarded have a low tolerance for frustration and give up easily. The falseness of this conception is emphasized in a film of children in our Cleveland preschool (14). One sequence focuses on a boy putting on his sock. For several minutes, the child struggles and struggles to get the sock around his toes. Both he and the audience are greatly relieved when he succeeds. The sequence is important because it demonstrates this retarded child's patience and tolerance for frustration. Because the handicapped may refuse to participate in activities which are too advanced for them, we tend to ignore the areas in which they *do* struggle to succeed. Determination may actually be strengthened—rather than weakened—by the fact that it often takes the retarded longer to achieve a goal. The aperiodic achievement of the award increases motivation.

Despite all observable and research evidence, there are those who still consider mental retardation a stable, unchanging condition. Perhaps this view is partially supported by a desire for retardation to be easily predictable and static. Those who work with the mentally handicapped are, however, challenged by the complex nature of the problem.

Medical science has extended everyone's life expectancy. Since the severely handicapped can no longer be expected to live short lives, community responsibilities for adequate planning and services for the retarded are increased.

Students who wish to explore the field of retardation in greater depth are encouraged to read recent texts (15,16) or current handbooks (17,18).

REFERENCES

1. Mercer J: The myth of 3% prevalence, in Tarjan G, Eyman RK, Meyers CE (eds): *Socio-behavioral Studies in Mental Retardation.* Washington, DC, Monographs of the American Association on Mental Deficiency, 1973, pp 1-18.
2. Grossman HJ (ed): *Manual on Terminology and Classification in Mental Retardation.* Washington, DC, American Association on Mental Deficiency, 1977.
3. American Psychiatric Association Committee on Nomenclature and Statistics: *Diagnostic and Statistical Manual of Mental Disorders,* ed 3. Washington, DC, American Psychiatric Association, 1980.

4. Arndt S: A general measure of adaptive behavior. *Am J Ment Deficiency* 1981;85:554–556.
5. Itard JM: *The Wild Boy of Aveyron* (Humphrey G, Humphrey M trans). Englewood Cliffs, NJ, Prentice-Hall, 1932.
6. President's Commission on Mental Retardation: *MR 71: Entering the Era of Human Ecology.* Washington, DC, Department of HEW (No 5), 1972.
7. Solnit AS, Stark MH: Mourning and the birth of a defective child. *Psychoanal Study Child* 1961;26:523–537.
8. Sattler JM: Assessment of children's intelligence, in Walker CE, Roberts MC (eds): *Handbook of Clinical Child Psychology.* New York, Wiley & Sons, 1983, pp 132–157.
9. Meyers CE, Nilira K, Zetlin A: The measurement of adaptive behavior, in Ellis NR (ed): *Handbook of Mental Deficiency,* ed 2. Hillsdale, NJ, Lawrence Erlbaum, 1979, pp 431–481.
10. Stetson E: Educational assessment of the child, in Walker CE, Roberts MC (eds): *Handbook of Clinical Child Psychology.* New York, Wiley & Sons, 1983, pp 158–185.
11. Gottlieb J, Alter M, Gottlieb BW: Mainstreaming mentally retarded children, in Matson JL, Mulick JA (eds): *Handbook of Mental Retardation.* New York, Pergamon Press, 1983, pp 67–77.
12. Jacobson JW, Schwartz AA: The evaluation of community living alternatives for developmentally disabled persons, in Matson JL, Mulick JA (eds): *Handbook of Mental Retardation.* New York, Pergamon Press, 1983, pp 39–66.
13. Clelland CC: Mental retardation, in Walker CE, Roberts MC (eds): *Handbook of Clinical Child Psychology.* New York, Wiley & Sons, 1983, pp 640–659.
14. Freedheim DK: *Three Years Later: A Developmental Study of Retarded Children.* Film produced at Case Western Reserve University, Cleveland, Ohio, 1966.
15. Robinson NM, Robinson HB: *The Mentally Retarded Child,* ed 2. New York, McGraw-Hill, 1976.
16. Kessler JW: *Psychotherapy of Childhood,* ed 2. New Jersey, Prentice-Hall, in press.
17. Ellis NR (ed): *Handbook of Mental Deficiency,* ed 2. New Jersey, Lawrence Erlbaum, 1979.
18. Matson JL, Mulick JA (eds): *Handbook of Mental Retardation.* New York, Pergamon Press, 1983.

Chapter 15

ADULT DEVELOPMENT AND OLD AGE

DALE SIMPSON, M.D., Ph.D.

The concept of adult development springs from the realization that humans exhibit systematic changes throughout their life spans, not just in the first 20 years. Children and adolescents change dramatically as they age. Adults also change, although less rapidly and dramatically. The patterns underlying the changes of adulthood represent adult development.

Previous chapters have discussed human development in childhood and adolescence. The enormous changes which occur during the first 20 years of human life are very similar in all individuals. Perhaps this accounts for the fact that childhood has been the major focus for most theories of human development. In recent years, however, there has been increasing interest in human development during the remaining 60 years of the life span. A major portion of this chapter will be devoted to several influential theories of adult development.

Adult changes are very different from those of childhood. Adults resemble each other less as they grow older, i.e., they are shaped more by their culture than by patterns of biological development. As in childhood, age-associated changes of adult life appear unique to the period in which they occur, but these changes are greatly influenced by social forces and vary between cultures.

If the concept of human development is to remain meaningful for the entire life span, the process must be viewed in terms of the portion of the life span under consideration. Most theories of adult development divide the life span into stages which appear to have some internal consistency; the exact nature of these divisions has varied through history. New or altered notions of these stages may result from social and cultural change, rather than additional insight into a static phenomenon.

Childhood was first identified as a conceptually separate stage of life in the middle ages, when children were suddenly no longer considered "little adults" (1). The concept of adolescence first appeared in the late nineteenth century, and became widely recognized in the early twentieth century (2,3). As more people in western societies have begun to survive into their seventies, the years beyond adolescence have become fragmented into youth, young adulthood, middle age, the "young-old," and the "old-old" (4,5). This division of adulthood into different periods reflects the undeniable fact that aging changes both people and their roles in our culture; the exact nature of these changes is harder to define. Work on adult development is really just beginning. The following sections provide an introduction to several recent and important stage theories of adult development.

STAGE THEORIES OF ADULT DEVELOPMENT

The Greek philosopher Solon divided adulthood into six periods, each with its appropriate task, e.g., learning to use one's capacities to the fullest; becoming a husband and father; increasing in virtue. Although modern tasks may differ, Solon's divisions are not very different from those of more recent theorists. Carl Jung, Erik Erikson, D.J. Levinson, and Roger Gould have each attempted to conceptualize adulthood in terms of specific stages. The differences among their theories, as well as their similarities, illustrate the complex nature of adult development and aging.

Carl Jung

Recent descriptive studies of personality change with age seem to strongly support the theories of adult development proposed by Carl Jung. Jung was a student of Freud, and the first psychoanalyst to theorize specifically about adult developmental stages. He felt that adult development was divided into two major periods, with a crucial transition occurring around the age of 40 (6). Prior to this transition, most individuals engage in characteristic sex-differentiated activities. Men seek achievement and productivity, while women seek to be nurturant and express the emotional sides of their personalities.

Jung argued that both male and female inclinations or principles are present in all individuals, but only one is primarily expressed. Following the mid-life transition, each person seeks to increase the expression of the previously repressed inclinations. In particular, men become more inwardly directed, emotional, and nurturant. The male transition represents a shift to "inner orientation," in which a balance between opposing forces is sought, e.g., male versus female; youth versus age. This view is supported by the fact that only introversion—out of the multitude of personality characteristics empirically studied (locus of control; dogmatism; cautiousness; conformity, etc.)—has consistently been found to increase with age (5).

Jung argued that the mid-life transition is often difficult, and represents a major change in life-style. The outer-directed life-style typical of the young man is not possible for the older man, who must turn inward for his rewards. Women who establish such a "masculine" life-style early in life will face the same problem at mid-life. Jung's theories seem to have much empirical validity. Recent cross-cultural empirical studies of aging populations have consistently found that men switch from a coping style of active mastery to passive mastery; women exhibit the opposite change (3,7). Jung's emphasis on the significance of the mid-life crisis, and the need for a definite life-style change in old age has been studied extensively (8–11). Jung felt that the preservation of an inappropriate younger life-style into old age was a major cause of neurosis in those past middle age.

Erik Erikson: The Three Tasks of Adult Life

Of the various theorists of human development, Erik Erikson has had the most pervasive influence. Erikson is a psychoanalyst, whose work led him to propose a theory of human development across the entire life span. For Erikson, development occurs in a series of eight epigenetic stages. Five of these stages occur before the age of twenty; the remaining three cover the rest of the human life span. Each of Erikson's stages is characterized by a primary task or conflict, which must be faced and solved if development is to proceed. One can only advance to a particular stage by successfully completing the tasks of the preceding stages. Present development is built upon the past, and there is a fixed order of stages. These stages are epigenetic in the sense that they must occur in a specific sequence, and are, to some degree, biologically predetermined.

The first of the three adult stages centers on the need to achieve interpersonal intimacy in early adulthood. This stage follows the adolescent struggle to achieve a stable sense of self, a prerequisite for the establishment of interpersonal intimacy. Failure to achieve intimacy leads to isolation and self-absorption, with consequent arrested development.

The second adult stage, occurring at mid-life, involves a need for generativity. In Erikson's terms, "generativity" means doing or caring for others, particularly those of the next generation. A major danger of this stage is self-involvement and a rejection of the needs of others—which prevents advancement to the next and final stage of development.

Erikson's last developmental stage centers on the need to achieve ego integrity. Basically, "ego integrity" means the achievement of a stable sense of the meaningfulness of one's past life. Failure to achieve ego integrity leads to a sense of despair.

Greatly simplified, Erikson is saying that adults must first establish a relationship with another person, usually a spouse. This is followed by the raising of children and/or a career which can satisfy the need to help others. Finally, each older person must come to terms with the fact that their life is largely over and cannot be changed; death is approaching.

Erikson has presented his theories in a series of entertaining, insightful studies of historical figures such as Luther and Gandhi (12,13). While they illustrate their value in understanding certain individuals, the studies do not support the general applicability of Erikson's theories, particularly to adulthood. His theories of adult development tend to be very general, nonspecific, subject to various interpretations, and have proved difficult to test empirically (14).

This lack of an empirical foundation is a common shortcoming of developmental stage theories. The following two theories have been generated in a more descriptive, empirical fashion than those of Jung or Erikson. Thus, they represent a different approach to the problem of identifying meaningful periods in adult development.

D.J. Levinson: Eras and Adult Life Structures

The work of Levinson and his associates has been popularized through the best selling book, *Passages: Predictable Crises of Adult Life* (15). Levinson and his group have proposed an invariable set of stages, through which men pass between the ages of 18 and 45. These stages differ from Erikson's in that they are based on social or cultural, rather than internal developmental, events. Levinson's group derived their theory from a study of 40 men, ages 35–45, representing several professions. Using lengthy biographical interviews, the researchers attempted to detail each man's life and then identify underlying patterns.

Levinson and his coworkers break the life span into what he calls "eras," each lasting about 20 years. Within each era, the most significant events are the creation by the individual of stable life structures or patterns of living which are modified every six or seven years. Two life structures are typically constructed between the ages of 20 and 40. These are followed by a mid-life crisis at the transition between the era of youth and middle age. This transition is often a period of retrospection and questioning of the life structures constructed in the previous twenty years. Levinson's original study (16) concluded with the period from ages 45–50, although his group believed the alternating pattern of stable life structures and transitions persisted throughout life. The recognition that the stages of adulthood, to a greater degree than is true in childhood, are determined by the individual's interaction with society makes Levinson's theories seem important.

R. Gould: Stages of Adult Consciousness

Roger Gould's theories were first formulated in a study of group psychotherapy patients in Los Angeles, California (17). Following the original study, a questionnaire was administered to 524 non-patients from various professions (9). Gould's concept of adult development involves the growth of the adult consciousness which gradually replaces the childhood consciousness established in early life. Childhood consciousness consists of emotions such as "demonic anger," which is seen as uncontrollable and destructive, and unconscious (unrealistic) beliefs, such as a belief in absolute safety.

Gould divides the period from ages 16–45 into four stages, each with a primary developmental task. The first task involves leaving the family. The second task (ages 22–28) involves abandoning a belief in the power of others to solve all problems. The third task (ages 28–34) requires the recognition of the contradictory and partially incomprehensible nature of the self and others. The final task, prior to the age of 45, centers on the need to confront death and human mortality. Gould argues that the illusions retained from childhood to protect against recognition of danger, unfairness, cruelty, and evil in the world prevent the growth of an adult personality and, if not abandoned, can lead to stagnation.

Aging: The Study of Adaptation and Coping

Theories of adult development tend to be very general or diffuse in characterizing the last periods of life, if they deal with old age at all. Specific theories of personality change in old age do not usually involve stages. Rather, they concentrate upon the way individuals handle the changes which occur throughout the life span. Unlike most stage theories, the way in which the individual deals with the transitions—rather than what lies between the transitions—is the focus of study. Jung recognized that such transitions often placed great stress upon individuals. The nature of these transitions, and the manner in which they are handled by the individual and his culture, may be more interesting than the exact nature of the stages involved. While the stages may vary greatly between individuals and cultures, the ways in which individuals handle the transitions are fairly constant. There is an extensive body of research aimed at determining the major stresses in adulthood and their effects upon the individual. Much of this work involves the study of life crises, such as illness and death, which directly involve health professionals. The study of these crises adds additional dimensions to our knowledge of adult development.

The Mid-life Crisis

Throughout the literature on aging, there seems to be general agreement that the entrance into middle age is a period of crisis (6,8,9,11). Middle age is a period of biological and social changes. Women undergo menopause and experience an end to childbearing. Men begin to experience the early physical problems of old age. In a youth-oriented culture such as ours, middle age is often identified as the beginning of old age and eventual death.

In the early twentieth century, Arnold Van Gennep, an anthropologist, noted in his book, *The Rites of Passage* (18), that all societies seem to employ a three-part process in establishing the necessary transitions between social roles: 1. separation from the major group; 2. isolation while aspects of the new roles are learned; 3. return to the group. Social role transitions such as occur at puberty, marriage, birth, or death involve rites of passage which promote socialization into new roles. The process of higher education and professionalization, a prerequisite for entrance into many high-status roles, represents one such set of rites of passage in our Western culture.

Western culture is also characterized by the lack of such ritualized transitions from young adulthood into middle age, and middle age into old age. Rosow (19) has commented that in our culture, role transitions in the first part of life are associated with social gains, such as greater autonomy, responsibility, or status; the reverse is true for the second half of the life span. Individuals are poorly socialized into the role changes of old age. Rather than being determined culturally, such transitions often occur abruptly in response to external events, such as illness or loss of a spouse. Such transitions produce great stress, and failure to adapt to these changes in late life often results in physical illness or death.

Liberman has carried out a series of studies to determine which factors predict successful coping with change in old age (20). He has found that the degree of stress is a function of the degree of change in life-style, and is not related to the subjective meaning of the change to the individual. Thus, the loss of a spouse may be a very significant event; however, if it is not followed by a major change in life-style, the individual has a good chance of adapting successfully. Furthermore, the perceived meaning of a change, such as retirement, was found to be much less relevant to predicting adaptation than the actual change in life-style which resulted. Liberman also found that coping mechanisms which reportedly function well in youth and middle age may be nonadaptive for the elderly (much as Jung might have suggested).

Successful adaptation in old age requires cognitive and physical resources. Thus, those individuals who were aggressive, irritating, narcissistic, and demanding were most likely to survive a crisis. Successful adaptation was also associated with a stable self-image, the ability to introspect, and a high level of hope (20).

Clinical Application of Theories of Adult Development

As psychiatry and psychotherapy have developed in this century, there has been a continual dialogue between clinical practice and theories of childhood development. Recently, there have been attempts to incorporate theories of adult development into psychotherapeutic theory (21). Given the uncertain state of our knowledge about adult development, these attempts are largely ambitious beginnings. Compared to childhood, adulthood is a period of great variability between individuals and cultures. The concept of adult development is increasingly being viewed from more of a social and cultural perspective. Society probably contributes enormously to the stages of adulthood and the nature of the transitions between stages. This socio-cultural relativism does not characterize the relationship between psychotherapeutic and childhood developmental theories; thus, theories of adult development may not make a comparable contribution to the psychotherapy of the individual. Theories of adult development may help us to understand the relationship between the individual and his culture, but we do not know whether such an understanding has clinical implications.

Psychopathology in Old Age

The incidence of formal psychopathology in old age represents an alternative source of information about the nature of the individual aging process. Although there seems to be little difference between the psychopathology of the early and middle portions of the adult life span, old age does appear to be associated with a number of distinct syndromes. Dementia is the most common psychiatric illness of old age. Over 50% of elderly patients in psychiatric facilities have a primary diagnosis of dementia (22). (See Chapter 3, Delirium and Dementia.)

Depression, the next most common psychiatric illness in elderly patients (23), is frequently associated with physical illness or major life change. Older patients do not usually complain of sadness or feelings of depression; they complain of physical symptoms or problems with concentration of memory. This can make it difficult to differentiate between the diagnoses of dementia and depression. Of the various treatable causes of syndromes presenting like dementia in the elderly, depression seems to be the most common.

A 1955 British survey of late-onset psychiatric illness in the elderly reported three major syndromes or illnesses: dementia; affective illness; paraphrenia or paranoid disorders (24). Roth used the term "paraphrenia" to refer to a syndrome of paranoid psychosis resembling paranoid schizophrenia, but with onset late in life. The term continues to be used in reference to chronic paranoid psychoses which occur exclusively in later life. Paranoid symptoms are common in the elderly, and can also be associated with dementia or affective illness (25,26). By far, the largest group of elderly schizophrenics is composed of those who manifested the disease prior to age 35 and continued to be symptomatic (27). However, cases of schizophrenia not previously diagnosed account for perhaps 10% of geriatric schizophrenics.

REFERENCES

1. Aries P: *Centuries of Childhood: A Social History of Family Life.* New York, WW Norton, 1962.
2. Gillis JR: *Youth and History.* New York, Academic Press, 1974.
3. Jordan WD: Searching for adulthood in America, in Erikson EH (ed): *Adulthood.* New York, WW Norton, 1978.
4. Keniston K: Youth and its ideology, in Arieti S (ed): *American Handbook of Psychiatry.* New York, Basic Books, 1974.
5. Neugarten BL: Personality and aging, in Birren J, Schaie KW (eds): *Handbook of the Psychology of Aging.* New York, Van Nostrand, 1977.
6. Jung CG: *Modern Man in Search of a Soul.* New York, Harcourt Brace, 1933.
7. Gutmann DL: Parenthood: Key to the comparative psychology of the life cycle?, in Datan N, Ginsberg L (eds): *Life Span Developmental Psychology.* New York, Academic Press, 1975, pp 232–245.
8. Erikson E: *Toys and Reason: Stages in the Ritualization of Experience.* New York, WW Norton, 1977.
9. Gould R: *Transformations: Growth and Change in Adult Life.* New York, Simon & Schuster, 1978.
10. Levinson DJ, Darrow CN, Klein EB, *et al.: The Seasons of a Man's Life.* New York, Alfred Knopf, 1978.
11. Rosenberg S, Farrell MP: Identity and crisis in middle aged men. *Int J Aging Hum Dev* 1976;7:153.
12. Erikson E: *Young Man Luther, A Study in Psychoanalysis and History.* New York, WW Norton, 1958.
13. Erikson E: *Gandhi's Truth.* New York, WW Norton, 1969.
14. Gruen W: Adult personality: An empirical study of Erikson's theory of ego development, in Neugarten BL, *et al.: Personality in Middle and Late Life.* New York, Atherton, 1964, pp 1–14.
15. Sheehy G: *Passages: Predictable Crises of Adult Life.* New York, EP Dutton, 1976.
16. Levinson DJ, Darrow CM, Klein EB, *et al.:* The psycho-social development of men in early adulthood and the mid-life transition, in Ricks DF, Thomas A, Roff M (eds): *Life History Research in Psychopathology.* Minneapolis, University of Minnesota Press, 1974, vol 3, pp 243–258.
17. Gould R: The phases of adult life: A study in developmental psychology. *Am J Psychiatry* 1972;129:521–531.
18. Van Gennep A: *The Rites of Passage.* Chicago, University of Chicago Press, 1960.
19. Rosow I: *Socialization to Old Age.* Berkeley, CA, University of California Press, 1974.
20. Lieberman MA: Adaptive processes in late life, in Datan N, Ginsberg LH (eds): *Life Span Developmental Psychology.* New York, Academic Press, 1975.
21. Colarusso CA, Nemiroff RA: *Adult Development A New Dimension in Psychodynamic Theory and Practice.* New York, Plenum Press, 1981.
22. Gurland B, Mann A, Cross P, *et al.:* A cross-national comparison of the institutionalized elderly in the cities of New York and London. *Psychol Med* 1980;9:781–788.
23. Lehman HE: Affective disorders in the aged. *Psychiatr Clin North Am* 1982;5:27–44.
24. Roth M: The natural history of mental disorder in old age. *J Ment Sci* 1955;101:281.
25. Small GW, Jarvik LF: Paranoid disorder in the aged. *Psychiatr Clin North Am* 1982;5:119–120.

26. Varner RV, Gaitz CM: Schizophrenic and paranoid disorders in the aged. *Psychiatr Clin North Am* 1982;5:107-118.

27. Gurland B, Cross PS: Epidemiology of psychopathology in old age. *Psychiatr Clin North Am* 1982;5:11-26.

Chapter 16

NEUROSIS
RICHARD B. CORRADI, M.D.

Neurosis is the emotional legacy of the human developmental experience. Its origins lie in the conflict between our nature and our nurture. It is the "nature" of human development, both biologic and psychologic, to proceed according to an innate groundplan, with maturational achievements specific to each stage of growth (1,2). Our "nurture," the environmental and interpersonal influences on the developing child, may either facilitate or impede the innate maturational potential. The impediments are the stuff of neurosis; they are the childhood experiences which thwart mastery of stage-specific psychological tasks. The result is a focus of conflict, an unresolved emotional problem which has been temporarily sealed over in the maturational progression but is prone to subsequent reactivation. Events in later life that touch upon important childhood conflicts may revive the original troublesome emotions. The revived anxiety is now experienced as out of context, neither entirely appropriate to the current event nor connected to its earlier sources. Perceived as alien and mysterious, such anxiety is not easily resolved. A nonspecific kind of containing action results, with various defensive maneuvers utilized to ward off distressing emotions whose real origins are outside of awareness. The early-acquired patterns of defensive maneuvers which protect against anxiety are applied repeatedly, and become consolidated as enduring personality traits. It is the relative failure of these maneuvers, consequent to a stress-induced revival of childhood conflicts, which leads to neurotic symptoms.

DEFINITION AND DIAGNOSIS

The American Psychiatric Association's *Diagnostic and Statistical Manual of Mental Disorders* (DSM-III) (3) defines a *neurotic disorder* as "a mental disorder in which the predominant disturbance is a symptom or group of symptoms that is distressing to the individual and is recognized by

175

him or her as unacceptable and alien (ego-dystonic); reality testing is grossly intact; behavior does not actively violate gross social norms (although functioning may be markedly impaired); the disturbance is relatively enduring or recurrent without treatment and is not limited to a transitory reaction to stressors; and there is no demonstrable organic etiology or factor." In DSM-III, the neuroses are included among affective, anxiety, somatoform, dissociative, and psychosexual disorders, with each neurotic disorder classified according to its predominant symptomatology. This is a strictly descriptive classification, without any etiologic implications.

This chapter will deal with the underlying psychic mechanisms of neurosis, an explanatory rather than descriptive approach. Neurosis will be discussed in terms of the *neurotic process* which, according to psychoanalytic theory, is common to all of the neurotic disorders. According to this orientation, psychogenetic and psychodynamic etiologic considerations are intrinsic to the very concept of neurosis, while the variety of its symptomatic expression is of secondary importance.

Anxiety

The concept of anxiety provides a meeting ground between descriptive and explanatory (process) views of neurosis. Its phenomenology allows descriptive classification of the neurotic disorders; dynamically, it is viewed as a signal of internal psychological conflict. As a subjective emotion with its physiologic concomitants, anxiety is the *sine qua non* of neurosis; the major characteristic of the genus "neurosis." The various subgroups, or species, of neurosis are classified according to the symptomatic way in which the anxiety is manifest. Anxiety may be experienced directly, without modification (anxiety disorders); it may be modified so that other symptoms assume prominence (e.g., phobic disorders, conversion disorder, obsessive compulsive disorder). For the subgroups of neurosis in which anxiety is modified, psychodynamic theory holds that unconscious psychological defense mechanisms are utilized to "control" the core anxiety. These mechanisms themselves are relatively unsuccessful and give rise to the distressing symptoms characteristic of each neurotic subgroup.

Neurosis versus Psychosis

Since anxiety is a ubiquitous symptom in mental illness, the genus "neurosis" must be distinguished from the genus "psychosis." Clinically, this is done on descriptive grounds. In the neuroses, there are no gross distortions in reality perception and interpretation; a delusion is pathognomonic of psychosis and incompatible with a primary diagnosis of neurosis.

Additionally, there is an important etiologic difference between psychosis and neurosis, although in our present state of knowledge it has more research than clinical utility. While environmental influences are themselves sufficient to produce personality traits, certain character pathology, and neurosis, such is not the case with the so-called "functional" psychoses (schizophrenia and the major affective disorders). Psychological and environmental factors may precipitate the latter, but probably only in the presence of a genetically mediated biologic predisposition. Thus, a unitary hypothesis of mental illness is not tenable. A psychosis is not a "severe" neurosis, nor should psychosis be thought of as existing on a continuum of severity with neurosis or character pathology.

Neurosis and Personality Disorders

Personality encompasses an individual's characteristic style of thinking, perceiving, and behaving, particularly in the interpersonal context. Psychodynamic theory views personality traits as resulting from early conflict resolution, solidifying with repeated usage in anxiety situations, and finally becoming incorporated as autonomous functions of the self. The personality *disorders* designate constellations of traits that are inflexible and significantly maladaptive (See Chapter 17, Personality Disorders).

The "dosage" and timing of the childhood stressors which produce psychopathology are important. Those which predispose to neurosis only impede complete mastery of specific developmental tasks; they neither arrest the emotional developmental process nor produce irreparable personality defects. In the latter case, as with profound maternal deprivation in the first year of life or with severe abuse or neglect later, the outcome may be significant character pathology, e.g., borderline personality states—rather than neurosis. Generally, the earlier and more profound the childhood stressors, the greater the propensity for fixed characterologic psychopathology. According to the traditional analytic concept of psychosexual development, personality disorders are derived from significant preoedipal fixations during the oral and anal developmental periods; a neurotic outcome is associated with unresolved conflicts from the later oedipal period. Such a neat distinction is an oversimplification, and subsequent writers have extended the concept of personality development as occurring throughout the life cycle (2,4). However, the classical psychosexual developmental model has given us a rich understanding of character formation and has correctly emphasized the overriding importance of the infantile maternal environment.

Descriptively, the DSM-III personality disorders are generally characterized by behavioral disturbances, gross social maladaptation, and significant problems in interpersonal relationships. Psychopathology tends to be egosyntonic, with symptomatology "acted-out" rather than experienced as intrapsychic distress. To the extent that symptoms are expressed behaviorally rather than producing personal anxiety, personality disorders are much more resistant than neuroses to psychotherapeutic intervention. While certain neurotic behaviors may also be personally maladaptive, the important components of the personality are basically intact and the individual is capable of learning more adaptive coping skills.

THE NEUROTIC PERSONALITY

A clinical neurosis should not be confused with a neurotic symptom. Minor neuroticisms are universal and usually cause only occasional inconvenience, e.g., stage fright, minor compulsive traits, anxiety in certain social situations, isolated phobias. In contrast, symptoms in a clinical neurosis are the tip of the neurotic iceberg—surface manifestations of internal psychological conflict which profoundly affects the personality. Symptoms (e.g., disruptive phobias, obsessions, or compulsions; conversions; persistent dysthymia or free-floating anxiety) indicate that unsuccessful psychological maneuvers are being used to contain or control a more pervasive conflict. People with a clinical neurosis rarely present with an isolated symptom; "typing" the neurosis on the basis of the most prominent or disabling symptom is an oversimplification. Before considering the psychodynamic mechanisms which produce neurotic symptoms, it is important to describe the kind of personality organization which frequently underlies a *clinical neurosis* and provides a fertile soil for its development.

The *neurotic personality* (5) is inflexible, unspontaneous, and constricted. Personal relations are often characterized by a monotonous repetition of self-defeating attitudes and behaviors. The most valued relationships suffer the most. Demands upon important people are unrealistic, highly symbolic, overly dependent, and ambivalent, i.e., people with neurotic personalities often behave as though attempting to redress grievances by reenacting childhood dramas in adult situations. This unconscious, repetitious attempt to master historical problems can markedly limit their behavioral options. They may respond to contemporary situations with old feelings, even when there is only a trivial or symbolic similarity to the childhood conflict. For example, a man with an anxiety neurosis would repeatedly respond to normal marital conflict by attempting to placate and cajole his wife; he would unjustly blame himself for the "unpleasantness," and subsequently experience acute anxiety and guilt. In therapy, he realized that repression of his anger was related to the old risk of losing his mother's love if he angered her. He was then able to free his marital interactions from the unconscious fear that anger would result in abandonment and helplessness. The compulsion to repeat and master infantile conflicts is a basic psychological phenomenon that underlies both neurotic personality characteristics and neurotic symptoms.

The unconscious nature of the repetition points up another characteristic of the neurotic personality—i.e., too much is unconscious. Such individuals are often out of touch with, or fear, their impulses, desires, fantasies, thoughts, and feelings. What may be natural to other people is often foreign to them. They may fear normal anger and regard it as having magical, destructive consequences. Sexuality is often forbidden, dangerous, and overly exciting. Thoughts and feelings are equivalent to deeds, and produce the same consequences. Normally, people consider fantasies as natural, acceptable, sometimes pleasurable parts of mental life, which often provide a safe, economical outlet for impulses. For the neurotic personality, fantasies are frequently forbidden, dangerous, or perversely erotic, and typically produce guilt. Feelings which most people find mildly uncomfortable but easily integrate into their lives—e.g., expectable anxiety, indecision, passivity, sad moods, aggressive feelings, etc.—are unacceptable. They produce too much anxiety or guilt, and trigger avoidance maneuvers which are more disruptive than the original dysphoric feelings.

Guilt is sometimes all-pervasive in the life of the neurotic personality. There may be a constant feeling of failure to measure up—to both self-imposed and external demands. Demands are often unrealistic, as illustrated by the unacceptability of natural feelings and fantasies. The inability to meet unreasonable demands produces harsh self-criticism. His self-esteem is very low; he also assumes that other people think as poorly of him as he does of himself. The behavior of a person with a neurotic personality is self-defeating. The defeats confirm his low self-opinion, and a vicious cycle perpetuates itself.

Paradoxically, defeat is often accepted more easily than success. Defeat is expected, deserved, and eminently just. Success produces guilt, and is considered evidence of fraud, e.g., "If someone loves me (or promotes me), it is because they don't know the real me; I have tricked or defrauded them because no one could be stupid enough to like me if they really knew me." The guilt associated with success is so severe that many such individuals unconsciously conspire to avoid success.

THE PSYCHODYNAMICS OF THE NEUROTIC PROCESS

Historical Aspects

Historically, the concept of neurosis as a psychodynamic process chronicles the development of Freud's thought. It is useful to place his contributions in a brief historical perspective. When Freud began his work, serious attention to psychiatric nosology had only recently begun. Kraepelin's great organizing statement (the categorization of psychosis into the two broad groups of affective disorders and dementia praecox) brought order for the first time to the problems of diagnosis, unifying a large number of what were considered disparate diagnostic entities. This set the stage for the scientific delineation of neuroses as mental disturbances distinct from the psychoses.

This relatively recent distinction had to await at least an attempt at a scientifically-based nosology. When all mental illness was thought to be due to demon possession, for example, the etiologic hypothesis logically determined the treatment approach; there was no need for subtle diagnostic distinctions.

In the late 19th and early 20th century climate of scientific determinism, in which Kraepelin and Bleuler established a system of psychiatric classification, the neuroses were considered the province of the neurologists. Jean Charcot (1835–1893), one of the most influential neurologists, conducted his famous clinical demonstrations of hysteria at the Salpetriere. Despite his belief that hysteria was due to an hereditary degeneration of the central nervous system, he dramatically demonstrated the effects of hypnosis on hysteria. In so doing, he attracted men like Janet and Freud to the field.

Although Pierre Janet (1859–1947) followed Charcot in considering the neuroses to be physically produced, he came very close to the idea of the "dynamic unconscious." His concept of "dissociation" was based on an hereditary constitutional "inferiority," which allowed certain nervous system and psychological functions to escape from the integrating dominance of higher CNS centers. The resulting loss of neurologic synthesis manifests as neurotic symptomatology. (Freud saw this phenomenon as exclusively psychological, and ultimately called it "repression.") Janet classified the neuroses into hysteria (which includes conversion and amnestic types) and psychasthenia (which includes phobic, obsessive-compulsive, and neurasthenic states, among others). This was a relatively sophisticated nosology, in light of his lack of knowledge of etiology and psychodynamics.

It is interesting that both Charcot and Janet considered hypnosis, which could "cure" hysterical conversion symptoms, as supportive of their thesis of a somatic etiology of the neuroses. They felt that only people with constitutional "degeneracy" could be hypnotized. It was Freud who realized that hypnosis was incompatible with a neurologic etiology of the neuroses—a major conceptual step in his psychodynamic formulations.

Freud's initial classification of the neuroses partially retained the notion of neuropathic etiology. He divided them into the *actual* neuroses and the *psycho*-neuroses (6). He thought the former (consisting of neurasthenia and anxiety neurosis) were due to the physiological effects of "unhygienic sex practices," e.g., masturbation and coitus interruptus; the latter (hysteria and the obsessional states) he believed were purely psychological. Later, of course, he came to regard sexual practices as having a psychological, rather than a somatic, role in the etiology of neurosis.

Theoretical Aspects

Freud used several theoretical hypotheses about the psychodynamics of the neuroses to explain some of the observable facts and the symptomatology. (The reader may wish to review the Introduction, Chapter 1, where some of these concepts are also discussed.)

The *structural hypothesis* (7) provides a convenient way of conceptualizing psychic processes. It involves an artificial, but useful, division of the psychic apparatus into functional units termed "id," "ego," and "super-ego." The *id* is the repository of the instinctual drives, the most psychologically important of which are the aggressive and the sexual (libidinal) drives. The id is entirely unconscious, i.e., outside of conscious awareness and inaccessible to ordinary cognition, and is, therefore, not bound by the laws of logic or reality. Thus, instinctual aggressive and libidinal drives are unfettered in relation to the id, and press for immediate discharge and gratification. The developmental analog of this is the, "I want what I want when I want it," position of the infant or young child. The id's characteristic logic (or illogic) is also analogous to the thinking of the prelogical child. It involves magic, e.g., the thought or wish is equivalent to the deed, condensations, distortions of concepts of time and causality, e.g., events which occur today can cause events which have occurred in the past, displacements, symbolic distortions, etc. A commonplace example of this kind of prelogical thinking is the dream, which is a manifestation of instinctual drives and wishes, expressed in the magical, symbolic, condensed language of the id.

The term *"primary process"* (8) is applied to both of these characteristics of the id, i.e., the handling of drive energies in accordance with the immediate gratification or "pleasure" principle, and the prelogical thinking.

The *ego* is the mediator between the instinctual demands of the id and the demands of the external world or "reality." It modifies the pressing instinctual demands to conform with the particular societal sanctions, mores, and customs in which it has been inculcated. The immature, developing ego of the young child will often favor instinctual demands over the requirements of "society" (the parents), i.e., it will try to get away with what it can. In contrast, the mature ego has incorporated reality demands, making it unnecessary to actually test limits; its id control functions are automatic. Among the psychological devices at its disposal in regulating the id drives are the *mechanisms of defense* (9), e.g., repression, projection, identification, reaction formation, etc. These operate at an unconscious level.

The ego, in contrast to the "primary process" of the id, functions in accordance with the *"secondary process,"* both in its handling of drive energies and in its thinking. The drive energies are modified so that immediate instinctual gratification can be postponed if it seems appropriate or might result in a higher order of gratification later. The ego's thinking process follows the principles of Aristotelian logic—reality based; empirical; deductive. Although there are lapses, the mature ego is usually characterized by logical thinking. "Lapses" normally occur in sleep, when the ego "allows" primary process thinking in the form of dreams, perhaps because there is no danger of motor discharge of the drives. The process of creativity also involves a temporary lapse of the secondary process. Much creativity involves a suspension of logical, goal-directed thinking, allowing novel, primary process associations to be applied to ideas which seem logically unconnected. Dreams and creativity reflect "normal" manifestations of the primary process. They occur under the relative control of the ego and in the service of healthy ego function. One measure of severity of psychopathology is the degree to which the ego relinquishes the secondary process and is dominated by the primary process. The neuroses and certain characterologic disorders are intermediate in this regard; both functional and organic psychoses are the extremes in severity. The psychotic ego is unable to perform the defensive maneuvers necessary to impose the secondary process upon the id's drive derivatives.

In addition to mediating between the demands of the id and those of external reality, the ego is also subject to *superego* demands. The superego is that aspect of the personality which we recognize as "conscience," i.e., the internalized standards of thought and behavior to which people hold themselves accountable. When these demands are not met, the ego experiences the affect of guilt. Another aspect of superego is the ego ideal—i.e., those largely unconscious standards of thought and behavior to which the individual aspires. These may or may not be realistic and attainable. A person who feels he is not measuring up to the ego ideal experiences a painful loss of self-esteem.

Although the various aspects of the personality have been artificially separated in this structural hypothesis, they normally function in an equilibrium. Ideally, there is no conflict among the various faculties. The ego perceives reality demands appropriately, free from unconscious, residual infantile influences. It is cognizant of, and comfortable with, the id's instinctual processes and allows itself a reasonable measure of instinctual gratification. Sophisticated defenses, such as sublimation, operate automatically; thus, the ego's energies are not exhausted by primitive defenses. The superego does not make excessively harsh demands upon the ego, and permits reasonable drive satisfaction without guilt. The ego ideal is attainable and enhances self-esteem. In this ideal state, there are no clinical manifestations of conflict, i.e., neurotic symptoms or significant personality problems. It is difficult to separate this model psychic apparatus into its functional divisions of id, ego, and superego.

It is in the neuroses that these psychic divisions are clearly seen. When the personality is in internal conflict, the opposing forces are readily apparent. With this theoretical background, these conflicting forces can now be described.

Neurotic Conflict

A psychodynamic formulation of neurosis is based upon the idea of conflict between id and ego. An id drive (libidinal, aggressive, or both) presses for discharge, and for some reason (to be described below) is unacceptable to the ego. This conflict produces a painful emotional state—anxiety—which the ego attempts to dispel. Its first defensive maneuver is usually repression, i.e., an active barring of the unacceptable drive from consciousness, including the feelings, thoughts, and fantasies (drive derivatives) associated with it. The ego is freed from its anxiety with this conflict resolution, but it pays a price. Repression is usually not a one-time proposition. It involves an ongoing expenditure of the ego's energy ("countercathexis"), since the id drives continue to press for discharge and gratification. The energy used to maintain repressions is not available for other ego functions. Therefore, the more it is engaged in repression, the more depleted the ego becomes. Less energy is available to invest in intellectual and interpersonal pursuits which should normally be conflict-free. In other words, the personality which is bound up in intrapsychic conflict is constricted; it is robbed of some of its capacity to derive pleasure from work, play, and relationships with other people. This state of affairs constitutes the "neurotic personality."

While this may be a stable, albeit constricted, personality organization, repressions are vulnerable and frequently unsuccessful. When repression is not successful, the ego reexperiences the anxiety associated with the forbidden drives. The ego will then use other defense mechanisms in its attempt to control the anxiety. To the extent that these are successful, equilibrium is restored again—at the expense of ego constriction.

A *neurotic symptom* is evidence that the defenses are relatively unsuccessful. It represents a compromise formation between ego and id. The symptom is both a symbolic partial gratification of the forbidden impulse and the ego's defense against it. A case vignette may help in clarifying these abstract concepts:

> A young Marine recruit in basic training developed a paralysis of his right arm—an hysterical conversion symptom—the first time he tried to fire his rifle on the target range. Psychotherapy revealed that he was

struggling with powerful aggressive impulses which he feared he could not control. He was aware of intense anger toward his Drill Instructor, who had been a severely demanding (but not sadistic) taskmaster in the preceding weeks of basic training. The Drill Instructor was standing at the perimeter of the line of fire when the recruit developed his symptom. The paralysis of the patient's "rifle arm" represented a defense against a murderous impulse toward the D.I., which he could have carried out and feared he could not control. It was both a symbolic expression of the forbidden homicidal wish, i.e., "Look what I would do if I only could," and a very literal defense against it, i.e., "I can't do it because I can't move my arm."

In this case, we see a rupture in the integrity of the patient's personality; one aspect of his personality has set itself in opposition to another. When such an intrapsychic conflict exists, we see more clearly those personality forces which we call ego, id, and superego. The murderous impulse was derived from the id as a manifestation of the aggressive drive (it contained libidinal or sexual components also, as will be described later). The aspect of the personality which controlled the impulse was ego, and it did so, not only because of its own reality testing function, but also at the behest of the superego. Even the thought of murder—let alone the act—was repugnant to the patient's superego.

Some historical data about this patient will enable us to use his case to further illustrate the psychodynamics of neurotic symptoms. He was the product of a tumultuous developmental background. His alcoholic father was brutal and sadistic toward his family when drunk. Sober, he was withdrawn, distant, remorseful, and chronically mildly depressed. The mother usually tried to stay out of the father's way. She was manipulative and seductive with the patient, whom—unlike her husband—she could control. Out of this background, the patient developed a rigid, constricted, and compliant personality. He tended to "blend into the background" in all areas of life. Although bright, he achieved only mediocre grades in high school. His teachers considered him a shy, inhibited boy who always did as he was told. He was barely noticed among his classmates. He liked sports, but only participated in informal neighborhood games, never trying out for high school teams because he "lacked coordination." He gradually lost contact with his male friends when they became interested in girls and began dating. Although he double-dated on a few occasions in high school, he described himself as ill at ease around girls and lacking self-confidence. After high school graduation, his vague plans for college never materialized. He finally drifted into the Marine Corps after two years of performing menial jobs around his small town. He thought he could learn a trade in the service, but was unsure of his interests. He was immediately uncomfortable in the unfamiliar military setting. He was disturbed by the drinking, drug abuse, sexual freedom, and promiscuity in which his barracksmates urged him to participate. Rather than seek compatible friends, he withdrew into isolation.

Prior to the sudden onset of his hysterical conversion symptom, this young man's personality structure was typical of a "neurotic personality." From a *descriptive* point of view, we are impressed by his severe inhibitions, the lack of goals or direction in his life, the paucity of meaningful interpersonal relationships, his inability to achieve in work, the lack of pleasure and gratification in his life, and his lack of self-esteem. From a *psychodynamic* point of view, i.e., one which enables a psychological understanding of what is observed, we would say that his personality is dominated by conflict over his sexual and aggressive drives. From his history, we observe that few of the age-expectable outlets for natural aggression (sublimations) were available to him, e.g., participation in sports and academic achievement; competition with peers; ambition for the future; success in work. In the sexual sphere, he had not even begun the adolescent task of establishing relationships with women—much less had any successes. In other words, his personality constriction was due to repression, i.e., the ego thwarted the normal expression of instinctual drives by actively barring their derivatives from consciousness. Another mechanism of defense is revealed by his overcompliance, i.e., reaction formation, in which the ego negates the aggressive drive by reversing it. Identification, in which the ego assumes behavioral and other characteristics of another person, was another of his defenses. He identified with his father in two ways: 1. He feared the brutal, drunken father's lack of control over his aggressive impulses. He behaved as though he too would lose control if he allowed any expression of aggression; 2. As another means of defense against his own feared aggression, he identified with the sober father—becoming withdrawn, remorseful, and chronically mildly depressed. Thus, he entered the Marine Corps with a neurotic personality structure, in which most of his emotional energy was consumed in controlling feared instinctual drives. His overuse of repression as a primary defense mechanism robbed him of gratification and spontaneity, making him vulnerable to symptomatic decompensation.

What upset this personality equilibrium and led to the production of a neurotic symptom? His longstanding repressions failed in a situation which he felt was out of control. The military environment seemed to license the free expression of the drives and impulses he had struggled so long to control. His fellow Marines appeared to be freely acting out the sexual impulses which were forbidden to him. He was being trained to kill and he feared that his destructiveness, once unleashed, would know no bounds. He became acutely anxious when the id impulses threatened to overwhelm the ego's previously successful defenses. The situation became intolerable when the aggressive impulse attached to the D.I. in the form of a homicidal wish. The ego resolved the conflict with the hysterical conversion symptom. When he entered the base hospital, it was apparent that the symptom had served its purpose. He appeared remarkably calm and relatively unconcerned about his paralysis (*"la belle indifference,"* often seen in a conversion neurosis).

We can now recapitulate what has been said about the psychodynamics of neurosis, and add to the general formulation. A neurosis is a psychogenic disorder characterized by an unconscious conflict between id and ego, in the presence of the ego's intact reality testing. The conflict involves the id's sexual and aggressive drives, which are unacceptable to the ego. The ego's expenditure of energy in defensive maneuvers (the mechanisms of defense) to keep the drives repressed results in varying degrees of ego constriction and maladaptive behavior, which constitute the neurotic personality. A neurotic symptom is the result of an attempt to bind the anxiety caused when an id drive threatens to escape the ego's controls; Freud called this "the return of the repressed." Neurotic symptoms are only partially successful in binding the anxiety and are themselves distressing and emotionally painful *(ego-alien).* Neurotic symptoms are therefore not a solution to the intrapsychic problem, but a *compromise.* An analysis of the symptom reveals derivatives of all parties to the conflict—id, ego, and often superego. In other words, the symptom contains elements of partial drive gratification, the ego's defenses against it, and, often, superego condemnation of the drive. *"Primary gain"* refers to the relief from anxiety which the ego obtains at the price of the symptom. Some symptoms are more effective than others, e.g., the conversion symptom used in our case is much more efficient than an obsessive-compulsive symptom in controlling anxiety. *"Secondary gain"* refers to those environmental benefits which accrue to the ego as a result of the symptom. Our patient's secondary gain involved removal from the field of conflict (both literally and figuratively) and receiving the concern and attention of medical personnel. This gratified dependency needs which had not been met in his childhood. Primary gain is always more important than secondary gain in symptom production; significant secondary gain may, however, result in an extremely treatment-resistant symptom consolidation, e.g., "compensation neurosis," in which the prospect of tangible benefits strongly reinforces symptomatology.

NEUROSIS—PREDISPOSITION AND PRECIPITANTS

Thus far we have primarily discussed psychodynamics; now we will turn briefly to *psychogenetics.* "Psychogenetics" means that the psychopathology of adult neurosis has its genetic origin in the early experiences of childhood, i.e., the predisposition to neurosis is to be found in developmental conflicts.

In this context, "genetics" does not refer to genes or heredity; it is used in its broader meaning of "genesis"—the way in which something is formed. The very early years of childhood are crucial to personality development. During this time, there is a normal maturational sequence in which the libidinal and aggressive drives develop, the ego and superego are formed, and the quality of an individual's relationships with other people is established (See Chapters 6–11 on Development). The normal developmental flow may be adversely affected by environmental influences, e.g., losses; separations; deprivations; overindulgences, which stress the ego's ability to completely master them. When this occurs, areas of unresolved conflict remain, and may be reactivated in adulthood. The reactivation may be an ongoing characterologic process in which the individual, unconsciously, unsuccessfully, and inappropriately, reenacts the early conflict in an adult setting, as though still attempting to master it. The reactivation may also take the form of discrete neurotic symptoms. Our patient exemplifies both of these outcomes.

We will now add the concept of "psychogenesis" to our formulation of neurosis. An unresolved, repressed childhood conflict may be activated by an adult situation which the ego unconsciously perceives as similar. The perception of similarity is often tenuous and highly symbolic, i.e., based on primary process logic. The ego reacts as though it were still immature, infantile, and in danger of being overwhelmed by the id's instinctual drives. This danger is signaled by the development of anxiety, the hallmark of neurotic conflict.

Freud (10) pointed out that such *signal anxiety* occurs in situations which recapitulate childhood danger situations, i.e., fears of abandonment, loss of parental love, bodily injury (castration anxiety), and superego condemnation (guilt). If these developmental issues are not sequentially confronted and mastered, they may remain as possible sources of anxiety in later life. Freedom from the influence of these infantile dangers is one measure of mental health. People with problematic developmental histories may unconsciously structure their personalities to avoid experiences which revive painful emotions associated with these early issues. When such maneuvers fail, signal anxiety may occur.

When the ego tries to control this anxiety, the compromise of a neurotic symptom often results. Why does the neurotic adult ego behave as though it were an immature ego, and react to a harmless contemporary situation as though it were a potentially overwhelming childhood trauma? It does so because the repressed, unresolved childhood conflict has remained unconscious and, therefore, subject to the laws of the primary process. As we have discussed, the primary process is illogical, and characterized by magic, condensations, time and causality distortions, etc. There is, therefore, a timelessness to the unresolved early conflicts. They are not "worn down" by conscious reality testing over time, and can become reactivated by adult situations which have no *logical* connection to them—only a symbolic, displaced, or magical resemblance. Thus, the neurotic adult is as much under the unconscious influence of his unresolved infantile conflicts as when he was a child. Furthermore, when the repressions are compromised, he may reexperience the affects and other drive derivatives in their original intensity. Now, however, he is unaware of what is producing the anxiety and he attempts a "resolution" via a neurotic symptom.

We shall again use our patient to illustrate some of these rather complex concepts. Psychotherapy revealed that the psychogenesis of his neurosis lay in his early, highly conflicted relationship with his parents. From a very early time, he had great difficulty with the feelings of rage engendered by his father's brutality; he felt guilty and feared losing control of them, as his father frequently did. He used repression, reaction formation, and identification to control his anger. He also generalized his fear of his own aggression to a rather blanket inhibition of assertiveness and competitiveness—in academic achievement, sports, work, and relationships with women.

Another important genetic influence was his mother's seductiveness. The erotic feelings she engendered became particularly problematic during the oedipal phase of his development. During this period (ages 3–6), libido normally attaches to the parent of the opposite sex; the same-sexed parent is the object of rivalrous aggressive feelings. This "romance" has momentous significance to the young child, and the feelings are very intense. The little boy in this situation projects his anger on his father. He is certain that his father is also caught up in this rivalry, is enraged, and will retaliate. To avoid the retaliation—which is frequently imagined in a very concrete, primary process fashion as castration—the little boy relinquishes his incestuous strivings, represses his aggressive impulses toward the father, and identifies with him instead. The unconscious reasoning seems to be, "If I can't beat him, I'll join him—and get mine later." The identification with the father, or with the mother, in the case of the little girl, is the basis for the formation of the superego, which Freud called "the heir of the oedipus complex." Incomplete resolution of the oedipus complex is a very common component in the psychogenesis of neuroses.

His parents' characteristics thwarted our patient's satisfactory resolution of the oedipus complex. Their behavior seemed to reinforce the validity of his oedipal fantasies and fears. His mother's seductiveness signified the possible fulfillment of his incestuous wishes—thereby putting him in a position which was both exciting and terrifying. The father's brutality lent credence to his fear of castration. On the other hand, the father's sober periods of remorse and passive depression seemed to represent his abrogation in the rivalry for the mother. Hence, his environmental situation put him in an insoluble dilemma, making a satisfactory resolution of his oedipal conflict impossible. Instead of resolution there was massive repression.

We can now better understand the primary process "logic" underlying both his personality problems and his neurotic symptom. To the primary process, *any* success was equivalent to "success" with mother. Any achievement which involved assertiveness or competitiveness—in school, work, play, or relationships with women—unconsciously represented the unforgivable fulfillment of his oedipal fantasies of destroying his father and possessing his mother. (This particular constellation is so common, that Freud labeled it "success" or "fate neurosis.") He also made other important primary process equations: Women to whom I am attracted = mother; men with whom I am angry = father.

The latter equation precipitated his conversion reaction. The Drill Instructor became the object of the murderous rage, which was unconsciously directed toward the father because of his brutality. During the oedipal period, the rage was accentuated and took on an additional unconscious meaning; it required further repression because gratification of the aggressive drive also meant gratification of the libidinal wish about mother. The unconscious formula, "men with whom I am angry = father," was abetted because in the primary process the D.I. shared some of the father's characteristics. The logic of the primary process did not discriminate between the D.I.'s severe authoritarianism and the father's brutality. (After the D.I. visited him in the hospital, the patient realized that he could not deal with the anger toward him because it stirred up unacceptable, murderous impulses toward his father. The D.I. seemed warm, sympathetic, and genuinely interested in the patient's welfare. The patient then became depressed and guilty about his anger toward him.)

The connection between aggression and sexuality in the oedipal conflict makes it easier to see that the conversion paralysis also contained elements of a defense against a sexual or libidinal wish. This conflict was revived in our patient not only by his aggression toward the D.I., but also by the atmosphere of sexual freedom in which he found himself. His confusion between sexual feelings toward women in general and forbidden sexual feelings toward his mother were acutely intensified. For the first time in his life, he developed distressing guilt feelings about masturbation; they previously had been handled by the defense mechanism of isolation, in which the ego isolates from consciousness troublesome affects associated with a drive and its derivatives. He felt guilty because the connection between his masturbatory fantasies and his sexual wishes toward his mother threatened to escape repression and break into consciousness. Thus, the conversion paralysis was not only a defense against aggression, but also against sexuality, i.e., it protected him from masturbation and its attendant forbidden sexual feelings about mother. This illustrates another fact about neurotic symptoms: they are generally *over-determined*. A neurotic symptom may represent a defense against one or *both* instinctual drives; its genetic determinants may derive from a number of developmental conflicts. This is further illustrated by the interesting fact that our parents had accidentally sustained a fractured right humerus when he was seven years old. His convalescence represented a respite from the intense oedipal conflict of the period. There was a reprieve from the turmoil with his father; his mother supplied some of the previously lacking maternal affection. When the oedipal conflict was revived in a contemporary setting, he arrived at a similar solution—a functionless right arm —this time on a psychological rather than a physical basis. The unconscious memory of his broken arm's psychological utility may have helped determine his "choice" of symptoms.

TREATMENT OF THE NEUROSES

Treatment considerations must take into account the distinction between neurotic personality and neurotic symptoms. In general, it is easier to remove symptoms than to alter personality. Some short-term treatments which ignore unconscious mechanisms and concentrate on symptom removal, e.g., hypnosis for conversion reactions or behavior therapy for phobias—may be quite effective in some cases; they of course do not change the underlying personality structure in which the symptom developed. Also, occasionally the simple removal of one symptom may be followed by the development of another, sometimes more serious, symptom. This sometimes occurs upon the abrupt removal of conversion symptoms, which often yield easily to techniques which utilize suggestion. For example, our patient's symptom represented the ego's last-ditch effort to handle a conflict which had overwhelmed its usual defenses. Had the symptom been quickly removed by hypnosis, without any resolution of the underlying conflict, it probably would have been replaced by another symptom, especially upon his return to the precipitating environmental stresses. On the other hand, a general denigration of all symptomatic treatments of the neuroses is by no means justified. Relief from distressing symptomatology may sometimes permit the ego to restructure its defenses and restore psychic equilibrium. For reasons which are not well understood, significant and lasting improvement in personality structure may result from brief supportive psychotherapy. These cases probably represent resolution of important intrapsychic conflicts just below the patient's (and his psychiatrist's) level of consciousness.

The symptomatic therapies, including supportive psychotherapy, sometimes utilize the minor tranquilizers (e.g., benzodiazepines) as adjunctive antianxiety agents. Although mildly ameliorative in the treatment of brief reactive anxiety states, these drugs are much overrated and overused by non-psychiatric physicians (See Chapter 33, Psychopharmacology). Electroconvulsive treatment (ECT) is not useful in the treatment of neuroses, including depressive neurosis.

Intensive psychoanalytically-oriented psychotherapy (including psychoanalysis) is the optimal treatment when the goal is to restructure the neurotic personality, as well as give symptomatic relief. This treatment attempts to provide the patient with intellectual and emotional insight into the unconscious conflicts underlying neurotic symptoms and personality patterns, and elucidate their infantile genetic determinants. Free association, dream interpretation, and the analysis of the transference are the major tools of intensive "uncovering" therapies. These techniques all try to make unconscious, primary process material accessible to the conscious, problem-solving ego. The use of the transference is most important and distinguishes these therapies from the "supportive" forms of psychotherapy. Transference is the process whereby the therapist becomes the object of unconscious feelings, fantasies, and behavior from the patient's infantile past. There is nothing mysteriously Freudian about transference. As has been pointed out, the neurotic personality frequently regards important people in his life as though they represented people from unresolved childhood conflicts. When the psychiatrist becomes such a figure, he has an emotionally compelling *in vivo* context in which to make the patient aware of this repetitious pattern.

Analytic forms of therapy require major commitments of time, money, and motivation on the part of the patient. They also demand intelligence and a certain "psychological-mindedness" which allows for detached introspection (See Chapter 32, Therapies, for additional discussion of psychotherapy in the neuroses).

REFERENCES

1. Freud S: Three essays on the theory of sexuality, in *The Complete Psychological Works of Sigmund Freud,* st'd ed. London, Hogarth Press, 1953, vol 7, pp 125-245.
2. Erickson E: *Identity and the Life Cycle.* New York, WW Norton, 1980.
3. American Psychiatric Association Committee on Nomenclature and Statistics: *Diagnostic and Statistical Manual of Mental Disorders,* ed 3. Washington, DC, American Psychiatric Association, 1980.
4. Vaillant GE: *Adaptation to Life.* Boston, Little Brown & Co, 1977.
5. Horney K: *The Neurotic Personality of Our Time.* New York, WW Norton, 1937.
6. Freud S: Sexuality in the etiology of the neuroses, in *The Complete Psychological Works of Sigmund Freud,* st'd ed. London, Hogarth Press, 1962, vol 3, pp 261-285.
7. Freud S: The ego and the id, in *The Complete Psychological Works of Sigmund Freud,* st'd ed. London, Hogarth Press, 1961, vol 19, pp 3-66.

8. Freud S: Formulation on the two principles of mental functioning, in *The Complete Psychological Works of Sigmund Freud*, st'd ed. London, Hogarth Press, 1958, vol 12, pp 215–226.
9. Freud A: *The Ego and the Mechanisms of Defense*. New York, International Universities Press, 1946.
10. Freud S: Inhibition, symptoms, and anxiety, in *The Complete Psychological Works of Sigmund Freud,* st'd ed. London, Hogarth Press, 1959, vol 20, pp 77–175.

GENERAL REFERENCES

Brenner C: *An Elementary Textbook of Psychoanalysis*. New York, International Universities Press, 1973.
Ellenberger H: *The Discovery of the Unconscious*. New York, Basic Books, 1970.
Fenichel O: *The Psychoanalytic Theory of Neurosis*. New York, WW Norton, 1945.
Freud A: *The Ego and the Mechanisms of Defense*. New York, International Universities Press, 1946.
Freud S: Introductory lectures on psychoanalysis, in *The Complete Psychological Works of Sigmund Freud,* st'd ed. London, Hogarth Press, 1963, vols 15 and 16.
Horney K: *The Neurotic Personality of Our Time*. New York, WW Norton, 1937.

Chapter 17

PERSONALITY (CHARACTER) DISORDERS
RUTH S. MARTIN, M.D. and HOWARD S. SUDAK, M.D.

DEFINITION OF "CHARACTER" AND "CHARACTER DISORDER"

Every individual has a fundamental state of equilibrium, which consists of unique patterns of thought, feeling, and behavior. This equilibrium is the product of the ego's balance with the various forces impinging upon it. These forces originate in other agencies of the mind (e.g., drive forces in the id, judgmental pressures in the superego) and the external world. The ego functions which habitually equilibrate these forces are fundamental, because they establish and maintain the integrity of the individual's personality organization, i.e., they are an individual's character traits. The summation or synthesis of these traits forms the individual's unique character. Therefore, "character" can be defined as the typical, habitual mode of the ego's reaction toward the id, the superego, and the external world. ("Personality" is considered as synonymous with "character.") (1)

A character disorder (personality disorder) represents a pathological equilibrium. In this respect, it differs from other types of mental disorders (e.g., anxiety, schizophrenic, adjustment disorders), which result from a breakdown in the usual state of equilibrium. A character disorder does not involve a breakdown in the ordinary balance of forces in the mental organization. There is no condition of disequilibrium between the ego and the internal forces (id, superego) and external forces impinging upon it. There is no conflict—the psychological manifestation of a disequilibrium within the mind. Instead, the psychopathology lies in the composition of the ordinary equilibrium. Consequently, the usual baseline of thought, feeling, and behavior of an individual with a character disorder falls outside society's arbitrarily established normal range (1).

Certain features typify both normal and pathological character traits:
1. The rudiments of character traits are established during the first few years of life. They are forged by the ego's efforts to mediate the conflicts between

193

inner biological drive forces and environmental demands. They are a result of the resolution of infantile developmental conflicts. 2. Every individual's character is his own unique possession. 3. A corollary to the long-lived, unique nature of character traits is that they generally become increasingly fixed throughout life. 4. Character traits are generally ego-syntonic, in contrast to symptoms, which are ego-dystonic. That which is familiar, acceptable, and comfortable to the individual is ego-syntonic. That which is foreign, unacceptable, and painful to the individual is ego-dystonic. Ego-syntonic traits are essential components of the psychic equilibrium which they establish and maintain (1).

FORMATION OF CHARACTER

The etiology of character formation can be broken down into genetic predisposition and psychodynamic theories. Although this chapter will concentrate on the latter, studies of alcoholism and certain antisocial character disorders have indicated that genetics may play an important role (2). Monozygotic twins show a higher rate of concordance for criminality (over 50% in males in one study) than do dizygotic twins (22% in males) or other siblings (3). Also, the children of criminal or sociopathic parents show a relatively high incidence of the trait, even those raised from infancy by "normal" (nonsociopathic) adoptive parents (3). Other investigators found that the incidence of criminality in male adoptees was about 10% when neither the biologic nor the adoptive parents had criminal records. This is considerably greater than the incidence for non-adopted individuals, but is consistent with other findings on psychopathology in adopted children. If an adoptive parent, but neither biologic parent, was criminal, the incidence was only slightly greater (11%). If a biologic parent, but neither adopted parent, was criminal, the incidence increased to 21%. If both a biologic and an adoptive parent were criminal, the incidence rose to approximately 36% (3). Bohman et al. concluded that different genetic and environmental antecedents influenced the development of criminality, depending upon associated alcohol abuse. Alcoholic criminals often committed repetitive violent offenses; nonalcoholic criminals committed small numbers of petty property offenses. Nonalcoholic petty criminals tended to have biologic parents with histories of petty crimes, but not alcohol abuse. In contrast, the risk of criminality in alcohol abusers was correlated with the severity of their own alcohol abuse —but not with criminality in the biologic or adoptive parents (4).

Psychodynamic theories of character generally attribute character to the balance of drives versus ego, superego, and the external world. The ego's task in character formation is to mediate between internal (intrapsychic) and external (extrapsychic) forces—specifically, between the id and the environment. A later internal component requiring equilibration is the superego—the representative of the environment, internalized within the mind as a separate mental agency; the ego does, however, apply autonomous, innate functions to this task. As the ego works to establish equilibrium by resolving conflict states, it organizes and strengthens its own functioning. The conflict states which are thought to have the greatest impact upon character formation are those in infancy. Examples of infantile conflict states include: 1. a hungry infant who is not fed due to mother's unavailability; 2. a toddler who fears losing mother's love in the struggle over bowel control; 3. a pre-schooler who has an urge to masturbate and this conflicts with the anxiety associated with forbidden fantasies and parental disapproval. The undeveloped personality has no pre-tested methods of resolving such conflicts. Thus, the infantile ego invests a great deal of energy in the development of mediating methods which will appease both drive and environment. Through repeated trial and error, the ego establishes a characteristic set of functions which can be used to maintain equilibrium in the face of recurring conflicts.

Poor ego resolutions can result in self-defeating personality traits. For example, excessive or deficient nursing experiences can cause later oral problems (e.g., obesity, addictions, depression). Badly-timed toilet training can result in later anal problems (e.g., stubborness, withholding). However, character per se is neither "good" nor "bad." Character traits are necessary for psychic economy and efficiency. Without them, we would have to react anew to every situation, rather than responding in a standard, individualized manner. A person's character is a blend of genital and pre-genital aspects. A person without any obsessive/compulsive character traits would be unable to complete any task which became boring. An individual without any hysterical character traits might have a rather colorless or bland affect. Love-making is greatly enhanced by behavior derived from pre-genital sexuality, e.g., looking; being looked at; tasting; smelling. Pre-genital traits are only considered pathological if they are *disproportionate* to the total character.

CHARACTER DEVELOPMENT
FROM THE STANDPOINT OF THE SUPEREGO

Brenner (5) describes several components of psychic conflict: 1. drive derivatives or instinctual wishes from childhood; 2. unpleasurable affects associated or aroused by these wishes; 3. defensive or ego functions used to avoid, eliminate, or mitigate anxiety or depressive affect; 4. aspects of superego functioning, usually having to do with demands and prohibitions. Brenner believes that conflict causes compromise formation among its several components. He states that such a compromise formation may be a normal character trait, a pathological character trait, a neurotic symptom, or a neurotic character trait. Brenner also describes the superego as not just a component, but a consequence of conflict, i.e., a compromise formation. He believes oedipal conflicts play the largest role in superego formation; and, that most of these compromises concern morality. Brenner states:

> With the exception of mental defectives—idiots and imbeciles—everyone has a superego. Everyone must deal with his or her oedipal drive derivatives somehow, which is to say that the conflicts over oedipal drive derivatives must lead to compromise formations, some of which have to do with morality. Whether an adult be a criminal or an ascetic, whether he be acclaimed and admired or treated as a social outcast, whether he be a liar or truth-teller, saint or sinner, he cannot be without a superego. It is of very great importance to both an individual and to those about him, i.e., society, just what compromise formations make up his superego and one can justifiably classify each person's superego as normal or pathological on the same basis as one judges the normality or pathology of any compromise formation. If a person's superego functions in such a way as to create too much unpleasure and permit too little pleasure, if self-injurious and self-destructive tendencies are too strong, and/or if superego function leads to too much conflict with the environment, it is justifiable and appropriate to call that person's superego pathological" (5).

In contrast to Brenner's beliefs, superego pathology is more typically described and explained in terms of *defects* in the superego or "superego lacunae," e.g., a sneak, a con artist, or psychopath with a "tiny superego" but a normal ego and id. The person's reality testing is intact. However, the ego overemphasizes the pleasure, rather than the reality principle, and fails to profit from experience. Such individuals have difficulty postponing their gratifications, and easily substitute one goal for another. Since impairment of activity and motility, their primary defenses, may cause considerable anxiety, such patients often act up in jails or hospitals. Thus, their egos are not truly "normal." The superego of the psychopath can be considered inconsistent. In the pre-operational state, the pre-conscience conditions the individual to expect punishment under certain conditions. An adult, however, is expected to have an internalized conscience, which makes self-love conditional on certain behavior. Thus, there is no real superego until guilt is felt in the *absence* of anticipated external punishment.

Superego formation can also be examined from the point of view of the child, who acquires his family's covert, tacit, and explicit ideals and values. The Johnson-Szurek hypothesis explains the way a child learns to act out the unconscious wishes (or the unconscious superego lacunae) of his parents (6). For example, the parents of a teenage boy are very upset because he has a poor driving record, has lost his license, and is being thrown out of college for rowdy behavior. The parents appear civic-minded and responsible, until it is revealed that the father has just bought a new Porsche, boasts about going around corners at 50 miles per hour, and brags about cheating on his income tax. Clearly, the underlying message is that the only way to become a man is to break the rules. A second example is that of a teenage girl whose mother grills her about how far she went on her dates and appears to derive vicarious pleasure from such details. Every month she asks the girl if she got her period, and indicates that she expects her to become pregnant. In both of these examples, both child and parent are unconscious of wishes transmitted and received. Such messages are affectively super-charged via their covertness; consequently, they are very potent. Although we all learn to read between the lines to some degree, we are generally not aware of either transmitting or receiving such messages.

DIAGNOSIS AND DIFFERENTIAL DIAGNOSIS

According to DSM-III, all personality disorders are coded on Axis II. Personality traits are enduring patterns of perceiving, relating to, and thinking about the environment and oneself; they are exhibited in a wide range of important social and personal contexts. According to DSM-III, personality disorders are the result of personality traits which are inflexible and maladaptive, thus causing either significant impairment in social or occupational functioning or subjective distress. This diagnosis should only be made when the characteristic features are typical of the individual's long-term functioning, i.e., not limited to discrete episodes of illness. Besides being ego-syntonic, it is important to remember that personality disorders maintain the individual's mental equilibrium. All of the Axis I diagnoses (i.e., anxiety disorders or neurosis, affective disorders, schizophrenia, organic brain syndromes) arise from a breakdown in mental equilibrium.

Vaillant describes mental equilibrium in terms of a theoretical hierarchy of defense mechanisms (7). Immature defenses, which are most characteristic of personality disorders, include the following:

1. *Projection:* Attributing one's own unacknowledged feelings to others;
2. *Schizoid fantasy:* The autistic use of fantasy for comfort, control, and conflict resolution;
3. *Hypochondriasis:* The transformation of difficulties with others into exaggerated somatic complaints;
4. *Turning against the self* (passive aggression or sadomasochism): Anger towards others expressed indirectly and ineffectively via passivity, masochism, or sadism;
5. *Acting out:* Direct nonspecific expression of an unconscious wish or impulse to avoid being conscious of the impulse or its associated affect.

These immature defenses must be distinguished from both psychotic and mature defense mechanisms. The defense mechanisms characteristic of psychotic breakdown include delusional projection, psychotic denial, and distortion. These all relate to a loss of reality testing and are considered even less healthy than immature defenses. Vaillant describes the following neurotic defense mechanisms:

1. *Dissociation:* Temporary but drastic modification of one's sense of personal identity in order to avoid emotional distress;
2. *Isolation* (intellectualization, undoing): The thought is conscious but the associated affect is unconscious;
3. *Repression:* The affect is often conscious but the thought is unconscious;
4. *Displacement:* A redirection of conscious feelings and ideation toward a less cathected object;
5. *Reaction formation:* Ideation and affect are conscious, but opposite to an unacceptable, unconscious impulse.

Needless to say, the mature defenses are considered the most healthy, and are rarely seen in personality disorders. Vaillant's list of mature defenses includes altruism, humor, suppression, anticipation, and sublimation.

TABLE I
DIFFERENTIAL DIAGNOSIS BETWEEN NEUROSES
AND PERSONALITY DISORDERS

	Neuroses	*Character Disorders*
1. Locus of the conflict	Internal (Pt. suffers)	External (society suffers)
2. How the ego views the conflict	Alien, dystonic, autoplastic	Syntonic, alloplastic
3. Manifested by	Symptoms	Behavior
4. Duration of the conflict	Acute to Chronic	"Life-long" (that is, once past the stage in which the superego ought to have been formed)
5. Response to Psychotherapy	Excellent to poor	None (unless the ego-syntonic character disorder has become an ego-dystonic character neurosis)

TYPES OF PERSONALITY DISORDERS
AS DESCRIBED IN DSM-III (8)

(Note: In *all* of these disorders, the diagnostic criteria are characteristic of the individual's current and long-term functioning. They are not limited to episodes of illness, and cause either significant impairment in social or occupational functioning or subjective distress.)

Paranoid Personality Disorder (8)

Characteristically, patients with paranoid personality disorders are suspicious, mistrustful of people, and hypersensitive. There are many life situations in which an attitude of suspicion and distrust is appropriate. In a person with a paranoid personality disorder, however, such suspicion and hypervigilance is pervasive. There is a tremendous concern over hidden motives and special meanings. There can also be transient ideas of reference (i.e., people paying special attention to them or saying bad things about them), as well as pathological jealousy. People with paranoid personality disorders are difficult to get along with, and are often viewed by others as guarded, secretive, scheming, and litigious. Such people usually appear "cold" and "aloof," and are often quite proud of their "objectivity" and "lack of emotional involvement." They are also known to be hostile, stubborn, and unwilling to compromise. Occupational difficulties are common among these people, probably because they have difficulty relating to authority figures and co-workers. This disorder is most commonly diagnosed in men.

Diagnostic Criteria for Paranoid Personality Disorder

A. Pervasive, unwarranted suspiciousness and mistrust of people as indicated by at least three of the following:
   1. Expectation of trickery or harm
   2. Hypervigilance, manifested by continual scanning of the environment for signs of threat, or taking unneeded precautions
   3. Guardedness or secretiveness
   4. Avoidance of accepting blame when warranted
   5. Questioning the loyalty of others
   6. Intense, narrowly focused searching for confirmation of bias, with loss of appreciation of total context
   7. Overconcern with hidden motives and special meanings
   8. Pathological jealousy
B. Hypersensitivity as indicated by at least two of the following:
   1. Tendency to be easily slighted and quick to take offense

2. Exaggeration of difficulties, e.g., "making mountains out of molehills"
3. Readiness to counterattack when any threat is perceived
4. Inability to relax
C. Restricted affectivity as indicated by at least two of the following:
   1. Appearance of being "cold" and unemotional
   2. Pride taken in always being objective, rational, and unemotional
   3. Lack of a true sense of humor
   4. Absence of passive, soft, tender, and sentimental feelings
D. Not due to another mental disorder such as schizophrenia or a paranoid disorder.

Schizoid Personality Disorder (8)

Individuals with diagnosed schizoid personality disorders are most often described as "loners." Because these people seem genuinely incapable of forming social relationships, they have few close friends. They are usually considered withdrawn, seclusive, aloof, and indifferent to the feelings of others. In situations which usually evoke emotional responses, such persons would appear without affect. In addition to being rather vague, indecisive, and self-absorbed, such individuals seem to daydream excessively.

Diagnostic Criteria for Schizoid Personality Disorder:

A. Emotional coldness and aloofness, and absence of warm, tender feelings for others.
B. Indifference to praise or criticism or to the feelings of others.
C. Close friendships with no more than one or two persons, including family members.
D. No eccentricities of speech, behavior, or thought characteristic of schizotypal personality disorder.
E. Not due to a psychotic disorder such as schizophrenic or paranoid disorder.
F. If under 18, does not meet the criteria for schizoid disorder of childhood or adolescence.

Schizotypal Personality Disorder (8)

Various oddities of thought, perception, speech, and behavior are the essential features of this diagnostic category. It should be noted that the peculiarities are not severe enough to meet the criteria of schizophrenia, i.e., there is no evidence of looseness of association. These people might describe episodes of magical thinking, bizarre fantasies, recurrent illusions, or derealization. As defined in the DSM-III, no single feature is invariably present. There is also some evidence that chronic schizophrenia is more common among family members of individuals with schizotypal personality disorder than it is among those of the general population.

Diagnostic Criteria for Schizotypal Personality Disorder

A. At least four of the following:

1. Magical thinking, e.g., superstitiousness, clairvoyance, telepathy, "6th sense," "others can feel my feelings" (in children and adolescents, bizarre fantasies or preoccupation)
2. Ideas of reference
3. Social-isolation, e.g., no close friends or confidants, social contacts limited to essential everyday tasks
4. Recurrent illusions, sensing the presence of a force or person not actually present (e.g., "I felt as if my dead mother were in the room with me"), depersonalization, or derealization not associated with panic attacks
5. Odd speech (without loosening of associations or incoherence), e.g., speech that is digressive, vague, overelaborate, circumstantial, metaphorical
6. Inadequate rapport in face-to-face interaction due to constructed or inappropriate affect, e.g., aloof, cold
7. Suspiciousness or paranoid ideation
8. Undue social anxiety or hypersensitivity to real or imagined criticism

B. Does not meet the criteria for schizophrenia.

Histrionic Personality Disorder ("Emotionally Unstable Personality;" "Hysterical Personality") (8)

Individuals with this disorder are overly dramatic and love to draw attention to themselves. They often exaggerate and act out the role of a "victim" or "princess." Small provocations will evoke emotional outbursts, i.e., "temper tantrums." Characteristically, individuals with histrionic personality disorders are easily bored with daily routines and crave excitement. Their interpersonal relationships are impaired. Because they appear superficially appealing and likeable, they may form friendships quickly; once the friendship is established, however, they are more likely to be viewed as demanding, self-centered, and inconsiderate. When disappointed, these individuals are prone to manipulative suicidal threats and gestures, or other similar behaviors. Constant reassurance is sometimes needed to counteract these individuals' basic feelings of helplessness and dependency. This diagnosis occurs more frequently in females, who are typically attractive and seductive. As per the DSM-III, individuals with this disorder often experience periods of intense dissatisfaction and a variety of dysphoric moods. They are also felt to be easily influenced by others and impressionable. Frequent somatic complaints and feelings of depersonalization are common.

Diagnostic Criteria for Histrionic Personality Disorder

A. Behavior that is overly dramatic, reactive, and intensely expressed, as indicated by at least three of the following:
  1. Self-dramatization, e.g., exaggerated expression of emotions
  2. Incessant drawing of attention to oneself
  3. Craving for activity and excitement
  4. Overraction to minor events
  5. Irrational, angry outbursts or tantrums
B. Characteristic disturbances in interpersonal as indicated by at least two of the following:
  1. Perceived by others as shallow and lacking genuineness, even if superficially warm and charming
  2. Egocentric, self-indulgent, and inconsiderate of others
  3. Vain and demanding
  4. Dependent, helpless, constantly seeking reassurance
  5. Prone to manipulative suicidal threats, gestures, or attempts

Narcissistic Personality Disorder (8)

Extreme self-centeredness and self-absorption are characteristic of an individual with a narcissistic personality disorder. These traits may be accompanied by a grandiose sense of self-importance and a preoccupation with fantasies of overwhelming success—to the extent that actual ability and achievement are drastically overestimated. Such individuals are tremendously concerned with outward appearances, and may need constant attention and admiration. As described in DSM-III, this disorder stems from fragile self-esteem that responds to criticism or disappointment with feelings of "narcissistic" rage and emptiness. Obviously, such individuals have disturbed interpersonal relationships. In addition to their lack of empathy and sensitivity, they exhibit interpersonal exploitation. They are similar to those with borderline personality disorders in that close relationships tend to alternate between love and hate, with little else in between, i.e., splitting. This personality disorder is often accompanied by a depressed mood. During episodes of profound stress, transient psychotic episodes are common.

Diagnostic Criteria for Narcissistic Personality Disorder

A. Grandiose sense of self-importance or uniqueness, e.g., exaggeration of achievements and talents, focus on the special nature of one's problems.
B. Preoccupation with fantasies of unlimited success, power, brilliance, beauty, or ideal love.
C. Exhibitionism: the person requires constant attention and admiration.

D. Cool indifference or marked feelings of rage, inferiority, shame, humiliation, or emptiness in response to criticism, indifference of others, or defeat.

E. At least two of the following characteristics of disturbances in interpersonal relationships:

1. Entitlement: expectation of special favors without assuming reciprocal responsibilities, e.g., surprise and anger that people will not do what is wanted

2. Interpersonal exploitativeness: taking advantage of others to indulge own desires or for self-aggrandizement; disregard for the personal integrity and rights of others

3. Relationships that characteristically alternate between the extremes of overidealized devaluation

4. Lack of empathy: inability to recognize how others feel, e.g., unable to appreciate the distress of someone who is seriously ill.

Antisocial Personality Disorder ("Dyssocial Personality," Psychopathic Personality," "Character Defect," "Sociopathic Personality") (8)

Lying, stealing, fighting, truancy, and resisting authority are typical early childhood behaviors (before age 15) of adults with antisocial personality disorders. Such an individual's adolescent history might include early sexual behavior, excessive drinking, and use of illegal drugs. These behaviors continue in adulthood to the extent that the rights of others are usually violated. Work histories are very poor, and family lives are chaotic. This diagnosis is much more common in males; there is a 3% prevalence for American men, as opposed to less than 1% for American women. This disorder is usually extremely incapacitating because these individuals do not become independent, self-supporting, functioning adults; in fact, many spend most of their lives in institutions—mainly jails.

Diagnostic Criteria for Antisocial Personality Disorders

A. Current age at least 18.

B. Onset before age 15 as indicated by a history of three or more of the following before that age:

1. Truancy (positive if it amounted to at least five days per year for at least two years, not including the last year of school)

2. Expulsion or suspension from school for misbehavior

3. Delinquency (arrested or referred to juvenile court because of behavior

4. Running away from home overnight at least twice while living in parental or parental surrogate home

5. Persistent lying
6. Repeated sexual intercourse in a casual relationship
7. Repeated drunkenness or substance abuse
8. Thefts
9. Vandalism
10. School grades markedly below expectations in relation to estimated or known IQ (may have resulted in repeating a year)
11. Chronic violations of rules at home and/or at school (other than truancy)
12. Initiation of fights

C. At least four of the following manifestations of the disorder since age 18:

1. Inability to sustain consistent work behavior, as indicated by any of the following: a) too frequent job changes (e.g., three or more jobs in five years not accounted for by nature of job or economic or seasonal fluctuation), b) significant unemployment (e.g., six months or more in five years when expected to work), c) serious absenteeism from work (e.g., average three days or more of lateness or absence per month), d) walking off several jobs without other jobs in sight (Note: similar behavior in an academic setting during the last few years of school may substitute for this criterion in individuals who by reason of their age or circumstance have not had an opportunity to demonstrate occupational adjustment.)

2. Lack of ability to function as a responsible parent as evidenced by one or more of the following: a) child's malnutrition, b) child's illness resulting from lack of minimal hygiene standards, c) failure to obtain medical care for a seriously ill child, d) child's dependence on neighbors or nonresident relatives for food or shelter, e) failure to arrange for a caretaker for a child under six when parent is away from home, f) repeated squandering, on personal items, of money required for household necessities

3. Failure to accept social norms with respect to lawful behavior, as indicated by any of the following: repeated thefts, illegal occupation (pimping, prostitution, fencing, selling drugs), multiple arrests, a felony conviction

4. Inability to maintain enduring attachment to a sexual partner as indicated by two or more divorces and/or separations (whether legally married or not), desertion of spouse, promiscuity (ten or more sexual partners within one year)

5. Irritability and aggressiveness as indicated by repeated physical fights or assault (not required by one's job or to defend someone or oneself), including spouse or child beating

6. Failure to honor financial obligations, as indicated by repeated defaulting on debts, failure to provide child support, failure to support other dependents on a regular basis

7. Failure to plan ahead, or impulsivity, as indicated by traveling from place to place without a prearranged job or clear goal for the period of travel or clear idea about when the travel would terminate, or lack of a fixed address for a month or more

8. Disregard for the truth as indicated by repeated lying, use of aliases, "conning" others for personal profit

9. Recklessness, as indicated by driving while intoxicated or recurrent speeding.

D. A pattern of continuous antisocial behavior in which the rights of others are violated, with no intervening period of at least five years without antisocial behavior between age 15 and the present time (except when the individual was bedridden or confined in a hospital or penal institution).

E. Antisocial behavior is not due to either severe mental retardation, schizophrenia or manic episodes.

Borderline Personality Disorder (8)

This personality disorder is characterized by instability in several areas—interpersonal relations, mood, and self-image. No single feature is always present. It is believed that the borderline patient uses three primitive defense mechanisms to maintain equilibrium, i.e., splitting, projective identification, and identity diffusion. Splitting is the rigid polarization of positive and negative thoughts and feelings. For example, most people can experience two contradictory feeling states at one time; this is not possible for the borderline patient. It is very difficult for these patients to be angry with someone they love; one is either all "good" or all "bad." Projective identification is the induction in another individual of disavowed aspects of oneself, e.g., cruelty or envy. Splitting and projective identification often complement each other and foster a "split" view of the world. Identity diffusion involves uncertainty about personal image, e.g., gender identity, goals, values, loyalties, and even a transient confusion in the fundamental sense of self. The cause of the borderline personality disorder is unknown, although environment and heredity are important. Some psychiatrists feel that borderline personality is a subset of biologic depressive illness; others relate this disorder to schizophrenia. Psychoanalysts focus on the early mother-child relationship and the failure of these borderline patients to develop a coherent, stable sense of self. Classically, the defect is thought to be in the area of separation-individuation; the borderline's adult relationships are often termed "transitional," with reference to the "transitional object" of early childhood.

Certain behaviors during treatment also suggest a borderline diagnosis. When hospitalized, these patients tend to split the staff into "good" and "bad" factions, almost as if they are acting out the borderline patient's internal world. In unstructured situations (even treatment settings), short episodes of transient psychotic thinking are not uncommon. It is believed that the institution of firm, non-punitive confrontation and structuring results in the transient reintegration of the borderline patient's personality.

Diagnostic Criteria for Borderline Personality Disorder
  A. At least five of the following are required:
   1. Impulsivity or unpredictability in at least two areas that are potentially self-damaging, e.g., spending, sex, gambling, abuse, shoplifting, overeating, physically self-damaging acts
   2. A pattern of unstable and intense interpersonal relationships, e.g., marked shifts of attitude, idealization, devaluation, manipulation (consistently using others for one's own ends)
   3. Inappropriate, intense anger or lack of control of anger, e.g., frequent displays of temper, constant anger
   4. Identity disturbances manifested by uncertainty about several issues relating to identity, such as self-image, gender identity, long-term goals or career choice, friendship patterns, values, and loyalties, e.g., "Who am I?", "I feel like I am my sister when I am good."
   5. Affective instability: marked shifts from normal mood to depression, irritability, or anxiety, usually lasting a few hours and only rarely more than a few days, with a return to normal mood
   6. Intolerance of being alone, e.g., frantic effort to avoid being alone, depressed when alone
   7. Physically self-damaging acts, e.g., suicidal gestures, self-mutilation, recurrent accidents or physical fights
   8. Chronic feelings of emptiness or boredom

  B. If under 18, does not meet the criteria for identity disorder.

Avoidant Personality Disorder (8)
Patients with the diagnosis of avoidant personality disorder are overwhelmingly sensitive to rejection, humiliation, or shame. Most people care about the way in which they are viewed and/or assessed by others; those with the above diagnosis, however, are incredibly devastated by any sign of disapproval from others. As a result, close relationships are extremely limited unless these individuals feel they have unconditional approval. Occupational functioning can also be limited if interpersonal contact is required. An important distinction must be made between avoidant and schizoid per-

sonality disorders. The latter is also characterized by social isolation, but there is no desire for social involvement; rejection and disapproval are met with indifference.

Diagnostic Criteria for Avoidant Personality Disorder

A. Hypersensitivity to rejection, e.g., apprehensively alert to signs of social derogation, interprets innocuous events as ridicule.

B. Unwillingness to enter into relationships unless given unusually strong guarantees of uncritical acceptance.

C. Social withdrawal, e.g., distances self from close personal attachments, engages in peripheral social and vocational roles.

D. Desire for affection and acceptance.

E. Low self-esteem, e.g., devalues self-achievements and is overly dismayed by personal shortcomings.

F. If under 18, does not meet the criteria for avoidant disorder of childhood or adolescence.

Dependent Personality Disorder (8)

Patients with dependent personality disorders have great difficulty in assuming responsibility for their own lives. They passively allow others to take over major areas, and seem to be unable to function independently. Because these patients lack self-confidence, they are comfortable having others make major decisions. Individuals with this disorder are also reluctant to make demands on the people they depend upon; they are afraid of injuring the relationship and possibly having to become more self-reliant. As a result, these individuals subordinate their own needs to those of people they depend upon.

Diagnostic Criteria for Dependent Personality Disorder

A. Passively allows others to assume responsibility for major areas of life because of inability to function independently (e.g., lets spouse decide what kind of job he or she should have).

B. Subordinates own needs to those of persons on whom he or she depends in order to avoid any possibility of having to rely on self, e.g., tolerates abusive spouse.

C. Lacks self-confidence, e.g., sees self as helpless, stupid.

Compulsive Personality Disorder (8)

Individuals with this diagnosis are usually perfectionists, who are also "stingy" with their emotions and material possessions. Preoccupation with rules, details, and procedures interferes with their ability to see things as part of a broad overview. Poor allocation of time frequently causes these individuals to get bogged down in trivial details. Although efficiency and perfection are idealized, they are usually not attained. These individuals are also preoccupied with issues of control and submission. There is a general insistence that others submit to their way of doing things, although they themselves have an underlying resistance to authority. Work and productivity are valued, sometimes to the exclusion of pleasure, tenderness, and interpersonal relationships. Individuals with this diagnosis rarely give compliments or gifts; they are sometimes considered rather "stiff" or "formal." They also have difficulty taking vacations. Decision-making is difficult because they fear making a mistake, and have trouble sorting out priorities. This disorder is more frequently diagnosed in men; it must be distinguished from the Axis I diagnosis of obsessive compulsive disorder, in which true obsessions and compulsions are present.

Diagnostic Criteria for Compulsive Personality Disorder

At least four of the following are present:

1. Restricted ability to express warm and tender emotions, e.g., the individual is unduly conventional, serious and formal, and stingy
2. Perfectionism that interferes with the ability to grasp "the big picture," e.g., preoccupation with trivial details, rules, order, organization, schedules, and lists
3. Insistence that others submit to his or her way of doing things, and lack of awareness of the feelings elicited by this behavior, e.g., a husband stubbornly insists his wife complete errands for him regardless of her plans
4. Excessive devotion to work and productivity to the exclusion of pleasure and the value of interpersonal relationships
5. Indecisiveness: decision-making is either avoided, postponed, or protracted, perhaps because of an inordinate fear of making a mistake, e.g., the individual cannot get assignments done on time because of ruminating about priorities.

Passive-Aggressive Personality Disorder (8)

The name of this disorder reflects the assumption that these individuals are passively expressing a tremendous amount of underlying aggression. Individuals with this disorder habitually use certain maneuvers to oppose demands but they maintain a certain level of functioning. Such maneuvers, which are expressive of indirect resistance, can include procrastination, dawdling, stubbornness, intentional inefficiency, and forgetfulness. For example, an executive repeatedly gives his secretary work to complete that somehow rarely gets accomplished. The secretary misplaces the letters or files, forgets to take proper notes at meetings, etc. It is interesting that individuals with this diagnosis fail to realize that their behavior is responsible for their difficulties. Thus, the secretary described in the above example may lose his/her job and not understand why. Individuals with this diagnosis may also consciously resent authority figures; however, they rarely see the relationship between their passive-resistant behavior and their resentment.

Diagnostic Criteria for Passive-Aggressive Personality Disorder

A. Resistance to demands for adequate performance in both occupational and social functioning.
B. Resistance expressed indirectly through at least two of the following:
   1. Procrastination
   2. Dawdling
   3. Stubbornness
   4. Intentional inefficiency
C. As a consequence of A and B, pervasive and longstanding social and occupational ineffectiveness (including in roles of homemaker or student), e.g., intentional inefficiency that has prevented job promotion.
D. Persistence of the behavior pattern even under circumstances in which more self-assertive and effective behavior is possible.
E. Does not meet the criteria for any other personality disorder, and if under age 18, does not meet the criteria for oppositional disorder.

Atypical, Mixed, or Other Personality Disorder (8)

If an individual qualifies for any of the specific personality disorders, that category should be noted—even if some features from other categories are present. For example, an individual who fits the description of compulsive personality disorder should be given that diagnosis, even if some mild dependent or paranoid features are present.

When an individual qualifies for two or more personality disorders, multiple diagnoses should be made.

Atypical personality disorder should be used when the clinician recognizes the presence of a personality disorder, but lacks sufficient information to make a more specific designation.

Mixed personality disorder should be used when the individual has a personality disorder that involves features from several specific personality disorders, but does not meet all the criteria for any one diagnosis.

Other personality disorder should be used when the clinician judges that a specific personality disorder not included in this classification is appropriate, such as masochistic, impulsive, or immature personality disorder. In such instances, the clinician should record the specific other personality disorder.

TREATMENT OF PERSONALITY DISORDERS

For the most part, character disorders are refractory to any fundamental change through any known psychiatric or medical procedures. Partial exceptions to this statement may include psychoanalysis, intensive psychoanalytically-oriented psychotherapy, certain forms of group therapy, certain behavioral modification techniques, and some forms of pharmacotherapy. Psychoanalysis and intensive psychoanalytically-oriented psychotherapy are aimed at changing a "character disorder" into a "character neurosis." In other words, one is motivating the person to seek change by transforming the *ego-syntonic* behaviors into *ego-alien* behaviors. Sometimes such changes occur spontaneously during adolescent or adult development. When dealing with such individuals, one should always try to ascertain the cause of the change and the current desire for help. Also, in individual psychotherapy for character disorders, one also tries to focus on the side of the ego, rather than the superego. In other words, individual psychotherapy attempts to help these patients assume responsibility for their own actions. People with character disorders (especially the antisocial) have a great propensity toward externalizing blame and responsibility.

Many patients with personality disorders have no desire to change. Such patients require careful management and treatment which does not attempt any fundamental alteration of personality. Good management entails recognition and support of noted personality strengths. In other words, one needs to help the healthy part of the patient's personality function as well as possible.

Group psychotherapy can sometimes be helpful for certain types of personality disorders. Ego-syntonic disorders may sometimes respond to group or peer pressures, even when there is little or no motivation for change. Alcoholics, addicts, and delinquents might be helped by group psychotherapy. Further discussion of group therapy and behavioral techniques is included in Chapter 32.

Recent evidence indicates that some patients with personality disorders benefit from treatment with drugs. Compared with schizophrenia, affective disorders, and neuroses, however, there have been only a few controlled drug trials. Part of the difficulty lies in the diagnosis of particular personality disorders. The fact that the same type of behavior can be caused by diverse pathologies is another problem.

Hostility is a common symptom in patients with personality disorders, particularly the antisocial. At present, there is no conclusive evidence that minor tranquilizers (anti-anxiety agents) are effective in the treatment of hostility, aggression, sociopathic personalities, or other personality disorders. The effects of neuroleptics (anti-psychotic agents) on hostility, aggression, and impulsiveness in patients with personality disorders are also inconclusive. There are, however, published reports of several *uncontrolled* studies, in which the authors stated that neuroleptics exerted a beneficial effect on hostility, aggression, and impulsiveness. Despite the lack of conclusive evidence, many clinicians use neuroleptics in the treatment of personality disorders. A large number of favorable reports on the effects of Dilantin (DPH, diphenylhydantoin) in the treatment of aggression and hostility in delinquents and sociopathic personalities are also based on observations from uncontrolled studies. In controlled studies, DPH was shown to be no more effective than a placebo. Uncontrolled studies have suggested that stimulants can have beneficial effects upon aggressive and impulsive young delinquents. This idea was supported by a controlled study with methylphenidate (Ritalin), in which a group of patients with personality disorders did benefit from treatment; this group included patients diagnosed in childhood as having minimal brain dysfunction. Lithium has been used in several studies of patients with personality disorders, delinquents displaying violence and aggression, and patients with emotionally unstable character disorders. These studies show that maintenance treatment with lithium is a promising development in the treatment of personality disorders and delinquents whose main traits are explosiveness, impulsiveness, and a tendency to respond to small provocations with anger and aggression. Blood levels less than 0.6 meq/liters have been found to be ineffective (9).

There are many authors who advocate psychopharmacology for the treatment of the borderline personality disorder. However, few, if any, controlled, double-bind studies have been published. The following are some of the prevailing opinions about different classes of medications and the borderline patient. Minor tranquilizers are acceptable anti-anxiety agents—so "acceptable" that many borderline patients have become dependent upon them. Antipsychotic agents are useful during transient psychotic episodes with some borderline patients whose lives are extremely chaotic. Tardive dyskinesia is the major disadvantage to the long-term use of antipsychotics, even in low dosages. Tricyclic antidepressants are useful for some borderline patients who are depressed, especially those with anxiety and insomnia. It should be noted, however, that tricyclic antidepressants are quite toxic and must be prescribed with caution. Lithium carbonate is reportedly useful in borderlines with a prominent mood-cycling component to their symptom cluster and in some violence-prone patients. Lithium is also very toxic and risky to use in suicidal patients. Monamine oxidase-inhibitors (MAO) are currently prescribed for borderline patients with "atypical" depressions with phobic or avoidant components. MAO inhibitors require strict dietary restrictions and are very toxic with overdosage. It should be noted that most of the literature on borderline patients focuses on psychological and social treatments, especially psychoanalytically-oriented psychotherapy (10).

REFERENCES

1. McDonald M: Case Western Reserve University School of Medicine Psychiatry course syllabus, 1955.
2. Cadoret R: Psychopathology in adopted away offspring of biologic parents with anti-social behavior. *Arch Gen Psychiatry* 1978;35:176-184.
3. Cloninger R: The antisocial personality, in Guggenheim FG, Nadelson C (eds): *Major Psychiatric Disorders*. New York, Elsevier Biomedical, 1982, pp 169-178.
4. Bohman M, Cloninger R, Sigvardsson S, VonKnorring A: Predisposition to petty criminality in Swedish adoptees. *Arch Gen Psychiatry* 1982;39:1233-1253.
5. Brenner C: The concept of the superego: A reformulation. *Psychoanal Q* 1982;51:501-525.
6. Johnson A: Juvenile delinquency, in Arieti, S (ed): *American Handbook of Psychiatry*. New York, Basic Books, 1959, vol 1, pp 840-856.
7. Vaillant G: Theoretical hierarchy of adaptive ego mechanisms. *Arch Gen Psychiatry* 1971;24:107-118.
8. American Psychiatric Association Committee on Nomenclature and Statistics: *Diagnostic and Statistical Manual of Mental Disorders*, ed 3. Washington, DC, American Psychiatric Association, 1980, pp 307-330.
9. Kellner R, Rada RT: Pharmacotherapy of personality disorders, in David JM, Greenblatt D (eds): *Psychopharmacology Update: New and Neglected Areas*. New York, Grune & Stratton, 1979, pp 29-63.
10. Groves JE: Current concepts in psychiatry—borderline personality disorder. *New Engl J Med* 1981;305:259-262.

GENERAL REFERENCES

Goldstein WN: Understanding Kernberg on the borderline patient. *National Association of Private Psychiatric Hospitals Journal* 1982;13:21-26.

Guggenheim FG, Nadelson C (eds): *Major Psychiatric Disorders*. New York, Elsevier Bio-medical, 1982, pp 133-217.

Kolb, L, Brodie HKH: *Modern Clinical Psychiatry*. Philadelphia, WB Saunders, 1982, pp 593-615.

Johnson AM, Szurek SA: Etiology of antisocial behavior in delinquents and psychopaths. *JAMA* 1954;154:814-817.

Brenner C: *An Elementary Textbook of Psychoanalysis*. New York, Doubleday, Anchor Books Inc, 1957, pp 62-140.

Michaels JJ: Character structure and character disorders, in Arieti S (ed): *American Hand-book of Psychiatry*. New York, Basic Books, 1959, vol 1, pp 353-377.

Vaillant GE: Theoretical hierarchy of adaptive ego mechanisms. *Arch Gen Psychiatry* 1971; 24:107-118.

Chapter 18

SUICIDE

HOWARD S. SUDAK, M.D.

INCIDENCE AND STATISTICS

Statistics about suicide are notoriously misleading. Victims often take pains to make the death appear "natural" or accidental. Family doctors and coroners may report deaths as non-suicides to save the victim's family from stigma. It is safe to assume that statistics on suicide attempts are even less reliable.

The "official" figures are, nonetheless, staggering. Each year at least 20,000 Americans kill themselves, and an estimated 140,000 attempt suicide. Thus, more Americans have died from suicide in the past 20 years than were killed in both World War II and Korea (1).

The suicide rate generally increases up to age 75, and then tapers off; 18 to 25-year-olds make the greatest number of attempts. Women make unsuccessful suicide attempts about three times as often as men; men complete suicides about three times as often as women. The suicide rate in whites is three times greater than in blacks (2).

Suicide rates should be viewed in absolute terms, i.e., the number of successful suicides per 100,000 of a given population at risk. The overall national rate for successful suicide is about 10/100,000 (16.6/100,000 males; 4.7/100,000 females; 11.4/100,000 whites; 3.9/100,000 blacks). Suicides account for about 1% of total annual deaths (2).

Suicide is the tenth leading cause of death in all age ranges, and the second or third leading cause in college age populations (2). This does not, of course, mean that 18 to 22-year-olds are three times more likely than older people to suicide; it does indicate, however, that this relatively healthy population is not as likely to be dying from physical illnesses. A given number of suicides will thus rank higher in a frequency distribution of leading causes of death.

Over the past few years there has been increasing awareness of a markedly rising suicide rate in the young. Hellon and Solomon (3) dramatically illustrated this increase among youths aged 15–25. They also showed that this trend continues as any given group of cohorts ages. Their Alberta study was replicated using U.S. statistics by George Murphy and Richard Wetzel (4).

Offer and Holinger (5) feel that the critical factor is the ratio of adolescents to the total population. The higher the ratio (e.g., the post-World War II baby-boom accounts for the high proportion of adolescents to the total population in the 1960s), the higher the suicide rate. Their prediction of a current slight decrease, due to a lower ratio, appears to have been validated.

ETIOLOGY

Sociological Theories

Much of the sociological theory concerning suicide focuses on the individual's integration with his environment. In 1897, Emile Durkheim categorized three types of suicide (6): egoistic (lonely and withdrawn people, insufficiently integrated with their environment); altruistic (people "too integrated" with their environment, e.g., the soldier who falls on the grenade in a foxhole, thus sparing his comrades; ritual sacrifices); "anomie" (people who accustomed place in society is disrupted, e.g., by financial disasters, loss of love, illness).

Sociological studies range from correlations of incidence rates with changes in climate, business cycles, etc., to sophisticated studies involving "status integration." Gibbs' studies (7) indicate that meaningful data must be based on norms for very specific subpopulations. For instance, the general suicide rate is lowest for married individuals, higher for singles, still higher for the widowed, and highest for divorced individuals. In a population of 35 to 44-year-old white males, these rates are 16.7, 29.8, 81.7, and 112.6 per 100,000, respectively (7). A population of white males 75 years and older, however, has more married than widowed suicides (widowed—27.0; married—28.5; single—39.2; divorced—90.5/100,000) (7). This fits Gibbs' contention that the rates of suicide within a subpopulation vary inversely with its similarities to the surrounding population, e.g., it is more "normal" (usual) to be widowed than married in a population of 75-plus year olds; one would thus predict that the widowed groups would have lower suicide rates than the married groups.

Although the suicide rate for blacks seems universally lower than that for whites, the rate for Northern blacks in urban areas may exceed that for Southern whites (e.g., Seattle black rate = 10.2/100,000; Mississippi white rate = 9.7/100,000) (8). There are a number of theories about the disparate racial rates: "shame" versus "guilt" cultures, i.e., more depression in guilt cultures leads to more suicides; reciprocal relationship between suicide and homicide, i.e., groups that externalize aggression have high homicide and low suicide rates, internalized aggression causes more suicides and fewer homicides. This would appear to fit the data showing high suicide and low homicide rates in whites as compared to high homicide and low suicide rates in blacks. However, Hendin (8) showed that New York City black males between 20-35 are twice as likely as white males to commit suicide. This finding led him to posit a high "violence index" of both externally- and internally-directed aggression for this population.

The male/female rate disparities have been attributed to the latitude allowed females in our culture. Their freedom to vent feelings makes them more likely to act impulsively. Thus, they tend to make more suicide attempts than males, picking methods that are certainly less lethal. A male's suicide attempt is usually more deliberate, better planned, and more likely to succeed. Females' tendency to select non-disfiguring and non-painful methods (e.g., pills as preferable to guns, stabbing, jumping) means there is likely to be more time allowable after the act in which to avert death.

Aside from adolescents, the suicide rate has remained remarkably constant over the years. The 1900 and 1980 rates were about the same (10/100,000); however, the 1932 rate was 17/100,000 and the rates during the war years (1941-1945) were considerably lower than 10/100,000 (9).

Psychological Theories

Suicidal behavior is a symptom, not a disease or diagnosis. There are various ways to classify suicide: primary psychiatric diagnosis; demographic subgroups; bonafide attempts vs. gestures; successful vs. unsuccessful; methodology; etc.

Primary Psychiatric Diagnosis. Suicidal behavior is often colored by the primary psychiatric diagnosis. Schizophrenics may, for example, make very unpredictable, bizarre types of suicide attempts—particularly in the early, turbulant stages of the illness. Young, chronic schizophrenics also have a particularly high rate (10). Histrionic characters often make dramatic and impulsive attempts. Psychoses, neuroses, character problems, acute and chronic brain syndromes, alcoholism, addictions, etc., can all give rise to suicidal behavior. Psychotic persons account for 5-10% of total annual suicide attempts (1). A recent, as yet unconfirmed, study (11) showed the highest rates were for schizophrenic patients (411/100,000 year!). Bipolar depressives were next (318/100,000), but unipolars showed a rate of only 42/100,000.

The fact that most people who commit suicide are significantly depressed accounts for the very high rates among those with primary diagnosis of depression. According to classical psychodynamic theory, the individual reacts to a real, symbolic, or fantasized loss with feelings of deprivation and rage. A conflict is created by simultaneous positive and negative feelings about the lost object, e.g., spouse or parent. Those aggressive feelings which are unacceptable to the superego may be redirected toward the self. He/she may identify with the lost object and incorporate some of its characteristics—especially those that were most resented. Having internalized the lost object, they are symbolically killing it by committing suicide. Hence is derived Menninger's progression—the wish to kill, to be killed, and to die (12).

Suicide may also represent a conscious or unconscious attempt to punish someone, or an unconscious denial of the finality of death. A common fantasy is that the suicide victim will become reunited with previously deceased loved ones. Some adults, and children in particular, may have omnipotent fantasies in which their deaths cause the end of the world.

The dynamics of suicide may not be as dramatic in older and/or physically ill persons. Feelings of depletion, exhaustion, emptiness, and despair, often coupled with physical pain, may lead to a profound loss of self-esteem and the desire to live. Some authors (13) feel that suicide can be a realistic solution, even for those who are not old or debilitated. Loss of hope and the breakdown of defense mechanisms appear to contribute to the high suicide rate among the elderly. In fact, hopelessness, rather than sadness, may be the most relevant of all causal factors in suicide (14, 15).

Demographic Subgroups. Suicide impartially cuts across most socioeconomic and religious lines. Predominantly Catholic Austria and predominantly Protestant Denmark both have very high rates. There is some general evidence, however, that rates are slightly lower among Roman Catholics (1). Of course, the influence of religion depends upon personal religious beliefs rather than those of one's country (e.g., belief in an anthropomorphic deity; life after death).

Hendin (16) correlated suicide rates with certain "national characteristics" of the inhabitants of Sweden, Denmark, and Norway. He concluded that disparate childrearing practices and differing mores regarding open displays of emotions by males may be influential.

There are numerous studies of occupational groups. The high rates among physicians (approximately 70 per 100,000) (17) lead some investigators to conclude that depression is caused by the emotional or physical arduousness of the role. The comparably high rates for dentists and pharmacists suggests that the availability of highly lethal drugs is an important factor.

It appears simplistic to ignore selection factors in appraising data on suicides. The medical profession may attract a higher than average proportion of depression-prone individuals. Among physicians, psychiatrists are reported (18) to have the highest rates; pre-selection biases would seem more germane than arduousness in understanding high rates for this specialty. Some studies (17) do not show a disproportionate number of suicides in psychiatrists, however—and it is easy to create facile explanations to fit any data. For example, why should ophthalmologists have rates purportedly second to psychiatrists? The rates for women physicians have been reported to be particularly high as well (19). Physicians on probation are reported to have a suicide rate of 20% (20,000 per 100,000) per year (20). Cab drivers have rates seven times as high as truck drivers (1). Again, pre-selection of an abnormally high percentage of transients, unemployed persons, etc., may appear to account for this.

There is no evidence of any inherited tendencies toward suicide. Inheritance has, however, been linked to the development of certain psychiatric illnesses (e.g., schizophrenia, affective disorders), some of which carry an increased suicide risk. The increased risk associated with a family history of suicide may also be due to psychological, rather than genetic factors, e.g., identification with a parent who has suicided. There also seem to be "suicide-attempt" families, i.e., families whose members learn to respond to emotional upset with suicide attempts.

"Attempts vs. Gestures;" Successful vs. Unsuccessful Attempts. Suicidal behavior can also be classified according to intent and outcome. A patient who intends to die may be saved unexpectedly, e.g., the patient who shoots himself in the chest but misses the heart. Patients who exhibit "sub-intentional" or indirect suicidal behavior do not consciously wish to die (e.g., a cirrhotic patient who continues drinking; a diabetic who refuses to take insulin; a patient with coronary disease who continues smoking). Although the term "suicide" is defined as a deliberate attempt at taking one's own life, the concept of less than conscious or attenuated, suicidal behavior is, nevertheless, useful. Classifying suicidal behavior according to outcome, i.e., completed vs. unsuccessful, is also helpful; the two groups usually represent the suicidal acts of separate populations with different motivations and dynamics. There is, obviously, some overlap, e.g., when a suicidal "gesture" is inadvertently completed, due to dosage miscalculation or an anticipated rescuer who doesn't show up. Unsuccessful attempts generally utilize less lethal methods; they are made by people who are more impulsive, less depressed, and less fully committed to dying than those who succeed. Suicidal "gestures" are actions which seem to be dramatic, manipulative devices, calculated to punish others or gain attention and sympathy. The contempt associated with the term "gesture" is unwarranted for two reasons: 1. It can lull others into believing they needn't take the patient seriously. Such patients may go on to make serious attempts; 2. It ignores the fact that such patients are disturbed. They need as much help in gaining

control over their unconscious conflicts as those who make more serious initial attempts. Some investigators have now begun to use factor analysis in differentiating among the complex classification of attempts (21).

Methods. Men generally choose more violent means of death than women, e.g., firearms, jumping, hanging. Women often select "non-disfiguring" means, which are readily available, but less lethal—e.g., aspirin. Obviously, the method correlates with the outcome. One tends to be more wary of the patient who has made a well planned but unsuccessful attempt using a very dangerous method (e.g., carbon monoxide from a car exhaust) than of one who has taken a few aspirins. One cannot be certain, however, that subsequent attempts will maintain a low level of lethality. In fact, studies have shown that today's aspirin-taker may turn out to be tomorrow's bichloride of mercury ingester.

DIAGNOSIS

The most important factor in suicide detection is a high index of suspicion. The risk of suicide should be automatically appraised in every patient with signs of depression, e.g., worthless feelings, sadness, anhedonia, tearfulness, and vegetative signs (insomnia, anorexia and weight loss, constipation, amenorrhea). These signs may be quite subtle and indirect. In addition, psychoses and organic brain syndromes predispose patients to suicide. Other risk factors include: past history of suicidal thoughts or attempts; current suicidal thoughts or wishes; alcohol or drug abuse; family history of suicide. Any suicidal threat should be taken seriously and weighed carefully. Patients who talk about suicide may commit it. Over half of the successful suicides have seen their family physicians in the three months prior to their deaths—indicating that doctors can play a critical role in suicide prevention. Particular attention should be paid to evidence of loneliness, isolation, and *losses of any kind.* Parental deaths and unstable family histories may also help to alert the examiner (22).

After picking up a hint about suicide, one should probe further to appraise the risk. While fears of putting ideas into the patient's head are unwarranted, one should not be overly blunt. After the patient has acknowledged sadness, one may start with fairly innocuous questions, such as: "Does it sometimes get so bad you wish you hadn't been born?" or ". . . that you wish you were dead?" An affirmative reply should lead to further questions, such as: "Have you thought about suicide?" If so, ask, "Have you thought about a method?" These questions help to determine the patient's commitment to dying. Which pills would he/she use? Has the patient been saving them? Is the person afraid he/she might act upon the suicidal impulses? One should not be too easily reassured by statements such as, "I don't have the guts," or, "Suicide is against my religion." Statistical data regarding particularly high-risk groups should not encourage complacency about low-risk groups, e.g., a given young black female may indeed be suicidal, regardless of the statistics.

Some investigators are working on possible methods to calculate biochemical indices of suicide risk (23-25). Another group has reported a high correlation between high 17-hydroxycorticosteroid levels in depressed patients and successful suicide attempts (26). Recently, a third group (27) has discovered both higher cortisol and lower norepinephrine to epinephrine levels in suicidal subjects. This is particularly interesting since high norepinephrine to epinephrine ratios are supposedly characteristic of populations who express anger outward (e.g., assaultive prisoners); low ratios are characteristic of those who direct anger inward.

MANAGEMENT

Although the type of treatment ultimately depends upon the underlying disorder, certain general principles apply.

If suicide appears at all likely, prompt psychiatric evaluation should be obtained. This may require the help of the patient's family who, in any event, should be apprised of the risk.

Immediate hospitalization is indicated if an evaluation suggests that the patient is a danger to himself—even if this requires legal action. It is easier to make a decision about hospitalization if there has already been an attempt. Patients whose personal lives have been unchanged by a suicide attempt are at particularly high-risk.

Psychiatrists occasionally elect to manage a suicidal patient without hospitalization. Such a course requires a longstanding, trusting doctor-patient relationship, and is risky even then. Unfortunately, a laissez-faire attitude toward suicide has become fashionable. Its adherents believe that hospitalization to prevent suicide robs the individual of dignity; they claim that, "Freedom equals free-doom." Such a stance essentially removes the physician's responsibility to those whose depressions or other psychiatric disorders could be treated if they were prevented from carrying-out their suicidal plans. Those with refractory conditions who really want to kill themselves will eventually find a way; hospitalization may only buy a little time. Hospitalization does provide some protection for patients. Other advantages of hospitalization include: patient's removal from a precipitating situation; greater therapeutic freedom to explore the patient's basic problems and feelings; optimal conditions for beginning more definitive treatment, e.g., psychotherapy, drugs, ECT.

Precautions are necessary if a suicidal patient must be managed on a general hospital ward. Medications and dangerous objects must be inaccessible. The patient's belongings should be searched. Windows should be barred, and cords or other possible means of hanging removed. Such patients often require constant surveillance.

The risk of suicide does not automatically diminish with hospitalization. The risk actually may increase when the patient recovers enough energy to overcome the motor retardation of a depression and carry out suicidal impulses. The period following discharge is also dangerous.

ROLE OF SUICIDE PREVENTION CENTERS

The rationale for suicide prevention centers is based on two factors: 1. Patients are generally ambivalent about wishing to die; 2. Certain high risk groups can be identified, e.g., people who have previously attempted suicide. The nature and functioning of these centers are very diverse. However, they all offer 24-hour service and some sort of prompt treatment or referral. The center's services are also extended to relatives and friends of the potential suicide. It is difficult to determine whether these organizations actually serve the truly suicidal population. Even if their only tangible service is arranging prompt evaluation of borderline risk cases, the existence of suicide centers appears justified. In addition, other services may be provided, e.g., research; education; coordination of community facilities.

EXISTENTIAL AND PHILOSOPHICAL ISSUES

The recent increase in adolescent suicide rates (5) has generated a great deal of interest. Even if it is correct, the population model does not provide an etiological explanation. Possible hypotheses include: more adolescents competing for fewer available jobs in a success-oriented, high-pressure, violence-prone, gun-happy, frontier-mentality society; rising unemployment and falling governmental supports for the disadvantaged; the pressures of modern society, with particular reference to living under the threat of nuclear destruction; the breakdown of the family via separations and divorce; the erosion of religious institutions and values; breakdown of morality; abuse of drugs and alcohol; upsurge of radicalism. Any and all of these factors may play a role, but must be scrutinized in relation to available data. For example, most of the factors related to social unrest should affect blacks more than whites. Although the relative increase in rates is highest among blacks, there is still a black/white disparity. What protects blacks? It is interesting that the rate of suicide is higher in young adult black males than in older black males (in contrast to rates for white males). This finding has prompted speculation in the New York Times (28) that, once having made it to adulthood, the most suicidal black males have been weeded-out and the strong survive. Is reaching adulthood the most difficult challenge to a black male, making everything else relatively easier?

Whether or not one can ever consider a suicide attempt "normal" is another issue. If the concept of a "normal individual" includes denial and hope as important defense mechanisms, suicide is never "normal." For example, the suicide rate among terminally ill or chronic pain patients is higher than that of age-matched controls; it is remarkable, however, that the difference is not higher. Why wasn't the suicide rate among concentration camp inmates higher? Considering the increased numbers of older, chronically-ill persons, why are euthanasia dilemmas relatively infrequent? One reason is that people have a strong instinct of self-preservation. We also tend to deny our frailty and mortality, hoping against hope that things will change for the better. It is only when this "normal" denial breaks down and "normal" hope is diminished that people go on to suicide. Thus, from this perspective, "normal" individuals do not kill themselves.

It is also instructive to consider our attitudes toward death—particularly our own. Few people appear capable of contemplating their own mortality with much objectivity. Normal denial is crucial to our inability to realistically comprehend our mortality. For example, Elisabeth Kubler-Ross (29), one of the most eloquent spokespersons for the dying, has accurately indicted the medical profession for its failure to deal with dying patients realistically and openly. It is, therefore, ironic that, allegedly, her more recent view is that there is really no such thing as death per se. Based upon her ability to "sense" people's spirits or souls going off into space, and her talks with patients who have had "near-death" experiences, she posits that we all live on in some altered state after death (30).

The last issue to be dealt with is suicide's painful emotional legacy. Suicide occurs so frequently that each of us has been or will be touched by a relative or close friend killing himself. The burden of guilt, inexpressible anger, sadness, shame, hurt, relief, etc., can be devastating to the surviving family and friends—particularly the children. "Survivor's Groups," established in some major cities, may provide support for their members. Children of suicides should be evaluated to determine their need for psychotherapy to help them deal with their feelings. Mental health professionals need to be alert to the painful sequellae of suicide and attempt to alter them.

REFERENCES

1. Perr IN: Liability of hospital psychiatrist in suicide. *Am J Psychiatry* 1965;122:631-638.
2. Farberow N, Shneidman E: *The Cry for Help*. New York, McGraw-Hill, 1965.

3. Hellon CP, Solomon MI: Suicide and age in Alberta, Canada, 1951 to 1977: I. The changing profile; II. A cohort analysis. *Arch Gen Psychiatry* 1980;37:505-513.

4. Murphy GE, Wetzel RD: Suicide risk by birth cohort in the United States, 1949-1974. *Arch Gen Psychiatry* 1980;37:519-523.

5. Holinger PC, Offer D: Prediction of adolescent suicide: A Population model. *Am J Psychiatry* 1982;139:302-307.

6. Durkheim E: *Suicide*. New York, The Free Press, 1951.

7. Gibbs JP, Martin WT: *Status Integration and Suicide*. Eugene, Oregon, University of Oregon Books, 1964.

8. Hendin H. Black suicide. *Arch Gen Psychiatry* 1969;21:407-422.

9. Shneidman E: Suicide. *Psychiatric Annals* 1976;6:9-121.

10. Roy A: Risk factors for suicide in psychiatric patients. *Arch Gen Psychiatry* 1982;39: 1089-1095.

11. Morrison JR: Suicide in a psychiatric practice population. *J Clin Psychiatry* 1982;43: 348-352.

12. Menninger K: *Man Against Himself*. New York, Harcourt Brace & Co, 1938.

13. Lowental U: Suicide—the other side: The factor of reality among suicidal motivations. *Arch Gen Psychiatry* 1976;33:838-842.

14. Wetzel RD: Hopelessness, depression, and suicide intent. *Arch Gen Psychiatry* 1976;33: 1069-1073.

15. Wetzel RD, Margulies T, Davis R, *et al.*: Hopelessness, depression, and suicide intent. *J Clin Psychiatry* 1980;41:159-160.

16. Hendin H: *Suicide and Scandinavia*. New York, Grune & Stratton, 1964.

17. Rich CL, Pitts FN: Suicide by psychiatrists: A study of medical specialists among 18,730 consecutive physician deaths during a five-year period, 1967-1972. *J Clin Psychiatry* 1980;41:261-263.

18. Rose KD, Rosow I: Physicians who kill themselves. *Arch Gen Psychiatry* 1973;29: 800-805.

19. Carlson GA, Miller DC: Suicide, affective disorders, and women physicians. *Am J Psychiatry* 1981;138:1330-1335.

20. Crawshaw R, Bruce JA, Eraker PL, *et al.*: An epidemic of suicide among physicians on probation. *JAMA* 1980;243:1915-1917.

21. Beck AT, Weissman A, Lester D, *et al.*: Classification of suicidal behaviors: II. Dimensions of suicidal intent. *Arch Gen Psychiatry* 1976;33:835-837.

22. Adam, KS, Bouckoms A, Streiner D: Parental loss and family stability in attempted suicide. *Arch Gen Psychiatry* 1982;39:1081-1085.

23. Bunney WE, Davis JM, Weil-Malherbe H, *et al.*: Biochemical changes in psychotic depression: High norepinephrine levels in psychotic versus neurotic depression. *Arch Gen Psychiatry* 1967;16:448-460.

24. Fawcett J, Leff M, Bunney WE: Suicide: Clues from interpersonal communication. *Arch Gen Psychiatry* 1969;21:129-137.

25. Bunney WE, Fawcett JA, Davis JM, *et al.*: Further evaluation of urinary 17-hydroxycorticosteroids in suicidal patients. *Arch Gen Psychiatry* 1969;21:138-150.

26. Asberg M, Traskman L, Thoren P: 5-HIAA in the cerebrospinal fluid: A biochemical suicide predictor? *Arch Gen Psychiatry* 1976;33:1193-1197.

27. Ostroff R, Giller E, Bonese K, *et al.*: Neuroendocrine risk factors of suicidal behavior. *Am J Psychiatry* 1982;139:1323-1325.

28. Williams J: Why are blacks less prone to suicide than whites? *New York Times,* February 9, 1982.

29. Kubler-Ross E: *On Death and Dying.* New York, Macmillan Co. 1969.
30. Lindsey R: Special report: An early leader in comfort for the dying moves into spiritualism. *New York Times,* September 17, 1979.

Chapter 19

PSYCHOSOMATIC MEDICINE
AND CONSULTATION LIAISON PSYCHIATRY

DAVID P. AGLE, M.D.

The term "psychosomatic" has become part of our general vocabulary. While many individuals recognize that mental processes can influence body function, and that a sick body can produce mental distress, there is considerable confusion as to how this occurs. The objective of this chapter is to define and explore the relationship between body function and mental processes, and demonstrate its relevance to clinical practice.

Psychosomatic medicine includes a body of knowledge, research approaches, and clinical directions that encompass all factors contributing to disease. Although medical school curricula teach comprehensive care in principle, the biomedical focus with its emphasis on technological investigative and treatment techniques often predominates. The biopsychosocial approach of psychosomatic medicine, on the other hand, explores all avenues of investigation and treatment—organic, psychological, and social (1). Consultation-liaison psychiatry is the clinical application of these precepts of psychosomatic medicine.

The term "psychophysiologic" refers to bodily states or illnesses with significant psychological determinants. Initially, this label was only applied to a small group of diseases, such as peptic ulcer; clinical experience indicates that this focus is too limited. The DSM-III classification "Physical Disorders Affected by Psychological Factors" appropriately broadens this field to include a wide range of disorders (2).

MENTAL EQUILIBRIUM AND THE BIOLOGIC FUNCTION
OF THE AFFECTS

Psychophysiologic responses are vital to successful adaptation. They do not necessarily result in disease or imply psychological dysfunction. The human mind attempts to maintain a state of comfortable mental equilibrium through mechanisms that minimize uncomfortable affects such as anxiety. When these psychological responses to stress are not sufficient to maintain equilibrium, biologic processes are activated. The conscious perception of these responses is emotion or affect (3). It is at this point that peripheral body physiology is influenced through the autonomic and neuroendocrine systems.

The affects initially promote adaptation by functioning as signals. The uncomfortable affects warn about stress just as pain serves as a warning to protect the body's integrity. In addition to the signal function, the affects associated with stress are accompanied by physiologic changes to prepare the body for possible action. Eliciting physiologic arousal is one biologic function of emotion. The degree of physiologic response may vary from subtle changes (increased alertness) to more profound arousal (panic state).

This biologic preparation may be clinically assessed by physical examination and laboratory measures. For example, epinephrine release prepares the body for a possible physical exertion by liberating hepatic glycogen and free fatty acids to provide a reserve of calories. There may also be an outpouring of adrenocorticoid products and endorphins useful in preparing the body for tissue injury, repair, and analgesia.

Some studies suggest a distinction between responses of fear and anger (4,5). Fear is closely associated with epinephrine output, anger with norepinephrine preponderance. For example, fear is accompanied by a rapid tachycardia; in states of anger, the cardiac rate is more in keeping with the body's needs. Anxiety or fear is associated with a cold, sweating skin; in anger, the skin is usually flushed and warm. Ideally, these "fight-flight" reactions (6) promote adaptation by facilitating useful arousal and action.

Clinical Implications

Despite their utility, the biological concomitants of the affects may be detrimental to individuals with certain physical disorders. For example, the patient with coronary insufficiency may be susceptible to emotion and experience angina as a response to stress. Similarly, strong emotional responses may precipitate respiratory insufficiency in patients with chronic obstructive pulmonary disease (7).

PSYCHOGENIC INFLUENCES AND DISEASE CAUSATION

The observation that psychological stress may worsen certain established diseases is not controversial; evidence for psychogenic causes of physical disease is more complex. Disorders traditionally attributed to psychological factors include peptic ulcer, bronchial asthma, ulcerative colitis, some forms of hypertension, neurodermatitis, migraine headache, rheumatoid arthritis, and hyperthyroidism. In fact, these disorders are probably determined by multiple organic, psychological, and social factors. The importance of each factor must be determined for each individual patient. In addition, this traditional list of diseases is misleading because it is not complete. Psychological factors may contribute to the causes and courses of many physical disorders. There is a vast array of studies and theoretical approaches aimed at understanding psychogenic contributions to disease. Several of the important models of psychogenic disease causation will now be reviewed.

Stress Response Model

The concept of stress and its responses provides an important framework for understanding the contributions of psychological factors to disease (8,9). A psychological stress is an event or situation that is perceived as threatening and may produce mental discomfort. While hierarchies of universally stressful events have been developed, there are enormous individual variations in response. For example, a divorce may cause profound depression in one individual, while another considers it an exciting challenge for growth.

Since individuals' stress perceptions vary, the examination of subjective distress and measures of peripheral responses provide clinical tools for recognizing its presence. These measures of distress include observation of obvious affects ranging from mild anxiety to full-blown panic and the intensification of certain psychological defenses and coping behaviors. A central focus of research on stress has been measurement of autonomic arousal. Most theories of psychogenic contributions to disease are based on the idea that a chronic repetition of such body responses may, in a variety of complex ways, contribute to tissue dysfunction or damage.

Models of Psychogenic Causation

In the early phases of psychosomatic medicine, strong efforts were made to identify the specific psychological factors that caused specific diseases:

Personality Specificity. Dunbar (10) described typical personality profiles that increased the vulnerability to specific psychosomatic disorders. These views, popular in the 30s and 40s, failed to survive more rigorous scientific scrutiny in the early 60s. Interest in personality has now been reawakened by the correlation between Type A behavior (i.e., intense competitiveness; profound sense of time urgency) and coronary artery disease (11).

Conflict Specificity. Alexander (12) used psychoanalytic concepts to explain organic disorders. He theorized that the arousal of specific unconscious conflicts caused changes in autonomic discharge balance; these changes resulted in specific psychosomatic disorders. He suggested, for example, that the peptic ulcer patient is an outwardly independent person who is attempting to deal with a strong, unconscious dependency need. He thought this unconscious wish resulted in repeated episodes of excessive gastric secretion.

Attitude Specificity. Graham (13) identified characteristic attitudes of patients with specific diseases. For example, individuals with chronic urticaria typically develop lesions in response to mistreatment from others. Though resentful, their passive helpless attitude indicates their preoccupation with what has been done to them rather than appropriate reaction. Graham's belief that significant vasodilation of capillaries and arterioles accompanied this attitude state was based on physiologic skin studies.

Modern Experimental and Clinical Approaches

Though the specificity theories appear to have some clinical utility, attempts to validate them have had limited results (14). This failure generated a new group of hypotheses and research directions focusing on illness-related roles of life events, alexithymia, and operant conditioning.

Life Events and Nonspecific Triggers of Disease. Life event studies focus on stress as a nonspecific trigger of disease. Holmes and Rahe (15) have demonstrated significant connections between stressful life events and the onset of a variety of illnesses. Rees (16) found that the death rate of bereaved persons was seven times that of controls in the year following the death of a close relative. Such studies seem to demonstrate that a combination of life change and poor coping mechanisms can increase susceptibility to many diseases.

Alexithymia. Sifneos (17) has observed that many individuals who are predisposed to psychosomatic disorders are unable to express their emotions and unfamiliar with their subjective experience. In clinical situations, such patients customarily describe various life situations in painstaking, unemotional detail. Although the relationship is not well understood, this alexithymia syndrome is reported associated with increases susceptibility to psychosomatic illness.

Operant Conditioning and Biofeedback. Operant conditioning studies indicate that the variation in autonomic nervous system activity related to learning through life experiences can lead to organ dysfunction or structural damage. Miller's (18) experiments demonstrated that the autonomic nervous system can be influenced and taught via rewards and punishments. This work was the basis for the biofeedback therapeutic approach. By providing patients with information about visceral function and rewarding desired change, it is possible to stimulate therapeutic gains, e.g., lower blood pressure, widen bronchial diameters, decrease skeletal muscle tension. The long-term benefits of these approaches are as yet undetermined.

PSYCHOSOMATIC MANAGEMENT

The vast majority of patients with psychophysiologic disorders (i.e., psychologically affected physical disorders) are treated by non-psychiatric physicians. Only a few are referred for psychiatric treatment, usually because they are doing poorly under conventional medical management. Many, but not all, of these patients can benefit from psychiatric care.

The notion that repressed conflicts and affects lead to disease, as well as the alexithymia hypothesis, may lead to an oversimplified treatment approach. Problems are generally not limited to the expression of too little or too much emotion. For example, patients who have not developed useful defenses and coping behaviors have primitive affective responses to stress. Psychotherapy may help such patients develop more mature defensive responses and better control the emotional arousal that triggers or sustains particular psychophysiologic responses.

Other therapeutic approaches include behavioral modification, biofeedback, hypnosis (19), and relaxation therapy—all attempt to modify undesirable physiologic and behavioral responses to emotional stimuli. Determinations of relevant approaches for treating these disorders must be made on an individual basis. One patient with stress-related asthmatic attacks may respond to direct symptom relief through hypnosis- or biofeedback-induced relaxation. Another may require the learning of more useful defensive responses through psychotherapy.

CONSULTATION-LIAISON PSYCHIATRY

Consultation-liaison psychiatry is the clinical application of psychosomatic medicine concepts. Approximately 30–60% of patients on medical and surgical wards have psychiatric complications serious enough to interfere with their medical management (20). The consultation-liaison psychiatrist's responsibilities include all diagnostic, therapeutic, teaching, and research activities relevant to the psychological and social aspects of illness and medical practice (21,22). Since a detailed description of these activities is beyond the scope of this chapter, this discussion will be limited to diagnostic issues frequently confusing to the beginning student.

The "Functional" Complaint
A physical complaint is often considered psychological in origin if it cannot be explained after an extensive organic investigation. Wastebasket terms

such as "functional," pejorative diagnoses such as "crock" or more scientific-sounding labels such as "hysteria" are commonly misapplied to these patients; their problems are often diagnostic challenges requiring careful work-ups. Diagnostic accuracy is considerably increased by a careful search for psychological determinants of complaints rather than the simple exclusion of organic causes. A careful psychiatric assessment's failure to produce positive findings to explain the syndrome is, in fact, suggestive of a primary organic process. There are specific criteria for accurate psychiatric diagnoses.

Hysteria, Somatization Disorder, and the Conversion Disorder

The term "hysteria" has several technical psychiatric meanings, and is often used incorrectly. A "histrionic personality disorder" is one that includes at least some of the following traits: dramatic self-display; wide mood swings; deficiency in controlling and using affect appropriately; provocativeness; suggestibility; sexual dysfunction; demanding dependency (23). Past medical histories often detail multiple physical symptoms, frequent hospital admissions, and sometimes surgery. The more extreme form of this symptom complex is now called "somatization disorder."

"Conversion" refers to a psychological defense against stress and conflict, i.e., the use of bodily activities or sensations to express ideal symbolically (24). Conversions frequently, but not exclusively, occur in patients with histrionic personality disorders. They primarily involve voluntary motor or sensory perceptual systems. A conversion reduces emotional discomfort by displacement to a physical symptom; it does not cause basic structural change.

Several criteria are helpful in distinguishing between somatization and conversion disorders (25). Beginning before age 30, the somatization disorder includes a syndrome of chronic, recurrent physical symptoms of unknown organic etiologies. Diagnosis requires a minimum of 14 significant complaints in women, and 12 in men. Pseudoneurologic, gastrointestinal, female reproductive, psychosexual, "pain," and cardiopulmonary complaints are common.

The conversion disorder is generally limited to a single predominant disturbance or alteration in physical function with no known organic cause (26). Etiology is psychological. If pain is the only symptom, the diagnosis is "psychogenic pain disorder."

It is also important to distinguish between conversion reactions and physical conditions affected by psychological factors (psychophysiologic).

TABLE I

	Body Area	(Symbolism)	Reduces Anxiety	Primary Structural Change
Conversion Disorder	Innervated by voluntary and perceptual N.S.	Present	Yes	No
Physical Disorders affected by Psychological Factors (Psychophysiologic Disease)	Basically innervated by Autonomic N.S.	Absent	No	Yes

SUMMARY

These remarks are merely an introduction to psychosomatic medicine and consultation-liaison psychiatry. Knowledge of mind-body interactions is necessary to fully understand and treat a wide variety of physical disorders. Essential physician's skills include the ability to obtain this information through a biopsychosocial approach and use it in management planning.

REFERENCES

1. Engel GL: The clinical application of the biopsychosocial model. *Am J Psychiatry* 1978;137:535–544.
2. American Psychiatric Association Task Force on Nomenclature and Statistics: *Diagnostic and Statistical Manual of Mental Disorders,* ed 3. Washington, DC, American Psychiatric Association, 1980, p 303.
3. Engel G: Somatic consequences of psychological stress: II. Decompensated states; somatopsychic-pyychosomatic disorders, in *Psychological Development in Health and Disease.* Philadelphia, WB Saunders & Co, 1962, pp 381–401.
4. Ax AF: The physiological differentiation between fear and anger in humans. *Psychosom Med* 1953;15:433–442.
5. Cohen SI, Silverman AJ: Psychophysiological investigations of vascular response variability. *J Psychosom Res* 1959;3:185–210.
6. Cannon WB: *The Wisdom of the Body.* New York, WW Norton, 1932.
7. Dudley DL, Wermuth C, Hague W: Psychosocial aspects of care in the chronic obstructive pulmonary disease patient. *Heart and Lung* 1973;2:389–393.
8. Caplan G: Mastery of stress: Psychosocial aspects. *Am J Psychiatry* 1981;138:413–420.
9. Lazarus RS: Psychological stress and coping in psychosomatic illness, in Levi L (ed): *Society, Stress and Disease.* New York, Oxford University Press, 1981, vol 4, pp 162–168.
10. Dunbar F: *Emotions and Bodily Changes.* New York, Columbia University Press, 1954.
11. Friedman M, Rosenman RH: Association of specific overt behavior pattern with blood cholesterol level, blood clotting time, incidence of arcus senilis and clinical coronary artery disease. *JAMA* 1959; 169:1286–1296.

12. Alexander F: *Psychosomatic Medicine: Its Principles and Applications*. New York, WW Norton, 1950.

13. Graham DT, Wolf S: Pathogenesis of hives: Experimental study of life situation, emotions and cutaneous vascular reactions. *Ass Res Nerv Ment Dis Proc* 1950;29:987.

14. Lipowski ZJ: New perspectives in psychosomatic medicine. *Canada Psychiatr Assoc J* 1970;15:515-525.

15. Rahe RH: Epidemiological studies of life change and illness. *Int J Psychiat Med* 1975; 6:133-146.

16. Rees WD, Lutkins SG: Mortality and bereavement. *Br Med J* 1967;4:13-16.

17. Sifneos PE: The prevalence of 'alexithymic' characteristics in psychosomatic patients. *Psychother Psychosom* 1973;22:255-262.

18. Miller NE: Learning of visceral and glandular responses. *Science* 1969;163:434-445.

19. Borrows GD, Dennerstein L (eds): *Handbook of Hypnosis and Psychosomatic Medicine*. New York, Elsevier/North Holland, Biomedical Press, 1980.

20. Lipowski ZJ: Review of consultation psychiatry and psychosomatic medicine: II. Clinical aspects. *Psychosom Med* 1967;29:201-224.

21. Strain JJ, Grossman S (eds): *Psychological Care of the Medically Ill*. New York, Appleton-Century-Crofts, 1975.

22. Hackett T, Cassem HN (eds): *Handbook of General Hospital Psychiatry*. St. Louis, CV Mosby Co, 1978.

23. American Psychiatric Association Task Force on Nomenclature and Statistics: *Diagnostic and Statistical Manual of Mental Disorders*, ed 3. Washington, DC, American Psychiatric Association, 1980, pp 313-315.

24. Engel GL: Compensated states—conversion reactions, in *Psychological Development in Health and Disease*. Philadelphia, WB Saunders Co, 1962, pp 368-375.

25. American Psychiatric Association Task Force on Nomenclature and Statistics: *Diagnostic and Statistical Manual of Mental Disorders*, ed 3. Washington, DC, American Psychiatric Association, 1980, pp 241-244.

26. American Psychiatric Association Task Force on Nomenclature and Statistics: *Diagnostic and Statistical Manual of Mental Disorders*, ed 3. Washington, DC, American Psychiatric Association, 1980, pp 244-247.

Chapter 20

ALCOHOLISM

MARTIN MACKLIN, M.D., Ph.D.

From 5-15% of all people who drink alcoholic beverages are alcoholics. Estimates are based on the population at risk, i.e., excluding those who never drank because of age, religious conviction, or some other reason. Many different criteria have been used to diagnose alcoholism. For example, one house-to-house survey used consumption of 60 or more drinks a month as the basis for a prospective diagnosis. Other surveys have based the diagnosis on two or more symptoms of physiological dependence, such as morning shakes, blackouts, withdrawal seizures, or delirium tremens (D.T.'s).

Many physicians and mental health professionals find it difficult to diagnose alcoholism. It is hard to recognize the fact that a practice they view as socially acceptable may cause problems for someone else. The patient or colleague may claim they can cut down their drinking whenever they want to, or that they can and have stopped at will. Rather than be misled by them, the examiner should view such reassuring comments as evidence of a possible problem.

A person is generally considered alcohol dependent if his drinking is causing problems in his life. To be more specific, the DSM-III (1) requires that a patient show both, "A. Either a pattern of pathological use or impairment in social or occupational functioning due to alcohol use," and "B. Either tolerance or withdrawal." Many experts working in the field would make the diagnosis without the second criterion; according to DSM-III, a diagnosis based only on criterion A would be Alcohol Abuse. The distinction between psychological and physical dependence is also important—although it is difficult to find a person who is psychologically but not physically dependent upon alcohol. The AMA *Manual on Alcoholism* provides the following definition (2): "Alcoholism is an illness characterized by significant impairment that is directly associated with persistent and excessive use of alcohol. Impairment may involve physiological, psychological, or social dysfunction."

In addition to a careful history, several screening tests can be used to diagnose alcoholism. The easiest test is the four question CAGE questionnaire described by Mayfield, McCleod, and Hall (3). Each "yes" answer receives one point. Patients admitted to a psychiatric ward who were diagnosed as alcoholic by a multidisciplinary treatment team had scores of one or more 90% of the time, and two or more 81% of the time. Non-alcoholics had scores of one or more 21% of the time, and two or more only 11% of the time. A score of two or three is, therefore, a good indication of alcoholism. The questions are:

"1. Have you ever felt the need to *cut* down on your drinking?

2. Have people *annoyed* you by criticizing your drinking?

3. Have you ever felt bad or *guilty* about your drinking?

4. Have you ever had a drink first thing in the morning, i.e., an *eye-opener?*"

It is important to realize that alcoholism exists in all social and professional groups; no group is spared. Indeed, five percent of drinking physicians are alcoholics.

Some writers (4) prefer the more general term "sedativism" to alcoholism because many people seem to be addicted to sedative drugs in general. That is, an alcoholic may use a sedative drug, such as a benzodiazepine, or a narcotic instead of alcohol. Many physicians and nurses who display the behavior patterns seen in alcoholics are addicted to readily available drugs. This ability to substitute one drug for another is important to recognize for the proper medical treatment of addiction. An alcoholic can use any drug with sedative properties as an alcohol substitute. Thus, prescribing a tranquilizer or antidepressant for the symptoms of alcoholism or drug abuse will only result in making additional drugs available to the dependent individual.

GENETIC STUDIES

There are no genetic markers that specifically predict the likelihood of alcohol or other drug dependency. There are no specific laboratory tests that can be used to identify alcoholics. The only possible exception is the finding of a random blood alcohol of 300 mg/dl in an awake person. (For reference, the legal limit for driving is 100 mg/dl or less in most states.)

Swedish studies (5) involving 913 adopted women and 862 adopted men produced valuable conclusions. In addition to identifying several subtypes of alcoholism, they discovered that a "patrilineal subtype has an heritability of 90% from father to son." They also concluded that the primary source of female alcoholism is maternal inheritance. Environmental factors are considered less important.

Donald Goodwin (6) found that 27% of alcoholics had alcoholic fathers (as compared to only 9% of schizophrenics who had alcoholic fathers). Adoptive twin studies show a 50% concordance for alcoholism in monozygotic, and a 25% concordance in dizygotic twins. This evidence indicates the need for increased vigilance with respect to substance abuse by children of alcoholics.

Other interesting findings include: the genetic link between alcoholism and depression (7); and a genetic link between female anorexia nervosa/bulimia and paternal alcoholism.

FETAL ALCOHOL SYNDROME

The effects of alcohol on an unborn fetus are seen in the symptom complex called Fetal Alcohol Syndrome (FAS):
1. Mental retardation, with poor motor coordination and hypotonia;
2. Both pre- and post-natal growth deficiency in about 80% of cases;
3. Characteristic facial appearance—short palpebral fissure; small upturned nose and hypoplastic philtrum (the ridge between the base of the nose and the upper lip); sunken nasal bridge; epicanthic folds; thin upper lip; hypoplastic maxilla; growth retardation of the jaw.

While these abnormalities are not individually significant, together they produce a characteristic facies, which may be accompanied by other malformations. These symptoms have only been found in the offspring of mothers who have consumed alcohol during pregnancy. Paternal alcoholism is not associated with birth defects; but it is associated with decreased fertility.

Based on the incidence of FAS in mothers who drink small amounts of alcohol, the Department of Health and Human Services recommends total abstinence from alcohol during pregnancy. A statistically significant 91 gram decrease in birthweight has been noted in offspring of women who reportedly averaged 1 ounce of alcohol per day in early pregnancy. Ingestion of the same amount in late pregnancy was associated with a 160 gram decrease in infant birthweight.

METABOLISM OF ALCOHOL

Ethyl alcohol, a waste product of metabolism by yeasts, is metabolized further by the human liver. Because the seven calories in each gram of alcohol are not accompanied by other nutrients, they are termed "empty calories." In addition, alcohol and acetaldehyde interfere with the liver's activation of vitamins. If sufficient alcohol is ingested, adequate diet will not prevent liver disease, thiamine deficiency, and other physical and neurological complications.

Alcohol metabolism occurs primarily in liver cell mitochondria in the following sequence:

Ethanol ———> Acetaldehyde ———> Acetate

The first step is catalyzed by alcohol dehydrogenase, and the second by aldehyde dehydrogenase. There are two drugs available to block the second step—disulfiram (Antabuse), an irreversible blocker, and carbimide (Temposil), a reversible enzyme blocker. The combination of alcohol and one of these drugs causes an unpleasant reaction, the severity depending upon the amount of alcohol ingested. Mild reactions include flushing, tachycardia, tachypnea, vomiting, and headaches; severe reactions include shock and loss of consciousness.

The microsomal ethanol oxidizing system (MEOS), a second, inducible endoplasmic reticulum enzyme stystem, metabolizes alcohol and other drugs. This may account for a significant amount of the physiologic tolerance seen in alcoholics.

The action of this enzyme system, also known as mixed function oxidase or MFO, is especially significant when the alcoholic takes a drug such as meprobamate or a barbiturate. Acute alcohol consumption inhibits the metabolism of these drugs thereby prolonging their effect. On a day when the alcoholic is not drinking, these same drugs are metabolized at an increased rate. Since the MFO system metabolizes many other commonly used drugs, special care must be taken when giving potentially toxic drugs to an alcoholic.

ALCOHOLISM TREATMENT

Alcoholism is a chronic, relapsing illness, i.e., anyone who has achieved sobriety through treatment is always at risk for returning to a state of uncontrolled drinking and declining health. Any treatment program must, therefore, be based upon lifetime follow-up for every patient. The goal of every treatment program must be total abstinence from alcohol and other sedative drugs. Alcoholism has at times been considered a sign of moral weakness or a symptom of an underlying emotional problem. This attitude has led to legal punishment for public drunkenness. Psychiatrists have attempted to get alcoholics to stop drinking by providing insight into the determinants of the drinking behavior. Both efforts have failed. Alcoholism is a true addiction that must be treated as a primary illness. The emotional problems of many alcoholics are frequently the consequence of their drinking. These problems may respond to psychotherapy once sobriety has been achieved or they may be resolved by sobriety alone.

The most difficult step is initiating treatment for alcoholism. Many alcoholics refuse to acknowledge the problem. The physician continues to treat the alcoholic's liver disease, heart disease, or anxiety, without trying to treat the primary illness. Although it is not necessary for the alcoholic to hit bottom before accepting treatment, frequently a crisis must be precipitated, e.g., threatened or actual job loss; threatened or actual divorce; loss of license to drive or practice a profession; etc.

The first step in treatment is withdrawal. Hospitalization is essential for most patients. The compulsion to drink frequently makes it impossible to stop in an unsupervised setting.

Some patients are able to stay sober by going to Alcoholic's Anonymous (AA); others require inpatient treatment. Inpatient treatment, usually in specialized treatment hospitals, commonly lasts from two to four weeks. After their withdrawal from alcohol and sedative drugs, patients begin programs of education and therapy which focus on their dysfunctional behavior. Treatment usually includes group therapy five days a week, daily lectures, frequent AA meetings, and recreational activities. All of these activities focus on patients' dysfunctional behaviors and attempt to get them to redirect their energies to behaviors that do not involve substance abuse. Firm ties are established with AA and the sober community. Many patients find sobriety fulfills their need for psychotherapy; others may seek further help from psychiatrists or clergy. At times, it is useful to utilize disulfiram in conjunction with treatment of an alcoholic. It is particularly helpful for patients who need an extra daily reminder not to drink.

Psychodynamically, it is important to understand and deal with the common defenses used by alcoholics. This is true during diagnosis and treatment. The alcoholic often makes use of denial to obstruct attempts to begin treatment and to obscure the diagnosis. Projection is typically seen when the problems caused by drinking are blamed on others.

A 70% success rate is reported for inpatient treatment of alcoholics with stable families and jobs. Single, unemployed, and poor alcoholics have a recovery rate of about 20%. Additional treatment periods are sometimes required in order to achieve long-term sobriety. Young alcoholics frequently experiment with small amounts of alcohol or drugs after treatment. They may return for further treatment when their drinking again becomes out-of-control.

Since alcoholism is best treated as a chronic illness, there is no acceptance of the concept of cure. However, the American Medical Society on Alcoholism (AMSA) adopted the following definition of recovery in 1980:

'STATE OF RECOVERY'

A patient is in a 'state of recovery' when he or she has reached a state of physical and psychological health such that his/her abstinence from dependency-producing drugs is complete and comfortable. In practice, this judgment must be made on clinical grounds based on the most complete assessment possible of the state and seriousness of the initial illness and the quality and length of remission.

An alcoholic individual is in remission when he/she is free of the active signs and symptoms of alcoholism. This includes abstinence from the use of substitute sedative, stimulant, or hallucinogenic drugs during a period of independent living. After a period of remission, which may vary for the individual, a state of recovery is achieved.

Indices of State of Recovery from alcoholism generally include:

1. Sobriety; comfortable abstinence from alcohol and/or other dependency-producing drugs.
2. Improvement in aspects of physical health previously adversely affected by alcohol use.
3. Improvement in family relationships and/or resolution of conflict in close relationships.
4. Improvement in functional responsibilities and self care.
5. Progress towards resolution of related emotional difficulties.
6. Willingness to share the recovery state.

DIAGNOSIS AND TREATMENT
OF ALCOHOL WITHDRAWAL SYNDROMES

The alcohol withdrawal syndromes consist of a continuum of clinical symptoms caused by relative or absolute abstinence from alcohol, usually after a fairly prolonged bout of drinking. Symptoms may begin several hours to several days after cessation of drinking, or in response to a diminished intake of alcohol. These symptoms are due to the cessation of drinking following chronic intoxication, not to vitamin or nutritional deficiencies. The clinical picture may range from benign tremulousness and irritability, to hallucinations and seizures, to life-endangering delirium.

Minor Withdrawal Syndrome

Alcohol withdrawal is most commonly manifested by coarse tremulousness, hyperexcitability, motor restlessness, and gastrointestinal symptoms of nausea and vomiting. Increased autonomic activity results in tachycardia, fever and elevated blood pressure. The severity of the withdrawal symptoms usually depends upon the length of the period of drinking and the quantity of alcohol consumed. Transient alterations of consciousness, nightmares, and shortlived hallucinations may also occur. The majority of these reactions are brief (24–96 hours), and do not progress to delirium tremens.

Supportive treatment consists of minor tranquilizers. Therapeutic dosages of multivitamins, especially Vitamin B1 (thiamin), are frequently given. Thiamin is a specific treatment for Wernicke's disease, which results from thiamin deficiency secondary to chronic alcohol consumption. Considered a neurological disorder, Wernicke's has the symptom triad of ocular abnormalities, ataxia, and delirium. Although the ocular signs and ataxia respond rapidly to thiamin, the delirium is slow to recover. Wernicke's disease may merge into Korsakoff's disease or the alcohol amnestic disorder.

Prevention of delirium tremens and seizures is the goal in treating minor withdrawal states. The patient is also made more comfortable. A safe, useful withdrawal program uses 25 or 50 mg of chlordiazepoxide by mouth every two hours as needed. A single parenteral dose of prochlorperazine or other phenothiazine is useful to control vomiting. Dosage titration during the first 48 hours should aim to keep the heart rate below 100, the blood pressure below 160/100 mmHg, and oral temperature below 99.6 degrees F. Treatment may sometimes have to be extended an additional 48 hours, especially if the patient has been taking other drugs. The benzodiazepines prevent withdrawal seizures and delirium tremens; side effects other than sedation are rare (8).

Acute Alcoholic Hallucinosis

While alterations of consciousness and mixed sensory hallucinations may occur transiently in the milder withdrawal reactions, acute hallucinosis constitutes a distinct clinical entity. It is a "toxic" psychosis in which auditory hallucinations may be the primary—sometimes the only—manifestation. Acute hallucinosis may occur with only relative withdrawal from alcohol, i.e., while the individual is still drinking. In contrast to delirium tremens, the sensorium is clear, other than in judgment and insight. There is no disturbance in intellectual functioning. Recent and remote memory are intact and orientation is unimpaired. Attention and comprehension are normal. The auditory hallucinations are threatening and maligning, and often produce panic-like fear. They sometimes result in the formation of a systematized paranoid delusional system, which motivates the patient to take violent action against his imagined tormentors. Since the first manifestation of illness may sometimes be an assaultive episode, an incorrect functional diagnosis, e.g., paranoid schizophrenia—may be made if the history of an alcoholic bout is not elicited. While it may be possible for this psychosis to persist for weeks following the cessation of drinking, a prolonged course should raise the consideration of an underlying psychotic process.

Hospitalization is necessary to prevent the patient from acting upon his delusions and harming himself or others. Antipsychotic drugs are often used to help the patient gain insight into the nature of his hallucinations.

Delirium Tremens

Delirium tremens is estimated to occur in 10 to 20% of alcoholics who abruptly stop drinking in unsupervised settings. It is a serious medical illness with a mortality of 10 to 15%.

The sine qua non of the syndrome is delirium—a profound alteration in the state of consciousness. Orientation to time, place, person, and situation is severely impaired. Attention span and ability to concentrate are markedly reduced. Recent memory is severely impaired. Judgment and reality-testing markedly deteriorate. There is extreme psychomotor agitation and hyper-excitability, which can progress to exhaustion and hyperthermia. Hallucinations occur in the visual, tactile, olfactory, and, occasionally, auditory spheres. They are bizarre, extremely vivid, threatening, and terrifying. The visual hallucinations, often of bizarre animals and animate objects, are sometimes associated with tactile hallucinations. The patient may report both seeing and feeling insects and other imaginary threatening creatures. Shadows and ordinary items in the room take on a terrifying animation during these delusions; familiar objects and persons are misidentified. Agitation is so severe that sleep is difficult.

The patient's affect and behavior are usually consistent with the content of his hallucinations, i.e., extreme fearfulness and apprehension, even terror. Behavior is erratic, uncontrolled, and often violent. The patient may mistake a fifth story window for a door as he attempts to escape his threatening hallucinations. Occasionally the predominant affect is one of silliness and euphoria.

Physical examination discloses evidence of autonomic nervous system over-activity—flushed facies, injected conjunctivae, dilated pupils, coarse tremor. Pulse is rapid and blood pressure elevated; sweating may be profuse, and there is often an elevation in temperature. Speech may be incoherent or consist of irrational attempts to order the confusing array of perceptual stimuli. Deep tendon reflexes are usually increased, although they may be diminished in the lower extremities if neuropathy is present.

Onset of D.T.'s is usually sudden and may be ushered in by a convulsion or mild prodrome (cf. "Minor Withdrawal Syndrome"). A knowledge of the natural history of the disease is extremely important in treatment. Fifteen percent of cases run their entire course in less than 24 hours, and 80% terminate in less than 72 hours. Fatal outcome may be due to circulatory collapse or hyperthermia; in most reported series, however, deaths are due to intercurrent infections, trauma, or complications of chronic alcoholism.

Treatment of D.T.'s involves sedation, usually with relatively large doses of intravenous diazepam, and careful attention to all physical problems. Alcoholics may normally be fluid overloaded (9) when they stop drinking, but those with D.T.'s may be dehydrated because of vomiting, profuse sweating, and lack of fluid intake. Fluid management is, therefore, also important in the care of these patients.

Coda

Alcohol, the most commonly used drug, has been recognized for centuries for its ability to decrease social inhibitions in small doses. Because of this effect alcohol is popular not only at social functions but also at quasi-social functions such as business meetings. Another property of alcohol, its central nervous system depressant effect, accounts for its use after a tiring day to aid in relaxation. In the non-tolerant person, these effects take place at blood alcohol levels of about 50 mg/dl. This level can be reached with approximately 3 ounces of 80 proof liquor consumed on an empty stomach by a 70 kg man.

As the blood level of alcohol increases, the brain cortex shows effects progressively from frontal lobes to the occipital lobes. At blood levels between 60 and 100 mg/dl there is a progressive loss of judgement and a decrease in motor coordination. At 100 mg/dl the probability of being involved in an automobile accident is increased seven fold over the sober state. (This level is the legal level for driving in most states.) Approximately 5 ounces of 80 proof alcohol will produce this blood level in a 70 kg man.

As the blood alcohol level increases to 150 mg/dl the cerebellum becomes affected and balance becomes difficult. At 300 mg/dl the non-tolerant person is comatose, whereas the alcoholic may still be walking around or driving a car at this blood alcohol level. The LD-50 for alcohol is 500 mg/dl. Death is due to direct effects of alcohol on the brain stem.

The habituated or tolerant person shows all of these effects but at a higher blood alcohol level than in a non-tolerant person. Unfortunately, excessive consumption of alcohol is all too common. Physicians are constantly treating the consequences of alcoholism but not often enough diagnosing the underlying disease.

Increased awareness of the symptoms of alcoholism and the ability to tell others they need help are important skills to be mastered. The task is to stop the consequences of alcoholism.

REFERENCES

1. American Psychiatric Association Task Force on Nomenclature and Statistics: *Diagnostic and Statistical Manual of Mental Disorders* (DSM-III), ed 3. Washington, DC, American Psychiatric Association, 1980.
2. American Medical Association: *Manual on Alcoholism*. Madison, WI, American Medical Association, 1977.
3. Mayfield D, McCleod G, Hall P: The CAGE questionnaire: Validation of a new alcoholism screening instrument. *Am J Psychiatry* 1974;131:1121–1123.
4. Gitlow SE, Peyser HS (eds): *Alcoholism, A Practical Treatment Guide*. New York, Grune & Stratton, 1980.

5. Cloninger CR, Bohman M, Sigvardsson S: Inheritance of alcohol abuse: Cross-fostering analysis of adopted men. *Arch Gen Psychiatry* 1981;38:965–969.

6. Goodwin D: Genetics and alcoholism, presented at World Psychiatric Association, New York City, NY, October 31, 1981.

7. Andreasen NC, Winokur G: Secondary depression: Familial, clinical, and research perspectives. *Am J Psychiatry* 1979;136:62–66.

8. Sellers EM, Kalant H: Alcohol intoxication and withdrawal. *New Engl J Med* 1976; 924:757–762.

9. Knott DH, Beard JD: A diuretic approach to acute withdrawal from alcohol. *South Med J* 1969;62:485–489.

Chapter 21

DRUG ABUSE

RICHARD A. McCORMICK, Ph.D.

INTRODUCTION

As we learn more about the use and abuse of psychoactive substances, we become more aware of the complexity of the phenomena. If we're willing to look closely, all of us have frequent personal and professional encounters with substance use. Aside from being a $60 billion dollar business, substance use has a deep foundation in the history and biology of man. This chapter is a brief overview of the problem and its treatment; its emphasis is on the themes which weave through the phenomenon of substance abuse—complexity and change.

DEFINING THE PROBLEM

The components of the DSM-III (1) definition of substance abuse are:
1. A pattern of pathological use;
2. Impairment in social or occupational functioning caused by the pattern of pathological use;
3. A duration of at least one month to the pattern.
The pathological pattern does not necessarily require daily usage. It may be manifested by repeated, unsuccessful efforts to maintain abstinence or controlled use (1).

Related, but potentially independent, issues are the development of tolerance, where increasing amounts of the substance must be used to obtain the desired effect, or withdrawal, where an observable physical syndrome follows sudden reduction in usage. This separation of the concepts of abuse and dependence underscores the fact that it is possible to abuse a drug for which no tolerance or withdrawal effects have currently been established. This formulation also underscores the subjective factor in drug abuse. Although some chemicals may have properties which increase their abuse potential, acutal abuse is an interaction between the user and the chemical. The World Health Organization (WHO) defines drug dependence as:

> A state, psychic and sometimes also physical, resulting from the inter-
> action between a living organism and a drug, characterized by behavioral
> and other responses that always include a compulsion to take the drug on
> a continuous or periodic basis in order to experience its psychic effects,
> and sometimes to avoid the discomfort of its absence. Tolerance may or
> may not be present. A person may be dependent on more than one drug.

While less pragmatic than DSM-III, this definition clearly underscores both the human-drug interaction and the search for psychoactive effects.

Man's search for psychoactive effects is a common denominator across time and cultures. Societies have historically recognized the potency of this interaction, and have sought to control its impact through rituals and cultural prohibitions. For centuries, Indians inhabiting the Amazon region have ritualized the use of the coca plant. Women powder the coca leaf, mix it with ashes (alkaloid base), and present it to the men. The men suck the powder to produce an energized euphoric experience that lasts for hours, ending in a gradually increasing state of relaxation. The peyote cactus is ritualized by native American Indian tribes; eastern cultures use cannabis derivatives.

The desire for psychoactive experiences is also clear across species. Animal laboratory studies have established that a variety of animals have drug preferences similar to those of humans. Given the choice, rhesus monkeys will self-reinforce themselves with cocaine to a degree detrimental to their health. Mice will work feverishly for opiates. As we learn more about neuroanatomy and neurochemical processes, we see that man's enchantment with psychoactive chemicals has, at least in some cases, a biological base. Man uses chemicals to mimic internal reactions to endogenous substances, such as endorphins.

The current use of psychoactive substances is widespread and ingrained. In a 1975 national sample of young men in their twenties, the National Institute of Drug Abuse found extensive usage of psychoactive drugs (Figure 1) (2). National studies of adolescent drug use show that 4% reported experimental use of marijuana and 3% reported use of other illicit drugs in 1962; by 1980, the figures were 68% for marijuana and 33% for other drugs (3,4).

The age of first use of drugs is decreasing. In 1975, 13% of high school seniors reported that they had first been exposed to marijuana before the eighth grade; by 1979, 23% reported such early exposure. The use of inhalants, often the first drug used, has steadily increased over the past decade in elementary school age children.

FIGURE 1
LIFETIME USE

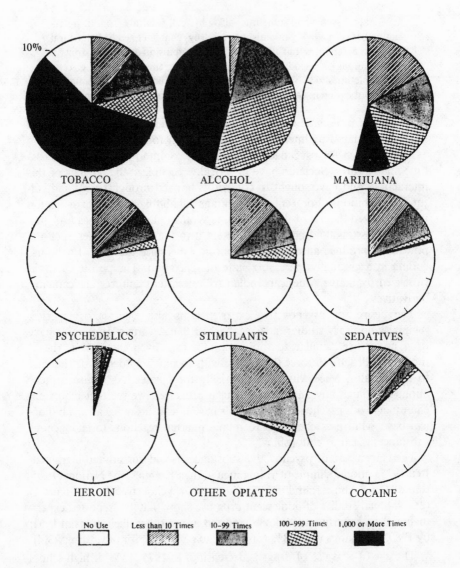

O'Donnel *et al.* "Young Men and Drugs"
NIDA, 1976 (Public Domain)

Evidence of the ingrained use of psychoactive drugs is no further away than the nearest TV set. From an early age we are bombarded by a series of advertisements with a common theme: No matter what your problem is—social, emotional, shyness, acne, unpopularity—there is a chemical over-the-counter solution. The young, shy, unhappy adolescent is converted through the miracle of time lapse TV photography—and an appropriate mouthwash —into a homecoming queen.

Clear cultural controls over the use of psychoactive substances are diluted and replaced by more variable, impersonal, social and legal prohibitions. Individuals who come from subcultures or family systems which have retained strong religious beliefs and traditional values have a lower probability of eventual abuse (5).

A fragmented technological society results in a more stressful environment—ironically, both for those who are and are not successful. Part of the technological ethic is the continual attempt to improve the efficiency and potency of matter. This has led to increasing refinement of naturally occurring psychoactive chemicals and the synthesis of more potent analogues—e.g., shift from wine to distilled spirits; the processing of opium into heroin; the refinement of the coca leaf to cocaine. In general, the greater the refinement of a drug, the higher its abuse potential. This can be accounted for on the basis of psychological and physiological factors. As in the case of the coca leaf, natural psychoactive drugs will generally produce a protracted, slowly rising and slowly subsiding, euphoric experience; cocaine, the refined derivative, will produce a shorter, more abrupt euphoric experience which peaks quickly at a high level and dissipates quickly to a level of dysphoria which is unpleasant. The constant search for the recurring peak euphoria accounts for much of the serious abuser's compulsion for use. The more frequent utilization of large amounts of more potent substances also significantly contributes to the development of physiologic addiction. Once this has occurred, the drive to avoid withdrawal symptoms further solidifies the abuse pattern.

Evidence for a biological predisposition to substance abuse is currently presumptive. Most studies have been in the area of alcoholism, where intergenerational incidence and limited studies of concordance rates in twins reared apart raised the possibility of a limited genetic factor (6). Substance abuse is also common in drug abusers' families of origin (7). Studies on potential metabolic imbalances are provocative, but complicated by difficulties in differentiating the secondary effects of long-term abuse from pre-existing irregularities (8).

The most parsimonious theories of the etiology of substance abuse take into account the interaction of a number of variables, none of which is likely to be sufficient in itself, and none of which, other than exposure to drugs at some point, is likely to be totally necessary. In capsule form, an interactive model may postulate that individuals vary, from birth, in both the stability and absolute level of arousal. Exposure to sufficient stress may further destabilize the individual; the required amount of stress depends upon the organism's original stability. Exposure to psychoactive chemicals, especially at an early age and during a period of destabilization, may result in their being used to compensate for the interactive effects of predisposition and presenting stress. Experimental use may then progress to abuse. The availability of other social supports and options decreases the stress and the probability of dependence upon psychoactive solutions.

PATTERNS OF ABUSE

Information on current patterns of abuse comes primarily from clinical and experimental data on the over 300,000 patients reportedly being treated for drug abuse. This does not include patients being treated for primary alcoholism, since the fields of drug abuse and alcoholism have been historically separate. The rationale behind this dichotomy is quickly being eroded by the trend toward poly-drug abuse. Data from the National Youth Poly-Drug Abuse Study (9) indicated that 86% of teenage abusers regularly used from four to seven different classes of drugs, including alcohol. The rate of serious alcoholism in opiate addicts exceeds 33%, and increases with the age of the addict (10).

The trend toward poly-drug abuse increases the complexity of the substance abuse problem. Poly-drug abusers demonstrate significant rates of diagnosable major psychiatric disorders, including depression (11), cognitive deficits (12), and personality disorders (13). Poly-drug abuse increases the risk of serious complications during withdrawal and the likelihood of accidental overdose (14).

Increased sophistication in the use of drugs to potentiate the desired effects of each other is a significant factor in the trend toward poly-drug abuse. This is exemplified in the increasing use of alcohol by cocaine abusers, to both depress the central nervous system so that cocaine use can continue and alleviate the dysphoria which often follows the cocaine euphoria. The trend toward the use of pharmaceuticals by heroin addicts is another factor. As the quality of street drugs ebbs, addicts turn towards more reliable pharmaceuticals. Addicts use analgesics, such as Dilaudid and Talwin, and pharmaceuticals from different classes, e.g., the stimulant Preludin. Finally, the poly-drug trend is fed by the ingenuity of abusers and entrepreneurs, who are constantly introducing new substances, derivatives, or combinations with desired (and saleable) effects.

The following summaries of abuse patterns for major classes of drugs are reflective of the problem's changing nature.

Analgesics

The quality of street heroin has increased cyclically in the past two years. Heroin of middle-eastern origin and unusual potency is available at comparatively moderate prices. Intravenous injection of good quality heroin produces a "rush," lasting about one minute. Tolerance develops over time, but dissipates following withdrawal; this creates the danger of overdose in the uninformed abuser who attempts to immediately return to prior levels of use.

Among pharmaceuticals, Dilaudid has historically been popular as a drug of abuse. Fentanyl and its street relative three methyl fentanyl ("china white") command high prices. The increased abuse of pentazocine (Talwin) is particularly alarming. Abusers boost the effect of pentazocine with tripelennamine or a variety of other drugs, including Phenergan, Compazine, Ritalin, and Preludin. Pentazocine abusers are often former or current heroin addicts, who also abuse a variety of other drugs (15). The pleasurable sensation is described as more energized than the heroin experience. Medical complications include a high incidence of drug-induced paranoid psychosis, probably due to the Talwin, and convulsions, probably secondary to overuse of tripelennamine. Alcohol abuse among opiate addicts can adversely affect treatment outcome and increase the probability of liver disease. Death rates are also higher among addicts who are problem drinkers.

Psychostimulants

Production quotas imposed by the Controlled Substances Act of 1970 have had a significant impact upon the availability of illicit amphetamines. Despite this fact, the abuse of psychostimulants has sharply risen in the past few years. Methylphenidate (Ritalin) and phenmetrazine (Preludin) are frequently diverted and abused, often in conjunction with analgesics. The use and abuse of cocaine has skyrocketed. The Drug Enforcement Agency estimates street sales of illicit cocaine in excess of $35 billion dollars per year, surpassing dollar sales for marijuana. Studies of patients in treatment (16) and recreational use (17) show increases, by a factor of three to seven times, in cocaine use and abuse during the past five years, with use being highest among young adults and students. Street cocaine sells for about $100–$200 per gram. Considering that a gram will yield between 50 to 100 "lines" or "coke spoons" for snorting, the popular conception that cocaine is strictly a rich man's drug is erroneous.

Serious abuse had primarily been restricted to intravenous cocaine hydrochloride. The recent popularity of kits which convert cocaine hydrochloride into ionized cocaine (freebase) has significantly contributed to the expansion of abuse. Once converted, freebase is either smoked or vaporized and inhaled. The result is a sudden intense euphoria which quickly subsides, generally leaving the user feeling irritable or dysphoric. The use of freebase is more likely to become compulsive than snorting cocaine, as the user seeks repeated rushes to avoid the after effects. Heavy freebase abusers may consume 20 to 50 grams or more a week. The development of a toxic psychosis, characterized by quickly developing suspiciousness, restlessness, and paranoia—very similar in character to amphetamine psychosis—is possible. Cocaine-related medical emergencies and deaths, generally from cardio-respiratory arrest, are steadily rising.

Sedatives and Hypnotics

Sedatives and hypnotics remain popular drugs of use and abuse, especially for the poly-drug abuser. They represent the clearest medical danger to the abuser. As tolerance develops, the difference between a psychologically satisfying and a lethal dose diminishes. The unpredictable synergistic effects of combinations of sedatives, including alcohol, further enhances the possibility of accidental overdose. Withdrawal symptoms from sedatives are potentially life-threatening.

The recent resurgence in the availability, misuse, and abuse of methaqualone (18,19) is particularly alarming. Educating physicians and pharmacists about the abuse potential of methaqualone has resulted in a decline in diversion through these sources. This has been more than offset, however, by increases in "counterfeit" pharmaceuticals, originating from European bulk producers or clandestine laboratories. Storefront "stress clinics" in some metropolitan areas have also been implicated in diversion of true pharmaceuticals. Counterfeit pharmaceuticals carry the added hazard of variability in potency and purity. This is particularly critical since the most common consumer of street methaqualone is the young, often somewhat naive, student. Wide variations in counterfeit methaqualone can result in accidental overdose for the consumer who unexpectedly receives a truly potent batch.

Controversy continues over the abuse potential of the benzodiazapenes (20,21). Considering their heavy utilization, the incidence of serious, singular abuse is certainly low. They are, however, often used by the poly-drug abuser, including the young, poly-drug abusing, primary alcoholic. Due to their sedative properties, they can significantly complicate the withdrawal process when they are used by alcohol abusers.

Phencyclidine

Following four years of steady increases, the use of phencyclidine (PCP) has apparently peaked; however, levels of use and abuse remain high. PCP was originally developed as an anesthetic. The brand name Seranyl was chosen because of the serene effect the drug has on animals, but its effects were too unpredictable for use with humans. The fact that PCP is easily and inexpensively synthesized accounts for its high availability and attractiveness, especially to naive youthful users. Adverse publicity has tarnished the drug's image, except among long-time sophisticated users. Because of its enormous advantage to the supplier, the drug still appears commonly in counterfeit pharmaceuticals and adulterated "look alike" capsules. It also remains a factor in the adulteration of low grade marijuana.

As with any drug which loosens perceptual processes, the effect of PCP is highly variable and heavily related to the user's mental set and the setting in which the drug is taken. Users report euphoria of an excitatory nature, hallucinations, and intense experiences of timelessness and isolation. The words of one regular, sophisticated user characterized the variety of possible effects: "Sometimes I use it to escape, sometimes just to have fun. It can do both." Contrary to the reports of long-time users who report minimal negative experiences, the documented incidence of severe adverse reactions to the drug continues to mount (22,23). Such reactions include severe agitation, aggressiveness, and drug-induced paranoid states, at times followed in a matter of weeks by severe depression. The shift from a positive to a negative experience can be sudden and insidious. Severe, life-threatening adverse reactions, such as coma and respiratory arrest, are related to large doses and chronic abuse. It is not uncommon, however, for the drug-induced psychosis to be associated with limited use. PCP and its metabolites remain stored in the body's fatty tissue. Release over time helps account for flashbacks, which are reported up to 30 days following use and are coincidental with the reappearance of metabolites in the urine.

Abuse of PCP is most often part of a poly-drug abuse pattern. Other disassociative anesthetics, such as Ketamine, are beginning to appear in the illicit market.

Inhalants

A recent comparative analysis of 162 inhalant users confirms earlier clinical impressions that they tend to be at risk for suicidal and violent behavior, exhibit cognitive deficits, are young (under age 17), and cut across all socioeconomic levels (24). Inhaling hydrocarbons, nitrous oxide, alkane gases, or toluene can lead to cardiac arrhythmias and death, often among very young (ages 13–16) individuals (25). Long-term inhalant abusers will often experiment with any available mind-altering substance.

Over-the-Counter Medication

Preparations containing non-controlled stimulants or depressants are commonly utilized by young users and abusers. These medications often contain the same ingredients as "look-alike" pills, which are sold as imitations of prescription pharmaceuticals. They generally contain non-prescription stimulants, such as caffeine or ephedrine, or mildly sedating substances such as antihistamines. Rare cases of drug-induced psychosis from over-the-counter medications have been reported. These include paranoid reactions from constant compulsive use of phenylephrine (Neo-synephrine) (26), Vicks Sinex, and Vapo-Rub (27).

TREATMENT APPROACHES

The 1970s marked the beginning of a new era in drug abuse treatment. Prior to the mid-1960s, awareness of the nature, scope, and prevalence of drug abuse was limited and funding for treatment was meager. Media coverage of potential drug abuse problems in returning Vietnam veterans, and awareness of the growing incidence of drug abuse among youth from all social classes, resulted in an unprecedented influx of resources into drug abuse treatment.

In addition to devising new treatments for drug abusers, treatments which had been utilized with other populations were transferred, with some modification, to this area of concern. Drug abuse treatment has now stabilized, and emphasis has shifted to the matching of treatment approaches with the patient's particular needs.

Patients generally appear for treatment only after their problems have reached crisis proportions. Problems of often staggering complexity are subsumed under the rubric of drug abuse. The patient may present with a combination of serious physical dependency, fractured interpersonal relationships and supports, no legal means of financial support, legal difficulties, and co-existing, diagnosable psychiatric conditions.

Effective treatment requires a comprehensive program of treatment and rehabilitation which will impact simultaneously or sequentially on all the patient's major needs and deficits. Specific interventions must complement and build upon each other. This section will outline some of the major treatment components of a comprehensive multimodal program. The core of such a program, analogous to the frame which holds together the working pieces, is a highly structured, action-oriented approach to the problem. Patients entering treatment are generally unable to effectively order their lives and act with due regard for the long-term consequences of their behavior. Program structure provides needed initial support in this regard.

Patients with heavy patterns of abuse will generally require the structure of an initial residential treatment stay. The use of explicit rules and behavioral contracting, combined with a specific schedule of mandatory activities and continual monitoring of compliance, imposes a structure which is gradually relaxed as the patient progresses and moves toward greater personal responsibility. There is a strong expectation that the patient will try new behaviors, and the system provides an immediate reward, i.e., peer approval, for complying with this expectation.

When an established residential substance abuse program is not available, ambulatory programs must capitalize on environmental opportunities for structuring and organizing treatment plans. Pharmacological interventions should be handled conservatively. A strong attempt should be made to involve the family in the treatment planning, implementation, and monitoring.

The first step in rehabilitation is the establishment of motivation for treatment. Rationalization and avoidance of responsibility are characteristic of the drug abuser. Initial motivation for treatment is usually the result of external pressure. Influential persons, including primary care practitioners, can play an important role in confronting the abuser with the legal, social, and physical consequences of continued abuse. The marshalling of such pressures through family-action techniques, where the patient's family, friends, and, in some cases, employer directly confront the patient's denial and manipulation in an organized meeting, is often necessary for success.

Detoxification

The gradual withdrawal from an addictive substance represents a critical step in the drug abuser's overall treatment and rehabilitation. Technical competence and caution are necessary to minimize physical discomfort and safeguard against physiological complications which may be life-threatening. Even the most technically sound detoxification, however, will generally be wasted if the procedure is not integrated into a long-term plan for reducing the patient's dependence on drugs of abuse. Decisions such as the rate of detoxification and the setting (inpatient vs. outpatient) must be consistent with factors such as the patient's history of treatment failures, progress in rehabilitation efforts, cross addictions, and social supports.

While the physician must rely on the patient's subjective report, both in establishing an initial data base and making adjustments during the detoxification process, it is important to utilize other sources for verifying or substantiating information. These will include:

1. Signs of withdrawal or intoxication;
2. Reports of other treatment personnel on psychological status and behavior;
3. Urinalysis for drug screening;
4. Presence of fresh needle marks;
5. Reports from significant others.

A continuing effort must be made to educate the patient about the importance of providing truthful reports during the detoxification process. A patient's personal agenda may cause him to either exaggerate or minimize drug usage. For example, a patient may exaggerate in order to maintain a euphoric state, or out of fear of excessive discomfort during the detoxification process. Patients may also exaggerate usage in order to maintain an image of importance and stature in the drug sub-culture. Patients may minimize their use of drugs to avoid external consequences from program rules or law enforcement sources. Even when the patient provides truthful information, it must be remembered that there is a large psychological component to the patient's perception of changes during the detoxification period. Data from other sources can aid the physician in sorting out the physical and psychological aspects of the patient's report.

A thorough physical exam should include sensitivity to conditions which may be masked by the ongoing analgesic effects of daily psychoactive drug use. The National Institute of Drug Abuse (28) recommends that the initial evaluation include:

1. A thorough drug and alcohol abuse history;
2. Complete information on current use of medically prescribed drugs to assess potential synergistic effects;
3. Special attention to possible renal, liver, and dermatologic complications of addiction;
4. Pulmonary and cardiovascular abnormalities;
5. Serological test for syphilis;
6. Obstetrical evaluation and test for pregnancy.

It is beyond the scope of this chapter to provide complete technical instructions on detoxification from all the drugs of abuse. Summary information will be provided on the most common classes of drugs requiring detoxification. Full technical details are available in the earlier referenced *National Institute of Drug Abuse Detoxification Treatment Manual.*

Opiate Detoxification

The patient abusing narcotics may be utilizing any combination of street heroin, illicit methadone, pharmaceutical morphine, codeine, Dilaudid, Talwin, or other analgesics, depending upon fluctuating availability factors. While generally not life-threatening, withdrawal symptoms are very aversive. They include nausea, cramps, muscular pain, and spasms. Symptoms generally diminish within ten days to three weeks, but heavy, long-time abusers report continuing anxiety, weakness, and aches for months following detoxification.

The history of opiate detoxification, dating back to the late 19th century, includes the use of opiates, such as heroin and methadone; other pharmaceuticals, including propoxyphene and propranalol; a host of procedures, including Vitamin C, acupuncture, and ECT. At present, methadone substitution is the most common approach, except in specific conditions where the use of clonidine is gaining favor.

Methadone has the general advantage of being a longer acting drug. This limits fluctuations in blood level and accompanying problems with withdrawal symptoms. It also facilitates detoxification on an ambulatory basis, since patients can generally tolerate a regimen of one dose per 24 hours. Beginning with a daily oral dosage of 10 to 20 mg, the dosage is adjusted until the patient seems stable. While reductions can occur at a rate of 15 to 20 percent of the daily dose, there is evidence to support as slow a detoxification as circumstances permit. FDA regulations require that detoxification be completed within 21 days, unless the patient meets the criteria for methadone maintenance. Patients who have been stabilized on methadone maintenance as part of a comprehensive drug abuse rehabilitation program do best with very gradual withdrawal, progressing at a rate of 3% per week—if possible, on a blind basis. The rate of slow withdrawal should be carefully coordinated with other information on treatment progress.

Originally developed as a possible nasal decongestant, and subsequently utilized as a treatment for hypertension, clonidine has recently shown promise as a detoxification agent for opiates (29). By suppressing noradrenergic activity, primarily in the locus coeruleus, clonidine greatly reduces withdrawal symptoms; however, patients still report insomnia, lethargy, and instability. Clonidine is administered in low doses (daily dosage of 0.3 to 1.2 mg on a t.i.d. or q.i.d. schedule) with careful attention to the drug's hypotensive effect. Detoxification should be accomplished within 14 days, since the drug's efficacy in alleviating withdrawal begins to decrease after that time. Clonidine has the benefit of being a non-addicting non-opiate which can be given outside of a structured methadone program. Perhaps the greatest potential use for clonidine is in easing the transition of selected patients from opiates to opiate antagonist treatment. Because clonidine does not act at the opiate receptors, changes which occur at these receptors have a chance to normalize during the detoxification process. This allows for a smooth transition to Naltrexone, without the intervening no-treatment period of seven to ten days needed to change a patient from methadone to the antagonist. Current research is exploring the use of lofexidine, a structural analog of clonidine which seems to have fewer side effects.

Sedative-Hypnotic Detoxification

Detoxification from depressants is complicated by the increasing tendency for abusers to use a variety of drugs with sedative properties. The major symptoms of withdrawal are similar for barbiturates, methaqualone, the benzodiazepines, and the other less commonly abused sedative-hypnotics. Symptoms vary, depending upon the specific drug abused, length of abuse, and individual differences in clients. They include tremulousness, irritability, anxiety, insomnia, cramps, and nausea. Grand mal seizures, which may occur between the third and seventh day of abrupt withdrawal, are observed in most patients who have been using over 900 mg of short-acting barbiturates per day for a matter of weeks, and in some patients maintaining smaller habits. Delirium has been observed, generally around the fourth day of abstinence, in high level abusers. Major withdrawal symptoms are generally observed in patients using methaqualone at dosages exceeding 600 mg daily, or valium in daily dosages exceeding 60 mg. There are less frequent observations of major withdrawal symptoms following abrupt withdrawal from long-standing therapeutic doses of benzodiazepines; symptoms may not appear until weeks after cessation of use.

Detoxification from sedative-hypnotics should normally be conducted on an inpatient basis, where close observation and medical supervision are readily available. While outpatient programs for successful detoxification have been reported, they require daily close contacts with the patient and utilization of family or volunteers for close supervision and information feedback to the treatment staff (30).

The most commonly accepted detoxification procedure calls for substituting a comparable dose of phenobarbital, a long-acting barbiturate, for the drugs of abuse. Thirty mg of phenobarbital is substituted for each 100 mg of secobarbital or pentobarbital, or for each 300 mg of methaqualone. The physician must rely on the patient's report in establishing the initial daily dose, bearing in mind the tendency of patients to overstate or understate their usage patterns. The upper limit of the initial daily dosage should generally not exceed 400 mg, and in no case exceed 600 mg. The total daily dosage is generally divided into three doses. The patient is observed over the first few days for signs of intoxication or withdrawal symptoms, and the daily dose is adjusted to a stabilizing level. The dosage is then reduced by 10% or 30 mg each day. The procedure should not be rushed. A dose of 200 mg I.M. is immediately given if withdrawal signs occur and the daily dosage is readjusted to 25% more than the current level. Detoxification from the benzodiazepines can generally be accomplished using the drug of abuse, since they have longer lasting effects.

Additional Detoxification Procedures

As noted previously, it is increasingly common for patients to abuse multiple drugs. Since the withdrawal symptoms of opiates and sedatives overlap, it is not advisable to attempt simultaneous withdrawal of the two classes of drugs. Generally, the patient should be stabilized on opiates and first withdrawn from the sedative-hypnotics. The procedure can be reversed if clinical conditions make it more advisable to first proceed with opiate withdrawal. Caution must be taken with patients who are seriously abusing alcohol as well as other drugs. Fifteen mg of phenobarbital for each ounce of alcohol consumed daily should be added to the initial calculation in sedative detoxification. In mixed alcohol/opiate dependent patients, withdrawal from alcohol should proceed first, generally utilizing Librium.

Withdrawal from stimulants and other commonly abused drugs, such as phencyclidine, will generally be addressed in the clinical setting as an addendum to the management of adverse reactions to their concentrated abuse. Protracted abuse of stimulants may precipitate an acute paranoid psychosis. The psychosis develops through stages of unusual attention to details, hypervigilance, increasing suspiciousness, and, ultimately, gross distortion in perception, agitation, and hallucinations. In this psychotic state, the patient may be assaultive, striking out in what he perceives as a necessary self-defense. Withdrawal is managed by placing the patient into an environment low in stimulation, and providing continuing reassurance, opportunity for sleep, and adequate nourishment. Moderate doses of haloperidol can be used with severely agitated patients, but should be reduced as soon as target symptoms subside.

Phencyclidine toxicity can result in highly variable symptomatology, which seems only partially dosage-related. High dosages may result in coma or convulsions. Once vital functions have been stabilized, the amount of phencyclidine in the system can be reduced through urine acidification and, if clinically indicated, gastric suction. In patients who are not comatose, management is similar to that employed with stimulants, i.e., isolation, reassurance, reduction of stimulation, and moderate dosages of haloperidol. Although the toxic psychosis resulting from phencyclidine use is more common in the chronic user, it has been observed in first time users. Paranoia, auditory and visual hallucinations, and highly erratic, potentially destructive behavior are possible. The toxic psychosis will generally subside within seven days, often sooner. Observation should extend beyond the immediate cessation of symptomatology, since symptoms may plateau and suddenly recur within a matter of hours.

Withdrawal from stimulants or phencyclidine may result in a severe rebound depression, which frequently occurs days after other symptoms have subsided. Since suicidal ideation may accompany this depression, it is imperative to monitor the patient or notify significant others following withdrawal.

Psychotherapy and Counseling

The drug abuser is characteristically responsive to peer group pressure and support. Group psychotherapy can be an effective means of eliminating defensiveness and reestablishing trust and adaptive interpersonal behaviors. In order to survive in the drug culture, many drug abusers learn to interact in a guarded, manipulative, and shallow manner. Effective social skills which may have existed prior to heavy drug use are often eroded by the drug abuser's need to deny and lie to those closest to him or her. A significant number of drug abusers never really develop the ability to form effective, enduring relationships; they may, in fact, have entered into chemical euphoria to escape from these unmet needs. As the group grapples with issues of trust and establishing closer relationships with people, a flurry of defensive activity—especially deflection to non-personal issues—can be expected. The group will have to deal with certain recurring themes, including depression, the expression of anger, personal control, and responsibility.

Continuous supportive counseling is advised in most cases of abuse. More intense psychotherapy should be selectively applied; this is particularly important with poly-drug abusers and others who have significant, concomitant emotional problems. While outcome research on the efficacy of individual psychotherapy as a treatment component is limited, preliminary controlled studies (31) indicate improved functioning for patients undergoing psychotherapy as part of a well-conceived treatment plan.

Family Therapy

There has been a surge of interest in the use of family therapy with drug abusers. A recent National Institute of Drug Abuse survey indicated that 69% of existing treatment programs provide some family therapy. This is an interesting and potentially beneficial departure from the earlier concentration on forming an exclusive "new family" for the patient within the treatment programs. Significant family involvement in treatment enhances the opportunities for structured, experiential problem-solving and emotional growth.

The drug abuser's family of origin is likely to display certain common characteristics. Minimal display of physical affection, especially on the part of the father, is striking. Although the family usually cares about the child, there is an inability to communicate caring; this may signify parental insensitivity to the child's emotional needs. It is not uncommon for one or both parents to have substance abuse problems.

The expression of anger in some families is often erratic and unpredictable. When the parent is abusing alcohol or other sedatives, the outbursts may be accompanied by physical abuse. Passive-aggressive behavior, which is not uncommon in these families, destroys meaningful communication, and must be addressed in the course of family therapy. The addict has lied and deceived family members to support his or her habit. Frustration is inherent in the relapses of the addictive cycle. Hope and trust are rekindled and extinguished over the course of years, each time increasing the anger of family members.

The drug abuser, and the recurrent crisis he or she creates, may be the force that has been keeping the family intact. Family therapy must consider implicit family pressures to maintain the patient's problem. Parents may attempt to use the addict as a scapegoat, by holding him responsible for all the turmoil in the family.

The increasing numbers of multi-family group treatment approaches offer special advantages as either a supplement to, or substitute for, individual family therapy. The multi-family group can provide family members with a needed source of support, and help soften the impact of the disruption associated with a drug abusing family member. In addition to sharing their frustrations in an accepting environment, families realize that their experience is not entirely unique. A mix of families with regard to the number of times the identified patient has relapsed and sought treatment helps people accept the chronic nature of the rehabilitation process. Families, especially those of young abusers, learn to keep their expectations within reasonable bounds without losing hope for eventual long-range changes.

Having other patients as allies in a group of families can diffuse a patient's defensiveness and permit confrontations not possible in individual family therapy. Family members can often deal with their guilt, which is associated with the patient's problems, and receive support and practical feedback.

A recent major outcome study on family therapy with the drug abuser documents the effectiveness of this modality (32).

Pharmacological Interventions

Pharmacological supports can play an important role beyond detoxification in the total treatment and rehabilitation of selected substance abusers. Their initial and continued benefits must be weighed against their potential hazard in a population already identified as having chemical dependency and misuse problems. Their effectiveness will be a direct function of the appropriateness of their match to a particular patient's problems, as well as the overall structure and comprehensiveness of the treatment approach.

Narcotic Maintenance: Methadone, a long-acting synthetic narcotic, is utilized as a substitute for illicit narcotics by over 100,000 addicts in treatment. This modality is only available in programs authorized by the F.D.A., which also limits the use of methadone maintenance to patients seriously addicted to opiates. In the past, doses in excess of 100 mg a day were commonly used in an effort to "blockade" any additional euphoria from heroin use. The trend in recent years has been toward the use of more moderate dosages (30–60 mg). While many patients can be effectively stabilized on moderate dosages, which certainly facilitates eventual withdrawal, available research still supports the relative advantage of higher dosages, especially in the early stages of treatment (33). The efficacy of a methadone maintenance program for a particular patient depends upon a number of variables, which interact with the absolute dose of medication and vary over time. The variables include:

1. The patient's need for the structure imposed by frequent clinic visits, concomitant counseling, and urine surveillance;
2. Quality of "competing" street drugs;
3. Level of motivation;
4. Methadone's possible psychotropic effect in reducing aggressiveness and anxiety, and the patient's current need for such psychotropic effects (34).

Even rehabilitated patients who are free of illicit drugs, gainfully employed, and stabilized on very low dosages (5–20 mg), experience great difficulty when they attempt to totally withdraw from methadone. In these cases, the methadone may be filling a psychological need for security. It has also been hypothesized that these patients represent a sub-set of narcotic addicts with some endorphin-related imbalance, who are returned to a stable physiological state by small amounts of narcotics. This imbalance may either precede addiction or be secondary to long-term opiate use which has depleted the endorphin reserve.

Patients are initially seen daily. Depending upon program rules and prevailing state law, they may receive take-home doses as they progress through methadone maintenance treatment. Moderate dosages of methadone are generally tolerated well by patients in stable treatment regimens.

Methadylacetate (LAAM), a long-acting narcotic substitute is being investigated for use with narcotic addicts (35). LAAM is generally administered three times per week, which allows fewer visits to the clinic without necessitating take-home dosages. It is hoped that this will offset the increasing diversion of methadone into the illicit market, and the accompanying increase in methadone-related medical emergencies. Most patients have tolerated LAAM as well as methadone, and recent research indicates that adequate doses of LAAM are comparable in outcome to the higher doses of methadone (36). Propoxyphene (Darvon-N) has also been utilized for the maintenance of narcotic addicts, but has not been found as effective as methadone (37).

Naltrexone. Naltrexone, a long-acting, orally effective narcotic antagonist with no agonist qualities, is being investigated as a pharmacological support for maintaining abstinence from opiates. By blocking access of opiates to receptor sites, it prevents the addict from experiencing euphoria following narcotic use; some immediate rush may still be experienced. Naltrexone is generally administered over 5-7 days in increasing dosages to attain a maintenance dose of 100 mg every Monday and Wednesday, and 150 mg every Friday. Side effects seem minimal at these dosages (38). Because naltrexone will displace opiates at the receptor, the patient must be totally withdrawn from opiates to prevent immediate, aversive withdrawal symptoms. The difficulty in keeping most addicts drug-free for seven to ten days following the last detoxification dose of methadone has limited naltrexone's usefulness. The use of clonidine as a detoxification agent minimizes this problem and may expand the usefulness of naltrexone (39).

Research studies clearly establish that adequate dosages of naltrexone significantly decrease the use of opiates, but most addicts will discontinue use early in treatment (40). Naltrexone treatment is significantly correlated with long-term abstinence only when the patient remains in treatment for at least 12 weeks. The retention of the addict in naltrexone treatment and subsequent opiate-free status are related to the overall comprehensiveness of the treatment program. Naltrexone patients engaged in a "high intervention" program, including individual and group therapies, remained on medication over four times as long as other patients, and were significantly more likely to be opiate free on follow-up (41). Sixty percent of naltrexone patients in multiple-family therapy remained on medication for more than three months, versus 20% of those not in therapy (42).

Pharmacological Intervention for the Poly-Drug Abuser. Traditional abstinence-minded approaches are often not effective in treating the individualized problems of the poly-drug abuser. In addition to providing an escape, drug usage may be an attempt to self-medicate for underlying psychopathology. Consequently, there is an increasing need for differential diagnosis and flexible use of psychoactive drugs in a controlled, structured manner. Careful evaluation for signs of depression or psychosis is especially critical following detoxification from the primary drug of abuse.

Antabuse should be considered for drug abusers with serious alcohol abuse problems. Antabuse has successfully been administered to patients on methadone maintenance with no adverse reactions and no altering of the methadone's effect (43).

Developing New Skills and Interests

Using and procuring drugs becomes an all-consuming activity which provides most of an abuser's pleasure and financial support. In order to succeed in maintaining abstinence or control, a patient must acquire new means of support and satisfaction. Abstinence is partially a function of the abuser's ability to establish a sound, rewarding base of financial support. Many abusers must put aside an exciting, challenging style of procuring money, which has been heavily supported by the peer group and at least intermittently successful, in favor of a less stimulating, albeit more stable, job or training program—which the patient may not experience as very rewarding. The patient may also have fears of not being able to succeed at a particular vocational endeavor. Vocational counseling and placement services can play a critical role in helping to break the addictive cycle. Specific training in the skills necessary to find work, and ongoing support throughout the frustrations inherent in looking for work, are often necessary. The patient and therapist often assume that the competence and salesmanship which abusers display in their "hustles" can be transferred to seeking and finding employment. In fact, may abusers have very inadequate basic job-finding skills.

The abuser needs to learn new ways to deal with daily life stressors. For most abusers, abstaining from psychoactive drugs means giving up their solitary means of stress management. Learning methods for managing stress which rely on the use of personal resources also allows the abuser to experience success in self-control. Programs of relaxation training, biofeedback-assisted stress management, meditation, and physical exercise can be effective adjuncts to the treatment process.

Using drugs is an exciting and highly pleasurable activity. The abuser, particularly the young, active abuser, often needs assistance in developing new interests to fill part of the void created by abstinence. Exposing the patient to other thrill-seeking or mastery activities, such as mountain climbing, skydiving, or competitive sports, has been successful in some cases. Selected patients may require other special interventions, such as sexual counseling and assertiveness training.

SUMMARY

Changing patterns of abuse, in particular the trend towards poly-drug abuse, have made the treatment of the substance abuser an increasingly complex task. When treatment is comprehensive and properly matched to the problems of the patient, a respectable level of success is possible. In a carefully controlled follow-up study of heroin addicts, between 54 and 63% of patients completing comprehensive treatment were drug-free at one-year follow-up, as compared with 35% who received only detoxification. The first group also had fewer arrests and better school or work attendance (44). While follow-up studies are certainly important, they only tell part of the story. They sample a slice of time in what is usually a long-term recovery process marked by repeated regressions. Although this long process can be frustrating for patients and treatment personnel, the data do support the position that substance abuse is treatable, and has a generally good prognosis for long-term success with appropriate treatment.

REFERENCES

1. American Psychiatric Association Committee on Nomenclature and Statistics: *Diagnostic and Statistical Manual of Mental Disorders,* ed 3. Washington, DC, American Psychiatric Association, 1980.
2. O'Donnell JA, Voss HL, Clayton RR, et al.: *Young Men and Drugs—A Nationwide Survey.* Washington, DC, National Institute of Drug Abuse, 1976.
3. Miller JD: *Epidemiology of Drug Abuse Among Adolescents.* National Institute of Drug Abuse Research Monograph Series, No 38, 1980, pp 25–38.
4. Pandina RJ, White HR: Patterns of alcohol and drug use in adolescent students and adolescents in treatment. *J Stud Alcohol* 1981;42:441–456.
5. Rausch GC, Thompson WD, Berberian RM: Psychoactive medicinal and nonmedicinal drug use among high school students. *Pediatrics* 1980;66:709–715.
6. Goodwin D: *Is Alcoholism Hereditary?* New York, Oxford University Press, 1976.
7. Fauman MA, Fauman BJ: *The Psychiatric Aspects of Chronic Phencyclidine Use: A Study of Chronic PCP Users.* National Institute of Drug Abuse Research Monograph Series, vol 21, 1978, pp 183–200.
8. Gold MS, Pattash AL, Extein I, et al.: Evidence for an endorphin dysfunction in methadone addicts: Lack of ACTH response to naloxone. *Drug Alcohol Depend* 1981;8:257–262.
9. Beschner GM, Friedman AS: *Youth Drug Abuse. Lexington, MA, Lexington Books, 1979.*
10. Rounsaville BJ, Weissman MM, Kleber HD: *The significance of alcoholism in treated opiate addicts. J Nerv Ment Dis* 1981;170:479–488.
11. Rounsaville BJ, Weissman MM, Kleber H, et al.: Heterogeneity of psychiatric diagnosis in treated opiate addicts. *Arch Gen Psychiatry* 1982;39:161–166.
12. Grant I, Adams K, Corlin A, et al.: The collaborative neuropsychological study of polydrug abusers. *Arch Gen Psychiatry* 1978;35:1063–1074.
13. Lachar D, Gdowski C, Keegan J: MMPI Profiles of men alcoholics, drug addicts and psychiatric patients. *J Stud Alcohol* 1979;40:45–56.
14. Gottschalk LA, McGuire FL, Heiser JF, et al.: *Drug Abuse Deaths in Nine Cities: A Survey Report.* National Institute of Drug Abuse Research Monograph Series, no 29, 1980, pp 1–172.
15. Lahmeyer HW, Steingold RG: Medical and psychiatric complications of pentazocine and tripelennamine abuse. *J Clin Psychiatry* 1980;41:275–278.
16. Gay GR: You've come a long way baby! Coke time for the new American lady of the eighties. *J Psychoactive Drugs* 1981;13:297–318.
17. Smart RG, Liban C, Brown G: Cocaine use among adults and students. *Can J Public Health* 1981;72:433–438.
18. Smith DE: West coast and east coast drug abuse patterns, 1979–80. *Ann NY Acad Sci* 1981;362:22–28.
19. Gonzolez ER: Methaqualone abuse implicated in injuries, deaths nationwide. *JAMA* 1981;246:813–819.
20. Smith RJ: Study finds sleeping pills overprescribed. *Science* 1979;204:287–288.
21. Marks J: *The Benzodiazepines—Use, Overuse, Misuse, Abuse.* Lancaster, England, MTP Press Ltd, 1978.
22. Barton CH, Sterling ML, Vazire ND: Phencyclidine intoxication: Clinical experience in 27 cases confirmed by urine assay. *Ann Emerg Med* 1981;10:243–246.
23. Rappolt RT, Gay GR, Farris RD: Phencyclidine (PCP) intoxication: Diagnosis in stages and algorithms of treatment. *Clin Toxicol* 1980;16:509–529.

24. Korman M, Trimboli F, Semler I: A comparative evaluation of 162 inhalant users. *Addict Behav* 1980;5:143-152.

25. Garriott J, Petty CS: Death from inhalant abuse: Toxicological and pathological evaluation of 34 cases. *Clin Toxicol* 1980;16:305-315.

26. Snow SS, Logan TP, Hollender MH: Nasal spray 'addiction' and psychosis: A case report. *Br J Psychiatry* 1980;136:297-299.

27. Blackwood GW: Severe psychological disturbance resulting from abuse of nasal decongestants. *Scott Med J* 1982;27:175-176.

28. Czechowicz D: *Detoxification Treatment Manual*. Washington, DC, National Institute of Drug Abuse, 1978.

29. Gold MS, Pottash AL, Sweeney DR, *et al.*: Clonidine hydrochloride: A nonopiate treatment for opiate withdrawal. National Institute of Drug Abuse Research Monograph Series, no 27, 1979, pp 233-239.

30. Hawthorne JW, Zabora JR, D'Lugoff BC: Outpatient detoxification of patients addicted to sedative-hypnotics and anxiolytics. *Drug Alcohol Depend* 1982;9:143-151.

31. Woody G, O'Brien CP, McLellan AT, *et al.*: Psychotherapy for opiate addiction: Some preliminary results. *Ann NY Acad Sci* 1981;362:91-100.

32. Stanton MD: *The Family Therapy of Drug Abuse and Addiction*. New York, Guilford Press, 1981.

33. Goldstein A, Judson BA: Efficacy and side effects of three widely different methadone doses, in *Proceeding of the Fifth National Conference on Methadone Treatment*. New York, National Association for Prevention of Addiction to Narcotics, 1973, pp 21-44.

34. Siassi J, Angle B, Alston D: Comparison of the effect of high and low doses of methadone on treatment outcome. *Int J Addict* 1977;12:993-1005.

35. Ling W, Klett CJ, Gillis RD: A cooperative clinical study of methadyl acetate. *Arch Gen Psychiatry* 1978;35:345-353.

36. Whysner,JA, Thomas DB, Ling W, *et al.*: *On The Relative Efficacy of LAAM and Methadone*. National Institute of Drug Abuse Research Monograph Series, no 27, 1979, pp 429-434.

37. Woody GE, Mintz J, Tennant F, *et al.*: *Usefulness of Propoxyphene Napsylate for Maintenance Treatment of Narcotic Addiction*. National Institute of Drug Abuse Research Monograph Series, no 27, 1979, pp 240-246.

38. Report of the National Research Council Committee on the Clinical Evaluation of Narcotic Antagonists: Clinical evaluation of naltrexone treatment of opiate dependent individuals. *Arch Gen Psychiatry* 1978;35:335-340.

39. Washton AM, Resnick RB: Outpatient opiate detoxification with clonidine. *J Clin Psychiatry* 1982;43:39-41.

40. Judson BA, Carney TM, Goldstein A: Naltrexone treatment of heroin addiction, efficacy and safety in a double blind dosage comparison. *Drug Alcohol Depend* 1981;7:325-346.

41. Resnick RB, Washton AM, Stone-Washton N: *Psychotherapy and Naltrexone in Opiod Dependence*. National Institute of Drug Abuse Research Monograph Series, no 34, 1980, pp 109-115.

42. Anton RF, Hogan I, Jalali B, *et al.*: Multiple family therapy and naltrexone in the treatment of opiate dependence. *Drug Alcohol Depend* 1981;8:157-168.

43. Tong TG, Benowitz NL, Kreek MJ: Methadone-disulfiram interaction during methadone maintenance. *J Clin Pharmacol* 1980;20:506-513.

44. Bale RN, Van Stone WW, Kuldau JM, *et al.*: Therapeutic communities versus methadone maintenance. A prospective controlled study of narcotic addiction treatment: Design and one-year follow-up. *Arch Gen Psychiatry* 1980;37:179-193.

OPTIONAL READING

If more depth is desired on a particular topic, the following references are recommended:

Detoxification and Emergency Management
Czechowicz C: *Detoxification Treatment Manual.* US Dept of Health, Education, and Welfare publication No. (ADM) 78-738. Washington, DC, National Institute of Drug Abuse, 1978.

General and Pharmacological Information
Jaffe JH: Drug addiction and drug abuse, in Gilman AG, *et al.* (eds): *The Pharmacological Basis of Therapeutics,* ed 6. New York, MacMillan, 1980, pp 535-584.

Phencyclidine
Petersen RC, Stillman RC: *Phencyclidine: An Overview.* National Institute of Drug Abuse Research Monograph Series, no 21, 1978, pp 1-17.

Cocaine
Gay GR: You've come a long way baby! Coke time for the new American lady of the eighties. *J Psychoactive Drugs* 1981;13:297-318.

Effects on Fetus
Finnegan LP: The effects of narcotics and alcohol on pregnancy and the newborn. *Ann NY Acad Sci* 1981;362:136-157.

Chasnoff IJ, Hatcher R, Burns WJ: Poly-drug and methadone—addicted newborns: A continuum of impairment. *Pediatrics* 1982;7:210-213.

Chapter 22

PSYCHIATRY AND THE LAW

PHILLIP J. RESNICK, M.D.

Forensic psychiatry, once of interest to only the few psychiatrists who evaluated criminal defendants, now affects the practice of all psychiatry. The following areas of interaction between law and psychiatry will be discussed in this chapter:

1. Competency
2. Criminal responsibility
3. Malingering
4. Involuntary hospitalization
5. The prediction of dangerousness
6. Confidentiality
7. The right to treatment
8. The right to refuse treatment
9. Expert witness testimony

The medical term *"insanity"* was used in the 19th century to refer to a group of severe mental disorders. Today, *"insanity"* is strictly a legal term that has no counterpart in medicine. Insanity cannot be equated with psychosis under any circumstances.

The term *"insanity"* is confusing because it is used in such a wide variety of legal contexts. It may be most simply defined as a degree of mental disturbance that entails legal consequences. These consequences may be: 1. relief from criminal accountability; 2. loss of certain privileges which require a sound mind. The word *"incompetency"* is often used as a synonym for the second type of insanity.

In this chapter, *"insanity"* will only be used to refer to the absence of criminal responsibility. *"Competency"* will be used to designate that degree of mental soundness necessary to carry out acts of a juridical nature.

COMPETENCY

The degree of mental soundness required for competency varies according to the particular act in question. A person who is totally unable to care for himself may require a guardian of person; on the other hand, it is possible to only be incompetent with respect to a specific act, such as entering into a contract. The general criteria for competency are an understanding of the nature of the specific act, and an awareness of the duties and obligations entailed. Since adults are presumed by law to be competent, the burden of proof is on those who think otherwise. Proof of mental incompetency, for any purpose, requires the following evidence:

1. The person has a mental disease.
2. The disease causes a defect in judgment.
3. The defect in judgment causes a specific incapacity with reference to the matter in question.

A person who is so impaired that he is unable to take proper care of himself may be declared *incompetent*. A court-appointed *guardian of person* is then authorized to manage the *incompetent* person's finances and care. The guardian of person has the authority to give consent for surgery and placement in a hospital or nursing home. Physicians should always obtain written consent from the guardian before performing medical procedures on an *incompetent* person.

A *guardian of estate,* or conservator, may be appointed when a person's incapacity is limited to financial management. For example, impaired judgment, due to mental illness, may cause a person to be: 1. a spendthrift; 2. unwilling to spend money, even for necessities; or 3. unable to protect himself from those who might attempt to secure his property without adequate recompense.

Guardians of estate may advance patients small sums of money for personal purchases. Guardians are answerable to the Court for judicious use of the incompetent ward's funds.

Competency to give informed consent for medical or surgical procedures entails the capacity to understand:

1. The procedure requiring consent;
2. The attendant risks;
3. The likely result if the procedure is not performed;
4. The alternative approaches to the problem.

If a patient has not been adjudicated incompetent, but does not appear capable of giving consent, it is safest to delay elective surgery until guardianship has been obtained.

Testamentary capacity or competency to make a will, requires that the person understand that he is making a will and that he knows, without prompting, his natural heirs and the nature and extent of his property.

Entering into a contract requires a greater degree of competency than making a will; more judgment is necessitated by the involvement of an adversary interest. A contract is not valid if one of the parties did not have a true understanding of its terms. This lack of understanding must be due to mental disease, not simply lack of sophistication or technical knowledge.

Competency to marry requires that each partner understand a marriage is taking place, as well as the implications of marriage.

Competency to be a witness in a court proceeding requires the ability to recall events and understand what it means to tell the truth.

Competency to stand trial requires an understanding of the criminal charges, and the ability to cooperate with an attorney in preparation of one's defense. Competency to stand trial is based upon the defendant's current mental state; criminal accountability is based upon the defendant's mental state when the crime was committed. Despite the extensive publicity given to insanity trials, ten times as many defendants are judged not competent to stand trial than are found not guilty by reason of insanity.

CRIMINAL RESPONSIBILITY (INSANITY)

Criminal law is primarily based upon blameworthiness. Persons are usually only held criminally accountable for forbidden acts *(actus reus)* done with an evil intent *(mens rea)*. If a person commits a crime because of a mental disease that precludes moral blame, he may be found not guilty by reason of insanity. However, the mere fact that psychosis was present when the crime was committed does not assure an insanity finding.

Tests for the insanity defense vary according to the jurisdiction. The McNaughtan test requires that mental disease prevented the accused person from either knowing the nature and quality of his act, or that it was wrong (1). This information, sometimes known as the *right or wrong* test, has been criticized because it is limited to the defendant's cognition.

The *irresistible impulse* test relieves a person of criminal accountability if mental disease made him incapable of refraining from the criminal act. Some jurisdictions require proof that the defendant would have committed the act even if a policeman had been standing at his elbow. The inability to control the impulse must be due to mental illness, not merely a loss of temper or outburst of rage. This test of control introduces the issue of volition.

The Durham rule held that, "The accused is not criminally responsible if his unlawful act is the product of mental disease or defect" (2). This *product test* has not been in general use since 1972 (3).

The Model Penal Code test, proposed by the American Law Institute, states, "A person is not responsible for his criminal conduct if at the time of such conduct as a result of mental disease or defect he lacks substantial capacity to appreciate the criminality of his conduct or to conform his conduct to the requirements of the law" (4). This formulation includes both the *right or wrong* (cognition) and *irresistible impulse* (volition) tests in modified form.

Federal jurisdictions currently use variations of the Model Penal Code test. Most states use the *right or wrong* test, either alone or in combination with an *irresistible impulse* test.

Voluntary intoxication with alcohol or drugs is not ordinarily considered a valid basis for an insanity defense. There are, however, four specific situations in which intoxication may warrant an insanity defense:

1. Involuntary intoxication;
2. Delirium tremens;
3. Idiosyncratic alcohol intoxication (pathological intoxication);
4. Permanent psychosis due to alcohol.

For example, if LSD were placed in a defendant's drink without his knowledge, and he committed a crime during the resulting psychosis, he could plead insanity. Idiosyncratic intoxication, i.e., an unusually marked behavioral change due to a small quantity of alcohol, may serve as an insanity defense only if the defendant had no prior knowledge of this propensity. In each case of alcohol-induced mental illness, the defendant must still meet the other requirements of the insanity test.

In 1975, Michigan became the first state in the country to enact legislation giving juries the option of a *guilty but mentally ill* (GBMI) verdict, in addition to a finding of not guilty by reason of insanity (NGRI). Within one year of John Hinckley's insanity verdict in the shooting of President Reagan, seven additional states passed such legislation. Although the insanity defense is successful in only one-tenth of one percent of felony trials, the public perceives it as a major loophole in the criminal justice system. Some insanity verdicts leave the public feeling that justice has not been done. The goal of the legislators enacting GBMI statutes was to reduce NGRI acquittals. However, the number of successful insanity acquittals did not decrease in Michigan after the addition of the GBMI verdict (5). None of the GBMI statutes actually eliminate the insanity defense. Although Idaho and Montana did legislatively abolish the insanity defense in 1982, the constitutionality of those laws has not yet been tested in the Courts. Three prior attempts by states to abolish the insanity defense have been found unconstitutional.

MALINGERING

Malingering is the voluntary production of physical or psychological symptoms in order to pursue an easily identified goal. No other syndrome is so easy to define, yet so difficult to diagnose. Simulated insanity is as old as the history of medicine. Ulysses feigned insanity in order to escape the Trojan War. He yoked a bull and a horse together, plowed the seashore, and sowed salt instead of grain. The deception was detected by placing his infant son in the line of the furrow. When Ulysses turned the plow aside to avoid the infant, it was considered proof that his madness was not real.

Persons usually malinger mental illness for one of the following purposes: 1. The criminal may seek to avoid punishment by pretending to be incompetent to stand trial, insane at the time of the act, worthy of mitigation of penalty, or too ill (incompetent) to be executed. 2. Malingerers may seek to avoid conscription into the military, be relieved from undesirable military assignments, or avoid combat. 3. Malingerers may seek financial gain from social security disability, veterans' benefits, workers' compensation, or damages for alleged psychological injury. 4. Prisoners may seek to obtain drugs or be transferred to a psychiatric hospital, to facilitate escape, or do "easier time." 5. Malingerers may seek admission to a psychiatric hospital as a haven from the police, or to obtain free room and board.

The research literature on the detection of malingered mental illness is sparse. No research has demonstrated the ability of mental health professionals to accurately detect malingering. In Rosenhan's (6) work, eight pseudopatients were admitted to psychiatric hospitals alleging that they heard voices. Although they stopped claiming symptoms once they were admitted, their hospital stays ranged from nine to 52 days. All were diagnosed as schizophrenic. Rosenhan concluded that mental health professionals were unable to distinguish normality from mental illness. The study's methods, results, and conclusions have been severely criticized (7).

The following clues may be helpful in detecting malingered psychoses:

1. Malingerers may overact their part (8). "Every malingerer is an actor who portrays an illness as he understands it" (9). Malingerers sometimes mistakenly believe that the more bizarrely they behave, the more psychotic they will appear.
2. Malingerers are eager to call attention to their illnesses, in contrast with schizophrenics, who are often reluctant to discuss their symptoms (10). Some malingerers limit their symptoms to repeatedly mentioning one or two "delusional" accusations (11). One malingerer stated that he was an "insane lunatic" when he killed his parents at the behest of "hallucinatory voices that told me to kill in my demented state."
3. It is more difficult for malingerers to successfully imitate the form, than the content of schizophrenic thinking (12). Common errors include the beliefs that nothing must be remembered correctly, and that the more inconsistent and absurd the discourse, the better the decep-

tion. If the imposter is asked to repeat an idea, he may do it quite exactly; the genuine schizophrenic will often wander off on a tangent. The psychotic's train of thought is often abrupt and changes rapidly; the malingerer may show premeditation and hesitation in presenting a succession of ideas (13). Some malingerers give the appearance of profound concentration before they give absurd answers (11).

4. Malingerers' symptoms may fit no known diagnostic entity. Symptoms may have been selected from various psychoses. Instead of labeling such persons "atypical psychosis," malingering should be suspected.

5. Malingerers may claim the sudden onset of a delusion. In reality, systematized delusions usually take several weeks to develop (14).

6. A malingerer's behavior is not likely to conform to his alleged delusions; acute schizophrenic behavior usually does. However, the "burned out" schizophrenic may no longer demonstrate agitation over his delusions (15).

7. A malingerer may tell a far-fetched story to fit the facts of his crimes into a mental disease model. One malingerer with prior armed robbery convictions claimed that he robbed only upon the commands of auditory hallucinations, and gave away all the stolen money.

8. Malingerers are likely to have contradictions in their accounts of the crime. The contradictions may be evident within the story itself; they may also become apparent when the defendant's story is compared with the physical evidence. When a malingerer is caught in contradictions, he may either sulk or laugh with embarrassment (11).

9. Malingerers tend to present themselves as blameless within their feigned illness.

10. Malingerers are likely to repeat questions or answer questions slowly, to give themselves more time to make up an answer. This may be especially evident when they are pressed for details about alleged hallucinations or delusions. There may be frequent replies of, "I don't know." When asked whether an alleged voice was male or female, one malingerer replied, "It was probably a man's voice."

11. Malingering should be suspected in defendants pleading insanity if a partner was involved in a crime. Most accomplices of normal intelligence will not participate in psychotically motivated crimes. The clinician may explore the validity of such a claim by questioning the co-defendant.

12. Malingerers are likely to have nonpsychotic alternative motives for their behavior, such as killing to settle a grievance or avoid apprehension. A crime without an apparent motive, such as the killing of a stranger, lends credence to the presence of true mental disease. Genu-

ine psychotic explanations for rape, robbery, or check forging are unusual.

13. It is rare for malingerers to show perseveration. The presence of perseveration suggests actual organic damage, or an extremely well-prepared malingerer.

14. Malingerers may describe the content of their auditory hallucinations in a stilted manner. One malingerer charged with attempted rape stated that the voices said, "Go commit a sex offense." A malingering robber alleged that the voices kept screaming, "Stick up, stick up."

15. Malingerers are unlikely to show the subtle signs of residual schizophrenia, such as impaired relatedness, blunted affect, concreteness, or peculiar thinking.

16. Persons who have true schizophrenia may also malinger auditory hallucinations to escape criminal responsibility. These are the most difficult cases to accurately assess. Clinicians have a lower index of suspicion because of the history of psychiatric hospitalizations and the presence of residual schizophrenic symptoms. These malingerers are able to draw upon their prior experience with hallucinations and their observations of other psychotics. They know what questions to expect from psychiatrists. If they spend time in a forensic psychiatric hospital, they are likely to learn the exact criteria for an insanity defense.

INVOLUNTARY HOSPITALIZATION

Most states have three types of admissions to psychiatric hospitals. The first is voluntary admission. The percentage of voluntary admissions has substantially increased in the last two decades. This may be due to the increase in psychiatric units in general hospitals, as well as the lessening of the stigma associated with psychiatric hospitalization.

The second type of admission is based upon an emergency medical certificate signed by at least one licensed physician. This permits dangerous mentally ill persons to be involuntarily detained in a hospital for a brief period of time. These patients are entitled to a judicial hearing within several days, to determine whether further care is necessary.

The third type of admission is based upon a judicial certificate. A family member or other concerned person must first file an affidavit in Probate Court, alleging that the person is mentally ill and in need of hospital care. If, after investigation, the court believes involuntary hospitalization is necessary, a warrant of detention may be issued; the police then transport the individual to a psychiatric hospital.

Different states have different criteria for involuntary hospitalization. Some states define mental illness by statute for commitment purposes. A typical definition is: "Mental illness means a substantial disorder of thought, mood, perception, orientation, or memory that grossly impairs judgment, behavior, capacity to recognize reality, or ability to meet the ordinary demands of life" (16). All states allow involuntary admission if a person's mental illness makes him dangerous to himself or others. As representatives of society, legislatures must determine the standards which balance the loss of a potentially harmless mentally ill person's liberty against the risk of violence in the community. Courts have recently begun requiring evidence of threats or violent behavior to prove dangerousness. Some states also allow involuntary hospitalization if mentally ill persons are unable to care for themselves (gravely disabled), or are likely to benefit from hospital treatment.

Above all else, physicians are taught to do no harm. Physicians are accustomed to erring on the side of hospital admission in assessing questionable heart attacks. Thus, they are inclined to admit mentally ill patients if there is any doubt about their potential dangerousness. Involuntary admission, however, is not merely a medical decision; such admissions constitute a legal deprivation of liberty. Lawyers do not unquestioningly accept the beneficence of physicians' decisions. Civil rights attorneys demand that such patients be afforded the same panoply of civil rights as criminal defendants (17).

A physician conducting an emergency evaluation must decide whether a patient meets the criteria for involuntary hospitalization. The final decision to hold a patient against his will, however, properly rests with a judge at a subsequent hearing.

PSYCHIATRIC PREDICTION OF DANGEROUSNESS

Approximately 50,000 mentally ill Americans are preventively detained each year because of predicted dangerousness—despite the lack of epidemiological association between violence and mental illness in general, or schizophrenia in particular. Only psychiatrists and juvenile judges are empowered to lock up people who have not committed crimes; both do so in the name of treatment.

Dangerousness is not a psychiatric diagnosis like schizophrenia. It is a legal judgment based upon social policy. Psychiatrists have traditionally felt it is better to be safe than sorry in deciding whether to involuntarily hospitalize a potentially dangerous patient. If a released patient commits a violent act, newspaper headlines proclaim the mistake, The community rarely objects if a patient is kept in the hospital longer than necessary.

Psychiatrists have not demonstrated the ability to accurately predict long-term dangerousness; in fact, their predictive abilities are no better than social workers, judges, corrections officers, or high school teachers (18). No psychological test is able to predict violence. Psychiatrists over-predict violence by a margin of 65% to 95%. Statistical principles demonstrate that accurate predictions of infrequent events, such as dangerous behavior, require one to cast a wide net, which inevitably includes many false positives. Psychiatrists receive no systematic follow-up information after they make predictions of dangerousness. Consequently, experience is not helpful in improving predictive accuracy.

Violence-prone patients are likely to suffer from psychosis, depression, organic brain disease, or a personality disorder. It is usually easy to recognize the potential violence in psychosis by the presence of delusions and disorganized thought processes. Depressed patients may react to their despair by striking out at others. Mothers, in particular, may kill their children prior to a suicide attempt—either because of difficulty separating from them or misguided altruistic motives (19). Impaired controls lead to violence in persons with organic brain disease. They may have histories of temper tantrums, explosive rages, and "soft neurological signs."

Violence-prone individuals with personality disorders often sustained emotional deprivation and physical brutality as children. They demonstrate impulsiveness, poor control of aggressive urges, and a pattern of repetitive antisocial acts. They are likely to abuse drugs and alcohol, and drive automobiles recklessly. The violence usually has a paroxysmal episodic quality. Mental status examination may reveal glibness, lack of introspection, and a tendency to project internal difficulties onto the environment. There is a tendency toward superficial relationships and the dehumanization of others. Although individuals with these symptoms clearly have an increased risk of violence, they cannot be civilly committed because they do not meet the statutory definition of mental illness.

In assessing dangerousness, the history should include a careful assessment of the patient's past use of violence. Past violence is the single best predictor of future violence. Drug use should be explored; alcohol, amphetamines, and PCP are particularly known to diminish controls. Questions about the ownership of weapons are most often overlooked. The childhood triad of fire-setting, enuresis, and cruelty to animals has been correlated with adult violence.

The psychiatric examiner assessing dangerousness should be attentive to anger, coupled with a lack of empathy and concern for others. Patients who feel helpless are especially prone to violent outbursts. Violent fantasies in delusional patients should be fully explored. A pattern of violence associated with the sexual drive tends to be cyclical, and therefore has a poor prognosis.

Psychiatrists must be careful to balance the protection of society against the patient's loss of freedom. Although decisions about long-term dangerousness are extremely difficult, they must be made. Psychiatrists must approach this task with humility and share the decision-making with others concerned with the safety of society.

CONFIDENTIALITY

Confidentiality prevents physicians from revealing information about patients without their consent, unless required to do so by law or to protect the welfare of the patient or community. Willful betrayal of a patient's confidence may result in revocation of a physician's license.

Physicians are legally obligated to report child abuse, treatment of gunshot wounds, and specified contagious diseases. Physicians may violate confidentiality to avert a catastrophe. For example, a physician who diagnoses serious heart disease in a commercial pilot may notify the employer, even over the pilot's protests. The protective privilege ends when public peril begins.

Because of the highly personal nature of psychotherapy, psychiatric patients are especially concerned about confidentiality. Psychiatrists have been held liable for damages resulting from the revelation of confidential information to employers and spouses.

In most states, a psychiatrist who determines that his patient presents a serious danger of violence to another, incurs an obligation to use reasonable care to protect the intended victim from danger. Appropriate steps may include initiating hospitalization, warning the intended victim, or notifying the police (20). The rights of potential victims take precedence over the patient's right to confidentiality.

Privilege prohibits physicians from revealing information about patients in court. Privilege belongs to the patient, not the physician. If a patient waives privilege, the physician may be compelled to testify (21). Failure to obey a judge's order to testify may cause a physician to be held in contempt of court, which is punishable by a fine or imprisonment. The psychiatrist who complies with the judge's directions is immune from any liability.

About three-fourths of the states have statutes granting privilege to patient-physician communications. Privilege, however, is never absolute. The court must decide in each case whether the benefit of the evidence outweighs the damage caused by disclosure of the information.

THE RIGHT TO PSYCHIATRIC TREATMENT

The right to psychiatric treatment has been viewed from its inception as a pressure device to upgrade the quality of institutional care. In 1958, Dr.

Harry Solomon, President of the American Psychiatric Association, stated, "I do not see how any reasonably objective view of our mental hospitals today could fail to conclude that they are bankrupt beyond remedy" (22). At that time, the average length of stay for schizophrenic patients was 13 years. In 1960, Dr. Morton Birnbaum, a physician and attorney, attempted to elevate concerns about inadequate treatment to a principle of constitutional law (23). He suggested that "due process of law" precludes a mentally ill person who has committed no crime from being deprived of his liberty by indefinite institutionalization without treatment in a mental prison.

The concept of a right to psychiatric treatment was first judicially recognized in 1966, by the D.C. Circuit Court of Appeals (24). The ruling stated that hospitals need not prove that treatment will cure or improve the patient; there must, however, be a bona fide effort to treat. Later that year, the same court ruled that civilly committed persons were entitled to the least restrictive alternative necessary for their safe treatment (25).

Wyatt v. Stickney, the landmark right to treatment case, began as a class action suit in Alabama, where conditions at Bryce Hospital "shocked the conscience of the court" (26). For cleanliness, patients hosed each other down with scalding water. Patients remained on penicillin for a year after treatment for pneumonia, because no doctor saw them to discontinue it. There was a total lack of psychiatric treatment.

In *Wyatt,* Judge Johnson stated, "To deprive any citizen of his or her liberty upon the altruistic theory that the confinement is for humane and therapeutic reasons and then fail to provide adequate treatment, violates the very fundamentals of due process." *Wyatt* mandates that minimal "medical and constitutional" standards include:

1. A humane psychological and physical environment;
2. Qualified staff in numbers sufficient to administer adequate treatment;
3. Individualized treatment plans;

In 1975, the Supreme Court ruled that a non-dangerous patient may not be confined without treatment, if, with the help of willing friends or family, he is able to survive safely outside the hospital (27). Although this case forbade the confinement of non-dangerous persons without treatment, it did not require treatment for confined patients.

In 1982, the Supreme Court ruled that a severely mentally retarded person had a limited right to treatment (28). The Court held that an institutionalized person had a right to reasonable safety, freedom from unnecessary restraints, and sufficient training to ensure safety and facilitate his ability to function without bodily restraints. The reasoning in recent cases (27,28) suggests that the Supreme Court will not mandate a broad constitutional right to treatment.

Some states have responded to right to treatment suits with a massive discharge of chronic mentally ill patients. Unfortunately, this often occurred without the provision of adequate alternative arrangements for the patients' care. In New York City, 25,000 discharged mental patients live on welfare in rundown hotels—unsupervised, unmedicated, and uncared for.

THE RIGHT TO REFUSE PSYCHIATRIC TREATMENT

Prior to the 1970s, a societal attitude of paternalism allowed psychiatrists broad discretion in treating non-consenting, involuntary hospital patients. The civil rights and consumer movements have recently challenged this unquestioned authority. Concern has been fueled by periodic reports of serious abuses, such as the use of electroconvulsive treatment (ECT) to punish patients, or the administration of major tranquilizers to quiet non-psychotic patients.

Justice Cardoza has stated, "Every human being of adult years and sound mind has the right to determine what shall be done with his own body" (29). Whether involuntary patients demonstrate soundness of mind is certainly questionable. However, involuntary psychiatric patients in almost all jurisdictions are now presumed competent unless specifically adjudicated incompetent. In the past, it was considered sufficient to obtain informal consent for treatment from the next of kin. Today, psychiatrists face a greater risk of a successful law suit if they treat without the consent of the patient or a legally appointed guardian.

Most states provide detailed consent requirements for the use of ECT. If a patient is not competent to consent, some jurisdictions require prior court approval for ECT—except in life-threatening emergencies.

Since the mid-1970s, there has been considerable controversy over patients' right to refuse psychotropic medications. One court held that involuntary patients are constitutionally protected against being forcibly medicated unless there is a "substantial likelihood . . . of extreme violence, personal injury or attempted suicide" (30). Another court stated that due process protections are satisfied by written consent forms and the right to have medication decisions reviewed by independent psychiatrists (31). The Supreme Court has remanded each of these cases back to lower courts for new opinions in view of subsequent court cases. Most observers believe that the Supreme Court will leave ultimate decisions about medication to psychiatrists. Judicial decisions about the right to receive and refuse psychiatric treatment are likely to continue to modify psychiatric practice for the next several years.

THE PSYCHIATRIST AS AN EXPERT WITNESS

Medical reports or testimony are required in over fifty percent of all trials. The initial reaction to a request for psychiatric testimony may be anxiety or even panic. Psychiatrists are accustomed to assuming positions of authority in hospitals and their own offices. Anxiety may be provoked by the realization that this authority will be challenged by cross-examiners.

Psychiatrists are usually called upon as *expert,* rather than *fact,* witnesses. "Expert witnesses" are persons who possess facts directly related to some science or profession which is beyond the average layperson's scope of knowledge. Only expert witnesses are permitted to offer opinions. A treating psychiatrist may, however, be compelled to testify as a fact witness. A "fact witness" only states his direct observations, such as the information learned during an examination.

It is a fallacy to consider the psychiatric expert witness impartial. Once he has formed an opinion, it is only human for the psychiatrist to identify himself with that opinion, and hope for the success of the side which supports his conclusions.

Psychiatrists sometimes forget that their conclusions are only *opinions.* Juries are instructed that they are to determine how much weight to give the testimony of each witness. A jury has the right to disregard psychiatric testimony, even when it is uncontradicted.

Before beginning a psychiatric evaluation for legal purposes, the psychiatrist has an absolute obligation to explain the absence of confidentiality. Patient-psychiatrist confidentiality may or may not be respected in the courtroom. When asked to reveal personal information in court, a psychiatrist may suggest to the judge that it should remain confidential. The judge, however, is the final decision-maker.

Courtroom procedure is quite formal and ritualized. *Direct* examination will begin with the elicitation of the psychiatrist's qualifications. The psychiatrist will then be asked to describe his examination of the patient. He will be asked whether he has formed an opinion with reasonable medical certainty regarding the critical legal issue. "Reasonable medical certainty" simply means that there is a 51% or greater probability that a conclusion is correct.

The purpose of *cross-examination* is to discredit damaging testimony by demonstrating that the witness is a fool, liar, and nitwit. The psychiatrist's credentials may be attacked by showing a lack of experience or education. Questions may reveal that he has either not completed his board examinations or did not pass them at the first sitting.

The cross-examiner may attempt to show witness bias or personal interest. The adequacy of the psychiatric examination may be attacked because of its length, the absence of privacy, or the lack of corroborating information.

The patient's version of the events in question conflicts with other factual accounts approximately 40% of the time. Consequently, psychiatrists should never base their conclusions entirely upon the patient's statements. The clinical examination is highly vulnerable to attack. Substantial evidence of the fallibility of psychiatric conclusions has been compiled, e.g., the inter-examiner reliability of psychiatric diagnosis is only 60% (32).

The following suggestions should enhance the effectiveness of psychiatric expert witnesses:

1. Have a pre-trial conference. At this time, the inexperienced witness may be told what to expect.
2. Give your curriculum vitae to the attorney in advance. This will allow him to elicit your qualifications most effectively.
3. Know the specific legal issue and standard. Ask the attorney to enclose these in a cover letter to you, along with the background information.
4. Dress conservatively. A three-piece suit conveys more credibility than a loud sport jacket.
5. Leave the courtroom immediately after your testimony.
6. Attempt to display dignity, confidence, and humility.
7. Give short, clear answers in simple language. The boredom factor can cause you to lose the jury's attention.
8. Qualify your answer when necessary. If an attorney demands a "yes" or "no" answer, you may ask the judge for the opportunity to explain your answer.
9. Look at the jury and direct your remarks to them.
10. Don't be, or even appear to be, an advocate. It is your absolute obligation to tell only the truth on the witness stand, regardless of its effect upon the outcome of the case.
11. Don't ever talk down to the jury. If they feel patronized, they will not accept what you are saying.
12. Don't use psychiatric jargon. It is likely to be misunderstood or made to look ridiculous.
13. Don't appear arrogant. Nothing alienates a jury more quickly.
14. Don't attempt to be humorous. A trial is a serious matter.
15. Don't be a smart aleck or argue with the cross-examiner. The jury will ordinarily identify with the witness. If the witness gets smart, however, the jury will take the part of the cross-examiner, in the belief that he is just doing his job.
16. Don't lose your temper.
17. Don't answer any question you don't fully understand. Ask the attorney to rephrase the question or define his terms.

18. Don't guess at an answer. It is better to say you don't know or don't remember.
19. Don't ever refuse to admit the obvious. It makes the psychiatrist look either foolish or biased.
20. Don't let a zealous attorney push you into an opinion that is not your own.
21. Don't try to avoid answering questions about your fee or pre-trial conferences.
22. Don't be cowed by the judicial process; remember, you are the expert.

The area of law and psychiatry is in a state of flux. Each year, new court decisions further define patients' rights and regulate psychiatric practice. It is, therefore, necessary for each practicing psychiatrist to keep abreast of the laws in his own state.

REFERENCES

1. Daniel McNaughten's Case, 10 C.&F. 200, 210-211, 8 Eng. Rep, 718, 722-723 (1843).
2. *Durham v. United States,* 214 F.2d 862 (D. C. Cir., 1954).
3. *U.S. v. Brawner,* 471 F.2d 969 (1972).
4. American Law Institute Model Penal Code, Proposed Official Draft Sec. 4.01 (1962) [First Presented in 1955].
5. Smith GA, Hall JA: Evaluating Michigan's guilty but Mentally Ill Verdict: An empirical study. *Univ of Mich J Law Reform* 1982;16:77-114.
6. Rosenhan DL: On being sane in insane places. *Science* 1973;179:250-58.
7. Spitzer R: More on pseudoscience in science and the case of psychiatric diagnosis. *Arch Gen Psychiatry* 1976;33:459-470.
8. Wachspress M, Berenberg AN, Jacobson A: Simulation of psychosis. *Psychiatric Quarterly* 1953;27:463-473.
9. Ossipov VP: Malingering: The simulation of psychosis. *Bull Menn Clin* 1944;8:31-42.
10. Ritson B, & Forest A: The simulation of psychosis: A contemporary presentation. *Brit J Med Psychol* 1970;43:31-37.
11. MacDonald J: The simulation of mental disease, in MacDonald J (ed): *Psychiatry and the Criminal.* Springfield, IL, Charles C Thomas Co, 1976, pp 267-279.
12. Sherman M, Treif P, Sprafkin QR: Impression management in the psychiatric interview: Quality, style and individual differences. *J Consulting Clin Psychol* 1975;43:867-871.
13. Ray I: *Treatise on the Medical Jurisprudence of Insanity.* Boston, Little Brown & Company, 1871.
14. Davidson HA: Malingered psychosis. *Bull Menn Clin* 1950;14:157-163.
15. Davidson HA: *Forensic Psychiatry,* ed 2. New York, The Ronald Press, 1965.
16. Ohio Revised Code Section 5122.01.
17. *Lessard v. Schmidt,* 349 F. Supp. 1078, (E.D. Wis. 1972).
18. Ennis BJ, Litwak A: Psychiatry and the presumption of expertise: Flipping coins in the courtroom. *California Law Review* 1074;62:1-50.
19. Resnick PJ: Child murder by parents: A psychiatric review of filicide. *Am J Psychiatry* 1969;126:73-83.
20. *Tarasoff v. Regents of the University of California,* 551 P.2d 334.

21. *In re Lifschultz*, 2 Cal.3d 415, 85 Cal. Rptr. 829, 467 Pac.2d 557 (1970).
22. Solomon H: The American Psychiatric Association in relation to American psychiatry. *Am J Psychiatry* 1958;115:1.
23. Birnbaum M: The right to treatment. 46 *A.B.A.J.* 499, 1960.
24. *Rouse v. Cameron*, 373 F.2d 451 (D.C. Cir. 1966).
25. *Lake v. Cameron*, 364 F.2d 657 (D.C. Cir. 1966).
26. *Wyatt v. Stickney*, 344 F.Supp. 373 (1972).
27. *O'Connor v. Donaldson*, 422 U.S. 563.
28. *Youngberg v. Romeo*, 457 U.S. 307 (1982).
29. *Schloendorff v. Society of New York Hospital*, 211 N.Y. 125, 105 N.E. 92, 93 (1914).
30. *Rogers v. Okin*, 634 F.2d 650 (1980).
31. *Rennie v. Klein*, 476 F.Supp. 1294 (D. NJ 1979), affirmed in part 653 F.2d 836 (3rd Cir. 1981).
32. Ziskin J: *Coping with Psychiatric and Psychological Testimony*. Venice, CA, Law and Psychology Press, 1980, vol 3.

Chapter 23

PSYCHOLOGICAL SEXUAL DYSFUNCTION
STEPHEN B. LEVINE, M.D.

INTRODUCTION

This chapter is intended to provide a sophisticated introduction to psychologic sexual dysfunctions. Prior to 1970, clinical concepts about sexual life were dominated by psychoanalytic theory and practice. Professional knowledge in this area was largely restricted to a relatively small group of highly-trained psychiatrists. The publication of Masters and Johnson's books on sexual physiology and inadequacy (1,2) dramatically changed clinical thinking. New assumptions about sexuality and different styles of therapeutic interventions emerged. Professionals of diverse backgrounds became interested in the subject.

There is much evidence to suggest that sexual dysfunctions are quite prevalent (3-5). The dramatic changes in media coverage of sexuality have resulted in more people seeking help for sexual inadequacies. The ability to effectively deal with these requests depends upon the professional's knowledge of the complexity of sexual life. A discussion of these basic complexities will, therefore, precede the section on therapy.

There are three major influences on sexual problems: constitutional; psychological; organic. Constitutional influences are biologically determined forces which seem to be consistent individual characteristics (6). Constitutional influences are products of neurophysiologic organization, e.g., libido; ease of arousal. Neither their mechanisms nor the extent of their contributions are well understood. Psychologic influences include all the emotional, cognitive, interactional, and cultural factors which are known to determine and influence behavior. Organic influences include the many recognized physical factors that structurally or chemically interfere with sexual functioning, e.g., disease processes; medication; surgery. Although many psychological sexual dysfunctions involve all three of these influences to some extent, this chapter will focus on the psychologic factors.

WHAT ARE THE DYSFUNCTIONS?

Thus far there is no widely accepted, all-inclusive definition of the term "dysfunction." It is much easier to define sexual problems that are not dysfunctions. There are problems that are too global and fundamental to be considered dysfunctions. Three such categories of problems are the gender identity disorders (transsexualism, transvestism), the perversions or atypical sexual motivations (desire to hurt, be hurt, fondle a child, exhibit one's genitals, etc.), and homosexuality. Approximately ten percent of the population displays one or more of these developmental outcomes.

There are other sexual problems which are too "minor" to be considered dysfunctions, e.g., concern over having multiple orgasms; failure to achieve simultaneous orgasm; aversion to oral-genital stimulation; sexual boredom; aversion to masturbation. These problems may be quite disruptive and lead to dysfunction.

The sexual dysfunctions are the various inabilities to experience sexual arousal to orgasm with a partner in a smooth well-integrated fashion. The key phrases in this definition are:

"Sexual dysfunctions"—Anyone may have a sexual dysfunction—heterosexuals, homosexuals, the perverse, and those with gender identity disorders. The term "dysfunction" refers to the objective and subjective aspects of actual sexual interaction, rather than the broader psychological context of the relationship. For example, a transvestite with premature ejaculation is said to be dysfunctional because of his pattern of rapid, uncontrollable ejaculation—not because of his cross-dressing. The latter is an entirely different matter. The dysfunctions represent only a limited aspect of the range of human sexual problems.

"Various inabilities"—A large number of discrete sexual dysfunctions exist. These include problems of desire, arousal, orgasm, penetration, and emotional satisfaction. There are at least several varieties of problems within each of these categories.

"With a partner"—Although many serious inhibitions of sexual expression are manifested during solitary sex (masturbation), the vast majority of individuals seek help for difficulties experienced in interpersonal situations. The definition does not specify any partner—for one can be dysfunctional with one partner and not another. It refers to a partner—usually, though not exclusively, the socially appropriate partner, e.g., spouse.

"Smooth, well-integrated fashion"—The absence of dysfunction cannot be ascertained by simply asking whether orgasms occur with a partner. Many dysfunctional patients are orgasmic, but have to work so hard at sex that the experience is not pleasurable. Other orgasmic patients complain about a lack of desire or emotional satisfaction. Dysfunctional sex represents an uncoupling of the usually smooth integration of mental and physical pleasure. The patient is usually quite aware of this uncoupling. This broad definition of dysfunction is not entirely satisfactory. For example, some women with severe vaginismus, i.e., an inability to tolerate penile penetration of the vagina, can easily achieve orgasm with their partner through manual or oral genital stimulation. They are considered dysfunctional in spite of their orgasmic attainment. There are other problems with this definition. The definition does not specify a particular mode of orgasmic attainment. There is still some controversy about the "normal" pattern of female orgasmic attainment (7). No concrete distinctions between functional and dysfunctional, smooth, well-integrated, and uncoupled are offered. These distinctions vary according to each patient's subjective standards. Also, the definition does not specify a vantage point. It does not state who determines whether dysfunction exists, i.e., the alleged symptom-bearer or the dissatisfied spouse. Sometimes spouses disagree about the existence of a problem.

Aside from these seemingly picayune problems, the definition of sexual dysfuntion provides a very useful, but highly arbitrary, grouping of similar subjective and objective phenomena. The study of the dysfunctions branches off in many different directions, e.g., interpersonal, organic, intrapsychic, and cultural spheres. In the process, some previously mysterious aspects of sexual life are illuminated, facilitating the assistance of many distressed individuals (see Table I).

THE EVOLUTION OF THE NOMENCLATURE

All sexual problems used to be considered forms of impotence and frigidity. This limited nomenclature reflected the attitude that the multiple manifestations of dysfunction were of little importance. They were merely symptoms. The pathogeneses of psychological symptoms, according to psychoanalytic theory, involved compromise formations, i.e., the result of the mediation of conflicting wishes or feelings. Ample clinical material to support such an assumption is only available on some problems. Clinical interventions based upon this assumption typically involve uncovering the underlying conflict within the symptom-bearer. This clinical tradition largely ignored the spouse, and did not foster any efforts to define the separate pathogeneses of different symptoms.

A nomenclature formulated by Masters and Johnson helped to further delineate organic, constitutional, and different psychological influences on dysfunctions (2). It was somewhat cumbersome, however, and was modified

TABLE I
PATIENT TERMINOLOGY FOR THE FORMS OF SEXUAL DYSFUNCTION
CATEGORIES OF COMPLAINTS

Male	*Female*
1. *Complaints about Sexual Desire*	
Absent	Absent
Absent and I hate the thought of sex	Absent and I hate the thought of sex
Low	Low
Strong	Strong
Incompatible with partner	Incompatible with partner
2. *Complaints about Arousal*	
Can't obtain erection	Can't become aroused
Can't maintain erection	Can't stay aroused
Special requirement for arousal,	Special requirement for arousal,
e.g., article of clothing, fantasy	e.g., fantasy
3. *Complaints about Orgasm*	
Premature ejaculation	
Ejaculation too difficult to achieve	Orgasm too difficult to achieve
Ejaculation doesn't occur in the vagina	Orgasm doesn't occur during intercourse
Ejaculation doesn't occur	Orgasm doesn't occur with partner
in partner's presence	
Reduced or absent physical	Reduced or absent physical pleasure
pleasure from orgasm	from orgasm
Orgasm occurs, but ejaculation	
does not	
Painful ejaculation	
4. *Complaints about Penetration*	
Erection is bent and makes	Vagina "disappears" when penetration
penetration and thrusting	is attempted
painful or difficult	
Lack of feeling in penis	Lack of feeling in vagina
during intercourse	during intercourse
Erection or penetration is painful	Penetration and thrusting are painful
5. *Complaints about Satisfaction*	
Something (1-4) is wrong	Something (1-4) is wrong and is
and is causing me not to be	causing me not to be emotionally
emotionally satisfied	satisfied
Nothing else is wrong, yet	Nothing else is wrong, yet something
something is missing	is missing
Partner's sexual response	Partner's sexual response is not
is not satisfying	satisfying

several years later by H.S. Kaplan (8). She suggested basing the nomenclature on the two distinct physiologic phases of sexual response: vasocongestion and orgasm. The vasocongestive phase is characterized subjectively by arousal, and objectively by erection and vaginal lubrication. The orgasmic phase is a bodywide, autonomically-coordinated response triggered by a high level of arousal; it is manifested genitally by prominent pelvic contractions. The nonspecific and pejorative term "frigidity" was replaced by the terms "excitement phase dysfunction" and "orgastic phase dysfunction." This was an important step. Masters and Johnson's term "anorgasmia" did not distinguish between the anorgasmic woman who could not get aroused and one who was easily aroused, but unable to achieve orgasm. Within several years, many female excitement phase problems were recognized as consequences of inadequate desire; this was also true of some cases of impotence (9). This realization, in turn, led to the conceptualization of sexual functioning as having three interrelated components: desire (locus thought to reside within the limbic system); arousal (thought to be predominantly a parasympathetic response—at least in males); orgasm (thought to be a largely sympathetic response). The nomenclature of the American Psychiatric Association—*DSM III*—broadly classifies dysfunction as involving: 1. inhibited desire; 2. inhibited arousal; 3. inhibited orgasm (10).

Sex therapists, professionals specializing in the treatment of dysfunction, use their own, even more refined terminology. Their terms are quite specific in their exclusive focus on the form of the symptom. While this facilitates identification of organic problems and fosters effective communication among professionals, the terminology has its limitations. Sex therapists use the terms "primary" and "secondary" in a very unique way. "Primary dysfunctions" are those that are lifelong; those that are described as "secondary" have had their onset after a period of better sexual functioning. Thus, "primary orgasmic (phase) dysfunction" is the lifelong inability to experience orgasm with a partner in a smooth, well-integrated fashion—although arousal is accomplished. A "secondary orgasmic (phase) dysfunction" is a similar inability in a woman who used to readily achieve orgasm with a partner. Similarly, "primary impotence" (or "erectile dysfunction") is the lifelong inability to accomplish intercourse; "secondary impotence" is erectile dysfunction that begins after a period of normal potency. The separation of dysfunctions into primary and secondary categories has major implications for differential diagnosis.

Organic causes are most commonly found among secondary dysfunctions. The psychological causes of primary dysfunctions typically reflect incomplete maturation due to internal conflict. The partner is not usually an important factor in the pathogenesis. The psychological causes of secondary dysfunctions are much more likely to involve significant interpersonal contributions.

The vicissitudes of sexual function are such that many symptoms are inconstantly present. The adjective "situational" is used to describe those psychological problems which are only present with certain partners or conditions. For example, a man who experiences the inability to ejaculate during intercourse with his wife, but can ejaculate with his girl friend, may be described as having "situational inhibited orgasm." All situational problems are, by definition, forms of secondary dysfunctions. Dysfunctions can be inconstantly present with the same partner. For example, a woman with primary excitement phase dysfunction may become aroused on rare occasions. To be more accurate, such problems ought to be described as "predominant" dysfunctions—but there is a practical limit to the number of terms in any nomenclature. The purpose of adjectives such as "primary," "secondary," "situational," and "predominant" is to draw the clinician's attention to the causal factors. The current classification schema exists because it is useful. It will undoubtedly evolve further as the field becomes more refined.

THE SEXUAL EQUILIBRIUM

Most individuals engage in superficially similar sexual behavior, i.e., they kiss, caress, fondle genitals, and have intercourse. When discussed in clinical settings, however, important behavioral differences become apparent. Each individual has a relatively unique sexual style. This style can be divided into five basic components: sexual orientation; frequency and intensity of sexual desire; ease of arousal; means of orgasmic attainment; contextual requirements for emotional satisfaction (see Table II). There are innumerable variations of each component. For example, one's orientation can be exclusively hetero- or homosexual, or it can be bisexual; desire for orgasm may be infrequent and mild, frequent and mild, infrequent and intense, etc. Simple caressing may stimulate arousal in some, while others require genital stimulation. Some achieve orgasm through several modes of stimulation; others are only orgasmic through coitus in one position. Some require a loving context for their emotional satisfaction; others may derive satisfaction only outside that context. In spite of the fact that almost everyone experiences a decline in desire and ease of arousal over many decades of adulthood, the evolution of any individual's four components is unpredictable.

The formation of an ongoing sexual relationship is a crucial developmental step for both individuals. The couple's sexual life exists in a dynamic equilibrium produced by the interaction between eight unique component characteristics. Once the equilibrium is established, these characteristics may

TABLE II
ANY COUPLE'S SEXUAL EQUILIBRIUM

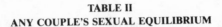

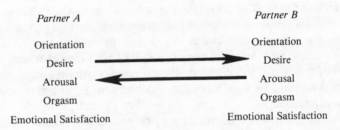

Partner A	Partner B
Orientation	Orientation
Desire	Desire
Arousal	Arousal
Orgasm	Orgasm
Emotional Satisfaction	Emotional Satisfaction

become profoundly interdependent. For example, a woman's arousal may become highly dependent upon the intensity of her partner's desire. A man's emotional satisfaction may require his partner's being orgasmic during intercourse.

Most individuals enter an equilibrium with some sexual inhibitions, i.e., internal forces which prevent erotic abandonment. Some utilize the equilibrium to develop their sensual capacities; others are incapable of exploring their sexual selves within the relationship. Sexual equilibria offer opportunities for the development of trust, personal growth, pleasure, and enrichment—as well as the risks of personal stagnation, relationship deterioration, and pain.

Couples with aproblematic sexual equilibria have variable sexual experiences. Sex is not always wonderful; in fact, it is sometimes relatively pleasureless. Sex is more likely to be described in superlative terms if each partner can achieve several basic characteristics: willingness to make love; relaxation; concentration on sensation (11). Most people cannot achieve these characteristics on every occasion. Personal, interpersonal, and external influences intervene and distract at least one partner. The quality of both partners' sexual experience declines as a consequence. This does not mean that sex is unpleasant. The brief, intense pleasure of orgasm can occur without the perfect combination of these characteristics.

In contrast, couples with dysfunctions experience much less variation of sexual pleasure and emotional satisfaction. Any physical pleasure is usually confined to one partner, and there is usually no emotional satisfaction. Dysfunctional sexual equilibria are characterized by persistent impairments of one partner's willingness, relaxation, and sensual concentration. Because these impairments are perceived by the partner as a lack of emotional involvement, they induce his or her own emotional withdrawal. Devoid of its essential ingredient—emotion, sex becomes mechanical. This general pattern is true for most dysfunctions. Premature ejaculation, for example, can have the same devastating effects on a sexual equilibrium as the inability to ejaculate or vaginismus.

A persistent dysfunctional sexual pattern initiates a large number of negative consequences in almost all couples:

1. *Spectatoring and performance anxiety:* Each new sexual encounter is marred by memories of the last unpleasant experience. Apprehension about the recurrence of the problem causes sensual abandonment to be replaced by watchfulness or "spectatoring." The couple's preoccupation with sexual performance, e.g., maintaining erection, not ejaculating, having an orgasm during coitus, interferes with their pursuit of pleasure.

2. *Avoidance of sex:* The intervals between sexual encounters lengthen as the couple avoids the pain of sexual "failure." Expressions of affection—such as hugs, kisses, love pats, also diminish because they might lead to "something."

3. *Poorer communication:* The couple doesn't mention sex as often. Discussions of anything important are avoided because they may include references to the sexual problem.

4. *Anger:* The symptom-bearer may blame the problem on the partner. The other partner may be angry about the loss of sexual pleasure. The anger may initially be displaced to a nonsexual topic, e.g., "I don't like the way you keep house!" Later, it may erupt in an ugly destructive manner—"You frigid. . . !"

5. *Search for an explanation:* The partners individually develop hypotheses which may be quite erroneous—"He (she) doesn't love me!" "My physical inadequacy (small penis, poor complexion, obesity) caused this."

6. *The symptom-bearer loses self-esteem.*

7. *Partner substitution:* Thoughts, fantasies, and dreams of partner substitution are normal wish-fulfillment processes. Some individuals respond to this "infidelity" with a surge of guilt. Some decide to act out the fantasy with another person to see if the symptom will go away—which often results in larger problems of guilt, disappearance of trust, poor communication, and anger.

8. *Masturbation:* A partner may initiate, increase, or revert to masturbation because it becomes more pleasurable than partner sex. This may cause individuals who view masturbation as a shameful secret to resent the partner even more.

9. *Hopelessness:* Individuals do not readily seek help for sexual problems. They only do so after trying many home remedies and waiting a long time for the problem to go away; by this time, they feel trapped and hopeless.

The sexual experiences of dysfunctional couples are often conspicuously painful. Persistently dysfunctional sex produces mechanical sexual behavior, emotional isolation, and relationship strain. These processes are nonspecific end results of dysfunctions. They explain the persistence of many dysfunctions, but do not account for the initial appearance of symptoms.

PSYCHOLOGIC CAUSES OF SEXUAL DYSFUNCTION

It is impossible, in a global sense, to pinpoint the exact psychologic causes of these problems. The decision to end an inquiry by saying, "This is the cause of the problem," is both individual and arbitrary. Some clinicians are satisfied by defining the immediate antecedents of a problem; some feel compelled to uncover remote, forgotten developmental processes. Still others seek causes in cultural, rather than individual, factors. Regardless of one's preference for types of explanations, each reasonable causal hypothesis provokes a host of further questions. The explanations for psychologic sexual dysfunctions are likely to be as diverse as those for any behavior pattern. The causes lie in a basically unfathomable combination of temperamental, familial, affectual, cognitive, and cultural influences. There are, however, answers to the question of causality which are useful in a practical sense.

MODEL FOR PURE SECONDARY DYSFUNCTIONS

Dysfunctions which appear after a long period of aproblematic sexual adjustment demonstrate that adequate sexual adjustment is no guarantee against future psychological dysfunction. The cause of these problems are illuminated by a consideration of three related dimensions.

Affectual Dimension
Many dysfunctional patients think they have inexplicable problems. They have often seen other physicians in hopes of finding some physical cause. Unrecognized affects, alone or in combination, are actually responsible for many of these problems, e.g., anxiety, guilt, anger, or sadness. It is surprising to realize that the difference between a person with a secondary dysfunction and one who is simply experiencing a vicissitude of sexual life may be the lack of awareness of the interfering affect and its significance. Both of these individuals overcame their dysfunctions after recognizing their interfering affects:

> A successful editor moved to a smaller town because of her husband's job opportunity. She had difficulty adjusting to a life without exciting cultural and business involvements. Her secondary excitement phase dys-

function began immediately before her move. She hadn't realized that her anger at herself and her husband, and her sadness over her losses, were interfering with her arousal.

A very eligible bachelor began dating several months after his wife's death. His initial attempts at intercourse with each of three women were unsuccessful. He had firm erections with his new partners until coitus was attempted. Thereafter, all he felt was anxiety, frustration, and embarrassment. When asked if thoughts of his wife intruded upon him during these intimacies, he replied, "No, never," and quickly added that his children were supportive of his dating. "Logically, there is no reason for me not to date—life must go on." He then cried throughout his lengthy description of their many beautiful years together and the horror of her slow painful death. At the end of the consultation he said, "Perhaps I did feel strange being with other women."

The "cause" of his impotence may have been his lingering sadness over his loss, plus his unrecognized guilt about being with other women. These feelings interfered with sensual concentration when coitus was attempted, causing anxiety, frustration, and embarrassment over his inability to "perform."

This man was a warm, trusting, articulate person whose brief dysfunction occurred during a painful life transition. Some transitions do not preserve interpersonal warmth and trust. The marital deterioration-divorce-new relationship sequence is often associated with dysfunction. Men frequently consult physicians for impotence, retarded ejaculation, premature ejaculation, lack of desire—seemingly at a loss to explain their problems. Many divorced men distrust all women and harbor a residual anger. They may openly acknowledge these feelings on some occasions, but do not seem to relate them to their sexual "failures." Far more men than women seek help for sexual dysfunctions during this transition. Women are more likely to intuitively connect their persistent wariness/residual anger with their sexual response problems. Men tend to think of their sexual response as a performance which should be isolated from the rest of their affectual lives.

Identifying the interfering affect is an important first step in understanding the cause of secondary sexual dysfunction. It is usually not a complete explanation. The interfering affects are often inextricably related to a series of conflicts.

Conflict Dimension

Conflicts which generate pure secondary dysfunctions usually stem from interpersonal sources. Unresolved differences between partners are a common cause of deterioration in sexual life. These differences are not necessarily related to sex, but they nonetheless lead to diminished desire, limited arousability, and dissatisfaction, even though the person may be orgasmic.

This sequence occurs in both men and women, but women are much more likely to develop the dysfunctional symptom. For the woman who feels victimized and powerless in the relationship, sexual unresponsiveness may be a way of maintaining self-esteem and dignity, and exerting power. Although she may masturbate to orgasm, she does not respond erotically during partner sex because she feels angry, too proud, or cheapened by his avoidance of the unresolved problem.

A 25-year-old woman found sex with her husband highly pleasurable throughout her engagement and early marriage. She was regularly orgasmic. Her husband, an extrovert with a "great gift of gab," began to irritate her because of a succession of unkept promises. This indicated to her that his image among his friends was more important to him than her feelings. Her libido and responsiveness declined dramatically and he began labelling her as frigid (rather than trying to comprehend his contribution to their problem). She insisted that her past good sexual adjustment was evidence that she was not frigid. After several years and one child, she became unsure and thought perhaps she really was frigid.

Some individuals clearly recognize the fact that their problem is basically interpersonal. Others, such as this woman, have doubts. Their interpersonal difficulties rekindle old conflicts about themselves, which add an additional burden to their situation.

This woman was raised between three homes in a chaotic fashion during most of her childhood and adolescence. Her perception that her husband insufficiently valued her was similar to her feelings about her divorced parents, who had traded her off between them many times. Old intrapsychic conflicts reappeared—"I'm a good person—No, I'm unloveable!" "I'm a unique, attractive person with many abilities—No, I'm kidding myself! Without parental love, I am nothing!" The interpersonal problem became intrapsychic and eroded her self-esteem. In this case, the old conflicts were so powerful that the patient could no longer determine which came first—her sexual unresponsiveness or her feeling of being devalued by her husband.

Dilemma Dimension

A third approach to pure secondary dysfunction is to focus on the patient's new circumstances. Dysfunction results when the patient perceives these circumstances as an overwhelming life dilemma. In this sense, affects and conflicts are simply manifestations of a larger personal dilemma. Individuals' lives proceed in unique ways, often becoming increasingly complicated (12). Poorly handled or unresolved past problems have a way of reappearing in more convoluted situations. Clinicians should not be surprised to learn that a dysfunctional symptom appeared in each of the following circumstances:

1. A man discovered that his wife had been having an affair for five years, and forgave her for the sake of the children.
2. A woman realized that she had been kidding herself about the quality of her marriage for many years; she then promptly forgot about it.
3. A man whose hopelessly demented wife had been in a nursing home for five years fell in love with another woman. He could not marry her because he refused to divorce and abandon his wife.

Such dilemmas do not just happen. They are subtly established by the person's responses to previous interpersonal or intrapsychic circumstances. When experienced clinicians speak of patients' sexual problems as being part of larger characterologic adaptations, they are usually referring to those personality elements that predisposed the patient to the final overwhelming dilemma. The man who quickly forgave his wife's five-year affair may have other difficulties, e.g., inability to face many serious relationship problems; longstanding sense of personal inadequacy. The woman who briefly realized she had no emotional bond to her husband "forgot" about it because she was terrified by the prospect of living alone. She might have responded differently if she had previously accomplished more in her life. The man with the demented wife was as trapped by his inflexible moral standards as by his wife's unfortunate condition.

Life is a continuous psychological process. Individuals utilize their strengths in dealing with adversity. These strengths are not always sufficient; their weaknesses are illuminated by the problems which develop. After a trans-urethral resection, a man panicked because he could no longer ejaculate. Too embarrassed to mention his problem to his busy doctor, his subsequent performance anxiety led to impotence. The doctor could certainly have warned the man that retrograde ejaculation would occur after the TUR. Had the man not been so intimidated by the doctor and embarrassed about discussing sex, he could have mentioned his problem. He would then have received the brief reassurance that might have prevented his impotence (13).

Certain life circumstances are at least initially overwhelming for almost all individuals—regardless of past accomplishments. The following occurrences will usually result in at least transient, if not permanent, dysfunction:

1. A woman recovers from a stroke with a visible hemiparesis. She is preoccupied with how grotesque she must appear to her husband.
2. A physician tells a man he can resume sex after his myocardial infarction—"but take it easy." (14).
3. A couple attempts to resume sexual relations after the wife's radical mastectomy and chemotherapy (15).

In summary, secondary psychological dysfunctions are caused by life circumstances that generate affects that appear in one form or another during sexual intimacy. The affects, the conflicts, the dilemma, and sometimes a problematic aspect of the patient's character, can be recognized in the course of a thorough psychological evaluation.

There are two important conceptual questions about pure secondary dysfunctions which usually remain unanswered, even after a thorough psychological evaluation: 1. Why did this particular symptom develop, i.e., premature ejaculation as opposed to erectile dysfunction; vaginismus rather than an arousal problem? The determinants of symptom choice in any individual are poorly understood. There are probably predispositions to specific symptoms stemming from past childhood experiences, neurophysiological organization, and character style. 2. Why was the patient able to withstand previous stresses without developing a dysfunction, i.e., what host factors contributed to the development of this dysfunction at this time? It is useful to consider the possibility that aging or an unrecognized organic factor may predispose some individuals to psychogenic dysfunction.

> A 25-year-old man who has trouble recognizing his anger may be fully potent with his wife two hours after a heated, poorly-resolved argument. The strength of his sexual desire and his responsiveness to tactile stimulation enable him to counter the effects of the negative affect state. Thirty years later, still physically healthy, he may be impotent two hours after a similar argument, because his desire and responsiveness to sexual stimulation are less powerful. If such a man happens to be on reserpine, his poor recognition of his anger may still be the cause of his impotence. The presence of the drug, however, may have reduced his sexual responsiveness even further.

A MODEL FOR PURE PRIMARY DYSFUNCTIONS

These dysfunctions are more difficult to conceptualize than those which are secondary. Research has thus far either yielded negative results (16) or been too limited in scope. Two assumptions usually prove helpful in thinking about the causes of lifelong problems. The first is that pure primary dysfunctions are the result of an individual's developmental failure to accept himself as a sexual person. This assumption allows the clinician to separate the problem from its many effects. It enables the clinician to see beyond the patient's illusions or rationalizations to the real issue of personal discomfort with sexuality.

> An articulate 50-year-old man has never been able to remain in the vagina for longer than 10 seconds without ejaculating. Although he has maintained this pattern with several other partners, he complains that the real problem is his wife's "semi-frigidity"—i.e., her dislike of sex, difficulty becoming aroused, refusal to engage in oral-genital behaviors.

> A 24-year-old woman has never had an orgasm with any of her four partners. She is frequently angry at her husband, but is easily aroused with him. As she approaches a high level of excitement, she becomes annoyed by his genital "fumbling" or his behavior during the previous few days.

If the responsibility for sexual comfort is considered a personal matter, there are three potential sources of psychological problems in any sexual equilibrium: his sexual comfort; her sexual comfort; their sexual interaction. The clinician can help patients assume responsibility for their own sexual discomfort and thus end the destructive scapegoating.

The second assumption is that the symptom-bearer's emotional difficulties are not entirely due to the sexual dysfunction. Primary sexual dysfunctions are often inextricably intertwined with other emotional difficulties —such as depressive episodes, neurotic symptoms, eating disorders, substance abuse, poor social skills. The sources of the dysfunction may be related to these other problems; the exact nature of this relationship, however, is often not clear. This assumption should prepare the clinician for the diverse emotional problems encountered in treating primary dysfunctions.

> A man had what his wife characterized as a "strange" involvement with his unhappy mother. The mother, who has been "dying" for at least twenty years of largely psychogenic illnesses, shares an unusual closeness with her son. He has forced himself to be sympathetic because he feels sorry for her. He listens to her complaints at great length, even though he frequently has to "blank out" his mind. Going away to college and moving to another city offered relief from the distress, except for his mother's frequent guilt-inducing phone calls. He has had unremitting severe premature ejaculation with two wives. A generally guilty, mildly depressed person, his business partners have repeatedly taken advantage of him. He complained he felt weak as a man.

> A 35-year-old woman has never been able to maintain arousal with a partner. She is readily orgasmic during masturbation, as long as she uses this fantasy: After a violent fight, the lover is so exhausted he can barely move. She stimulates him until he gets an erection and then quickly has intercourse. This fantasy seems to capture many aspects of this woman's style. She hates surprises and needs to be in control of everything. She does not permit herself spontaneous emotion. She maintains an unusually large distance between herself and others. Although this distance creates loneliness and depression, closeness leads to intolerable anxiety. She often provokes arguments whenever she feels sex is imminent. Her husband says she is fearful of sex, unwilling to satisfy his sexual needs, and unable to see her role in their interpersonal problems.

Discussions of the causes of primary dysfunctions are often couched in terms of two psychologic ideologies: 1. Primary dysfunctions are caused by intrapsychic conflicts (19). Thus, vaginismus, for example, might be caused by conflicts about being a heterosexual. "I want to be normal and experience penetration—I am afraid. I want intercourse badly—I am not ready. I feel it is wrong for me." Clinicians who bypass intrapsychic conflict as a cause because it is either too obvious or invalid use another ideologic language; 2. Primary dysfunctions are caused by negative conditioning about sex (20). Thus, vaginismus might be caused by past teaching that intercourse was evil, prior sexual assault, erroneous sexual education, etc. Confusion sometimes arises because the proponents of differing ideologies, e.g., psychoanalytic, behavioral, interactional, only·discuss their own causal concepts. Most clinicians, however, tend to borrow concepts from several ideologies. The role of conflict in sexual dysfunction is as obvious as the idea that the conflict was derived or conditioned by past events and interpersonal processes.

The study of the subjective experience of sex afforded by the primary dysfunctions provides an important introduction to the psychology of the self. Problems which are manifested by decreased self-esteem, damaged self-image, and failure to accomplish age-appropriate tasks are likely to share a causal relationship with primary sexual dysfunctions. All of these problems represent symptomatic expressions of impairments of the sense of self. For practical purposes, the causes of any primary dysfunction may involve one or more of the following.

Problematic Parental Relationships

Some individuals whose conflicts result in sexual discomfort have never really become psychologically independent of their parents. Persistent psychologically-limiting parental ties result from both the child's anxiety about being independent and the parental clinging which fosters guilt or lack of confidence.

A 23-year-old woman, married for eight months, was cured of her primary excitement phase dysfunction after six psychotherapy sessions and an all-night talk with her previously distant older sister. She realized that her guilt over being angry with her mother had caused the problem. She characterized her mother as an over-controlling, ignorant, and otherwise unlikeable person who never had anything nice to say about sex. The daughter's guilt was increased when she married and left her depressed mother only a year after her father's death. She learned that her sister also had similar perceptions and resentments, which had never been mentioned. In fact, the sister had experienced the same sexual difficulty early in her marriage. the sister's kind revelations enabled the patient to stop punishing herself and separate from her mother. "I don't have to be miserable just because my mother is!"

The role of intrapsychic conflicts stemming from parental relationships is exemplified by the premature ejaculator with the clinging hypochondriacal mother and the over-controlled woman who would only allow herself any sexual expression with powerless men. Such problems usually result from extended interactions, rather than single incidents. For example, the overly-controlled woman had a verbally and physically violent psychotic father. He had several hospitalizations before the parents divorced when the patient was four. Her sexual patterns may have resulted because her mother was too preoccupied with her unstable marriage to form a close relationship with her daughter. Her fear of men might have been generated by witnessing violent rages, being beaten by her father, or her grandmother's constant comments that men were untrustworthy creatures. The exact causes are never determined with certainty.

Maturational Unreadiness

Not all interfering intrapsychic conflicts are due to problematic parental relationships or negative conditioning. Individuals arrive at various developmental landmarks at different times, e.g., walking, reading, talking comfortably with adults, dating. Some adolescents are late bloomers. Some realize that their anxiety-ridden initial sexual intimacies are due to their immaturity. Others in similarly overwhelming circumstances may propel themselves into situations that prevent stable personal growth.

A 15-year-old girl's sudden perception of her older sister as her father's favorite caused her to begin having intercourse with a variety of boys on a casual basis. She was vaguely aware that there was a defiant, rebellious quality to this sexual behavior. In college, she sought help for the primary orgasmic phase dysfunction experienced with each of her 11 partners. She refused any exploration of the sources of her inhibition, insisting that she should only be taught how to be orgasmic. She was certain that sex was basically mechanical, and she just hadn't learned the technique properly.

A struggle for separation from parents, grief over dead or divorced parents, and denied need for parental nurturance are some reasons for an individual's persistence in seeking physical intimacy when faced with obvious maturational unreadiness. Readiness for sexual intimacy is extremely variable. The subcultural influences on the age of readiness are not yet understood (21).

Fear of Loss of Control

The sensation of being swept away is an integral part of the orgasmic experience. Most individuals first have this experience during masturbation.

They are subsequently able to tolerate the sensation without fear during partner sexual behavior. Many dysfunctional individuals have great fears about losing control, which cause them to inhibit their excitement. They are unable to specifically identify their fears and can only say that terrible things may happen, e.g., loss of bladder or bowel control, bursting of a blood vessel, death, loss of moral restraint, fear of hurting the partner. It is interesting that not all these men and women are inexperienced with masturbation. Their feared loss of control is specifically related to their inability to feel safe with a partner. Some possible causes of the inability to trust a partner are:

1. Familial or cultural teaching that sex is bad. The unidentified fear during sex is a disguised form of guilt.
2. Previous nonsexual relationships with undependable, impulsive persons.
3. Inexperience.
4. Familial silence about sex which conveys a negative message.
5. Obsessive-compulsive and paranoid personality styles.
6. Past prolonged difficulties in gaining control, e.g., over bedwetting, temper, sibling rivalry.

Individuals have varying sensitivities to cultural ideas. Why prohibitions against sexual expression are taken seriously by some and not by others remains unclear. A woman felt very foolish after seeking help for an orgasmic phase dysfunction. Her physician suggested she try masturbation. A devout Catholic, she distinctly remembered being taught masturbation was a sin. After discussing the doctor's recommendation with four friends from parochial school, she learned that each had begun regular masturbation in adolescence. They were all easily orgasmic with intercourse. Distraught, she asked her religious mother, who "confessed" to also being orgasmic under these circumstances.

Cognitive Deficiencies—Sexual Ignorance

The dysfunctional are apt to be ignorant in a number of sexual areas: female genital structures; partner's preferred means of stimulation; physiological concomitants of arousal; their own arousal potential during foreplay, genital play, and coitus. These cognitive deficiencies partly result from the lack of opportunity to learn about sexual matters. Sex education begins when toddlers first notice the differences between boys and girls. Later, questions about the origin of babies are answered. Other realities are also explained, e.g., homosexuality, sex before marriage, masturbation, contraception, etc. Families vary enormously in their willingness and ability to calmly discuss sexual matters.

Sexual ignorance does not, however, simply result from a lack of exposure; it may stem from a persistent need to not know. At any given time, the impact of sexual knowledge may be more than the child or adolescent can handle. Exposure to sexual information prior to maturational readiness may produce confusion, anxiety, and avoidance of the subject. Parental behavior that stimulates sexual feelings in children, witnessing of parental intercourse, and being used sexually by an adult have been repeatedly implicated in producing individuals with strong needs to not know about sex.

Unresolved Oedipal Complex

Psychoanalytic theory stresses that the development of a healthy personality depends upon the resolution of the child's inevitable sexual attraction to the parent of the opposite sex. All primary sexual dysfunctions may ultimately derive from persistent incestuous wishes. These unrecognized wishes may interfere with maturation. The process of maturation enables an individual to participate in sexual behavior without overwhelming anxiety. This formulation raises the question of which factors prevent the resolution of oedipal strivings. The answer to that question is likely to be unfocused because it may involve all the complex issues inherent in parent-child interactions.

THE APPLICATION OF THE MODELS
TO MORE COMPLICATED PROBLEMS

More complicated dysfunctional equilibria may be simplified by using the assumptions that primary problems represent discomfort with one's sexual self and secondary problems result from new life situations which generate unmanageable affects. Many complicated problems are mixtures of primary and secondary dysfunctions. For example, the models of causality suggest that both remote personal developmental, and recent psychological, factors would be important in the following situations:

1. A man with lifelong premature ejaculation becomes impotent.
2. A woman who had been easily aroused, but never orgasmic, is no longer able to become excited.
3. A couple seeks help because of the wife's newly-acquired aversion to being touched. He has frequently been unable to ejaculate with a partner; she has never had much sexual desire.

In such cases it is safe to assume that some new factor has been added to the symptom-bearer's lifelong discomfort with sexuality. Individuals may have more than one dysfunctional symptom. All symptoms may be primary, secondary, or some combination. The number of symptoms often increases when the couple is considered, rather than the individual. Some of the component problems in an equilibrium may simply be reactions to the partner's dysfunction, but many have individual personal origins.

TABLE III
INFLUENCES ON THE DEVELOPMENT OF PERSONAL SEXUAL COMFORT

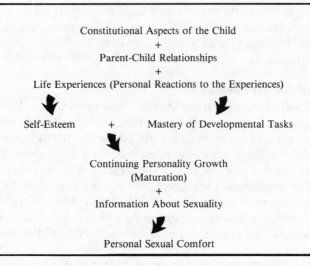

Constitutional Aspects of the Child
+
Parent-Child Relationships
+
Life Experiences (Personal Reactions to the Experiences)

Self-Esteem   +   Mastery of Developmental Tasks

Continuing Personality Growth
(Maturation)
+
Information About Sexuality

Personal Sexual Comfort

Table III is a schematic representation of the general influences on the development of sexual comfort. There are probably very few individuals who are genuinely comfortable during their initial sexual experiences, i.e., free of guilt, anxiety, or fear; many, however, can contain these negative affects without suffering an impairment of sexual physiology. The origins of all primary psychologic dysfunctions—from the profound incapacities of desire, arousal, and penetration to the more common, lesser impairments of the orgasmic phase—are thought to involve one or more of the factors included in Table III. Personal sexual comfort is not an absolute, either-or phenomenon; nor is it the only factor that enables sexual responsiveness. The interpersonal milieu can foster either individual comfort or discomfort. Table IV is a schematic representation of the possible interactional effects between the degree of individual sexual comfort and the quality of the nonsexual relationship. Table IV suggests that the quality of a sexual equilibrium may vary considerably over time, depending upon the rate of personal maturation and the degree of interpersonal support.

A synthesis of these figures is necessary to the understanding of the pathogeneses of many complicated sexual equilibria. Individuals who can comfortably accept and value their sexuality as an integral part of their beings are more likely to maintain their sexual responsiveness in a variety of life circumstances. They can provide emotional support if faced with a partner's dysfunction. Some individuals are only marginally comfortable with their sexuality. They have no symptoms under certain conditions, e.g., romantic

TABLE IV
NATURAL HISTORIES OF SEXUAL EQUILIBRIA

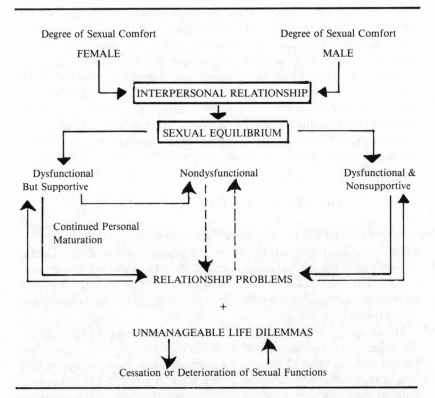

mood, no financial worries, no partner demands. Besides becoming dysfunctional under stress, they may have little capacity to provide emotional support if their partners are, or become, dysfunctional. Dysfunctional individuals who completely lack sexual comfort may be unable to help one another, in spite of their best intentions.

Two young, loving, sexually uneducated and inexperienced people marry. They find sex difficult to discuss before marriage—and difficult to "perform" afterwards. After several years, the husband has still not acquired ejaculatory control and the wife cannot achieve orgasm by any means. In their quest for better sexual adjustment, they have tried to follow the advice of prominent authors. When she spends more time stimulating him to help his control, he becomes nervous, fearing he will ejaculate. When she makes suggestions about touching her genitals, his feelings are hurt. When he does it her way, he either falls asleep from boredom or gets her so excited that she stops the clitoral stimulation.

When he stimulates her in his preferred fashion, he ejaculates before she becomes excited.

The behavioral interactions of dysfunctional partners add to the complexity indicated by the causal models. The insights of psychoanalytic theory and behavioral psychology can only partially illuminate the operation of the sexual equilibrium. The systems are very unique and dynamically responsive. Changes within individuals (e.g., maturation, depression, poor health, job failure) and their relationships (e.g., strengthening of the bond between the couple, suspicion of untrustworthiness) affect the equilibria. Systems theorists are beginning to formulate some of the principles of behavior systems (22,23). Although this field promises to further illuminate the nature of the sexual system, general principles cannot enable a complete understanding of individual lives.

THE SIGNIFICANCE OF THE SYMPTOMS

Any individual's or couple's current dysfunctional symptoms may have a significance that transcends the immediate causes of the problem. The significance of the symptom furnishes a more global explanation for the causal factors. The individual may never recognize the symptom's significance; if he does, this recognition may precede or follow the awareness of its immediate causes.

The answers to three questions can be helpful to patients and clinicians in determining a symptom's significance: 1. Why is the patient coming for treatment at this time? (Typically, the chief complaint has been present for a long time. What else has motivated the consultation?) 2. What was responsible for the initial appearance of the symptoms? 3. What factors maintain the existence of the symptoms?

> A plain, softspoken man with long-standing discomfort with his sexuality was brought in to be "fixed" by his attractive, aggressive, sexually comfortable wife. "If necessary, I am willing to spend thousands of dollars to have a good sexual life with him!" As his potency improved, however, she attempted to undermine the treatment. When confronted with the incongruity of her behavior, she lost all sexual desire. Months later she announced she did not love him and sought a divorce.

The husband had been periodically impotent during his entire five-year marriage. Apparently none of his previous partners had demanded anything beyond his standard quick intercourse in the dark without foreplay. His nervousness during sex seriously limited his wife's sexual expression. She felt she was losing her mind and could no longer stand the "pathetic" sex. During therapy, it became clear that his sexual anxiety was partly maintained by her endless demands for more of whatever he provided—sexually, materially, and socially. "I'm calm all day at the office. I feel myself getting tense on the way home." She eventually decided that her anger, lack of sexual desire, and general unhappiness was due to her mistake in marrying this nice, but for her inadequate, person. Her wish to have him fixed at any cost and her sense of losing her mind were probably attempts to avoid facing this realization. When it was all over, he confessed, "I always knew I wasn't good enough for her."

Clinicians and patients are equally incapable of defining love. They too wonder what role this intangible factor plays in the genesis and maintenance of psychogenic symptoms. Love seems to help some couples cope with a dysfunction with relatively little pain. On the other hand, the lack, or disappearance, of love may cause the problem for some people.

> A husband, distraught over his wife's distaste for sex, dragged her in for help. He had just read a book about "frigidity" that described her perfectly. He complained that she avoided sex whenever possible, didn't like foreplay, and required prolonged clitoral stimulation on the very rare occasions when she had orgasm. The wife acknowledged the accuracy of his descriptions. With the exception of their more pleasurable early experiences, she just could not tolerate the thought of sex. When seen alone, however, she quickly informed me that she is not "frigid" with her married lover of five years. She had loved this man even before her marriage. She loves sex with him and had no inhibitions—i.e., she readily engaged in oral sex and was easily orgasmic through hand and mouth stimulation or intercourse. Although she loved her husband "in a way," it just wasn't the same as her feeling for her lover.

Significant realizations such as "I don't love her (him); I made a mistake in this relationship; I have outgrown this person," although common, are not the only larger explanations for dysfunctions. Others include: "I cannot accept growing old and not having the power or beauty of my youth, I am not grown up. I do not approve of my own behavior; I am not working in the correct job; I am paying you back; I am depressed; etc."

All psychogenic dysfunction probably has some personal significance involving issues of commitment, life direction, or perceptions of one's role in intimate and social contexts. The behavior that initiates and maintains a symptom relates to its significance. Clinicians must be careful, however, to not draw premature conclusions about the significance of symptoms. Usually it is only appreciated after a protracted time period. On the other hand, they must not avoid considering these larger issues, since the problem's resolution may be expedited by the discovery of its meaning.

TREATMENT OF SEXUAL DYSFUNCTION

Most individuals who seek help for sexual dysfunctions have at least eight questions in mind: 1. Can I be helped? 2. What are my chances of getting better? 3. How quickly can I be helped? 4. Will hypnosis help? 5. How much will therapy cost? 6. Will therapy be upsetting? 7. Which type of therapy should I have? 8. Who is a good therapist? These are all reasonable questions. Unfortunately, they do not all have reasonable answers.

A number of interesting changes occur when these questions are rephrased from the therapist's perspective: 1. "Can I be helped?" becomes "What variables involving patients, therapists, and techniques determine successful treatment outcome?" 2. "What are my chances of getting better?" becomes "Given 100 individuals or couples with the same component dysfunctions, how many will improve with any given treatment modality? How many will be cured?" 3. "How quickly can I be helped?" becomes "What is the mean and range of duration of treatment for successfully treated problems?" 4. "Will hypnosis help?" becomes "Can I be cured without being actively involved?" The patient wants to know if a psychological problem can be dealt with like a medical problem, i.e., given to the doctor to "fix." Under what circumstances can such an approach be helpful? 5. "How much will therapy cost?" becomes "Should fees for sex therapies be individualized or should there be a standard fee for a set number of sessions contracted in advance, e.g., two weeks of daily therapy; 10 weekly sessions, etc.?" 6. "Will therapy be upsetting?" becomes "Can the patient deal with the pain involved in recognizing the causes and significance of the problem? Can therapy conceivably worsen the person's emotional adaptation? What are the risks of therapeutic failure?" 7. "Which type of therapy should I have?" becomes "Is there any evidence that one therapeutic approach is superior to another for any given problem?" 8. "Who is a good therapist?" becomes "What qualities should a competent sex therapist possess?"

Only some of these important questions have been subjected to careful analysis; there are no firmly established, scientifically redocumented answers (24). Opinions, however, abound.

Therapy for a sexual dysfunction, regardless of the technique employed, is more of an art than a science. It involves a relationship specifically designed to have a positive effect on sexual function. It is relatively simple to describe the principles and techniques of any therapy; it is impossible to describe the interaction in any therapeutic relationship. This section will present some of the newer techniques currently used in the direct treatment of specific sexual dysfunctions. It should be recognized from the onset, however, that there is only questionable evidence of their being more effective in the long run than more traditional therapies that focus on personal conflicts assumed to underlie psychologic sexual symptoms.

Sensate Focus Technique for Couples

This technique has been the source of both Masters and Johnson's fame as therapists and the rapid development of the field of sex therapy. Sex therapy is often erroneously equated with this elegantly simple aspect of an essentially psychotherapeutic process. Sensate focus is an experiential learning process that helps the couple overcome performance anxiety by exploring the dimensions of giving and receiving sexual pleasure. The couple learns to relax and concentrate on sensation; they discover new ways of providing pleasure and communicating more effectively (2,25).

Besides facilitating the accomplishments of these laudable goals, sensate focus is an excellent diagnostic tool for determining the sources of the barriers to better sexual functioning. Once these sources emerge and are evaluated, the focus of therapy is redirected towards overcoming the "new" problem. After this is resolved, the patient can proceed to the next step in the experiential learning process.

Sensate focus instructions are usually prefaced with a brief introduction by the therapist. My remarks include three major points:

1. I know you want to . . . (regain your potency, have an orgasm, gain ejaculatory control, etc.). The achievement of three basic psychological states during your sexual behavior is a prerequisite for attaining your goal. These states involve your willingness to make love, relaxation during lovemaking, and ability to concentrate on sensation. I cannot stress enough how important these basic psychological ingredients are to your sexual life; without them, neither of you will experience much sexual pleasure.

2. You should know that I consider sex as much more than penis-vagina intercourse. Sex is the sum total of a couple's physical interactions. Kissing and caressing are sexual activities that are important unto themselves. They are not merely a warm-up for intercourse.

3. When people who have no sexual problems make love, their behavior includes both giving and receiving sexual pleasure. At times the partners take turns giving and receiving; at times these behaviors occur simultaneously. Both activities are important because they make each partner feel competent, powerful, and valued. Between now and our next appointment, I would like you to try the following exercises exactly according to the instructions.

   a. No matter what may occur, there is to be no intercourse—just lovemaking.

b. Each of you is to take turns giving and receiving sexual pleasure. Each turn as a receiver must last at least 10 minutes. You should both be naked, in a comfortable bed, with some light in the room.

c. As the giver, you are to use your hands, lips, and tongue to kiss and caress your partner's whole body—front and back, top to bottom, with the exception of the breast and genital areas. Your responsibility is to provide your partner with pleasant sensations. Experiment: touch firmly, massage, touch lightly. Do not tickle. Touch parts of the body you usually bypass—buttocks, armpits, feet, between fingers. Watch your partner's responses—facial expressions, breathing—and do more of what seems enjoyable. As the receiver, you should relax and feel what is happening to you. Your concentration should be at the skin level when your partner is touching you. Make your partner aware of what is pleasurable—through words, sounds, smiles, movements, etc. Do not try to stimulate your partner during this experience. Just relax and receive the sensations. Feel free to use more than ten minutes. When this task is over, switch roles.

These are the easiest and most pleasant sensate focus instructions. They provoke little resistance, unless the partners are angry at each other or have deteriorated relationships. Such couples cannot "find the time" to follow instructions, i.e., in spite of their professed desire to be helped with their sexual problems, they are unwilling to participate in therapy. Couples with desire or arousal problems usually have difficulty relaxing and concentrating, in spite of their willingness to make love. Therapy focuses on the interfering thoughts, feelings, or conflicts. Once these factors have been discussed, the couple may notice increased relaxation and arousal.

The first set of instructions induces considerable arousal in many patients. The therapy session is spent discussing the sources of each partner's pleasure, and the personal meaning of the experience. Breast stimulation is then added. The couple is encouraged to continue their experimentation with various means of stimulation. They are warned not to try to replicate their previous behaviors because every experience is somewhat different and pleasure must be discovered anew.

Nondemand Genital Stimulation. The next set of instructions extends the earlier principles of giving and receiving pleasure to include the genitals. Genital touching is used to provide various modes of pleasure and communicate about what feels good. Genital anatomy is reviewed. Previous modes of genital stimulation and their related problems are discussed. Each partner is instructed to do what the other seems to enjoy, without trying to produce an orgasm. Oral-genital stimulation is recommended only if the couple finds it acceptable. Intercourse is still strictly prohibited.

When sensate focus goes well, it results in increased communication, caring, attention to each other's needs, and a sense of sharing a meaningful learning experience. These elements combine to produce a noticeable new sense of closeness or bonding, which helps individuals to face their own anxieties about the next stages.

Extravaginal Orgasmic Attainment. The couple is instructed to induce orgasm through hand or oral stimulation. After this has been repeatedly accomplished, intercourse is introduced—usually in the female-superior position.

The sexual tasks are modified according to each couple's needs and component dysfunctions. Some of the modifications for common dysfunctions are:

For Premature Ejaculation. The man is told that his previous strategy of minimizing arousal, though understandable, is exactly the opposite of what should be done. He must concentrate on penile sensation, allowing his partner to stimulate his genitals directly. When he feels himself approaching the stage of ejaculatory inevitability (1), he should signal her to stop the stimulation for at least thirty seconds, or until his urge to ejaculate has passed. She should then begin again. Repeated manual or oral-genital stimulation without intercourse quickly raises the man's tolerance level. When prolonged genital stimulation can be tolerated, the couple can begin the quiet vagina exercises, i.e., penis remains in the vagina for one minute without movement (female-superior position). When this is accomplished without the occurrence of ejaculation, the woman is instructed to move slowly. She must quickly return to the quiet vagina position if the man feels the escalation of the urge to ejaculate. In this manner, the couple learns to pace the thrusting according to the man's degree of arousal. When he can tolerate long periods of the partner's thrusting, they are encouraged to turn over and allow the man to pace himself. When this is accomplished, they are instructed to take turns giving and receiving pleasure during intercourse. Although another means of learning ejaculatory control—Seman's squeeze technique (26)—is better known, it is employed less frequently than the above stop-start technique.

For Female Orgasmic Phase Dysfunction. During nondemand genital stimulation a great emphasis is placed on the clitoris—its appearance, anatomy, and function as a physical site of intense sexual pleasure. The woman is encouraged to show her partner the types of stimulation which produce the greatest pleasure. She must assume responsibility for her own orgasm, i.e., the man can only stimulate her; she must lose her inhibitions and allow orgasm to occur. This often requires considerable encouragement from the therapist (27).

Masturbation exercises are often suggested for women who are not able, or have never tried, to induce orgasm through self-stimulation. They allow women to experience orgasm by themselves, before becoming involved in the more psychologically complex environment of partner sex. These exercises may accompany or precede the first set of instructions (28).

For Coitally Anorgasmic Women. Such patients are easily orgasmic through manual- or oral-clitoral stimulation, but not through coitus. It is probable that as many as one-third of adult women are not often orgasmic during coitus, but exact figures are not available (29). This condition may be a variation of normality or a mild, subtle, psychological disorder; in the past, it was incorrectly classified as "frigidity." The clinician should attempt to clarify the couple's reasons for concern, i.e., is the man uneasy because he can't satisfy his wife? Or, does the wife have a desire to be "normal?" Women are encouraged to move during coitus in any way that is pleasureable. They must learn that their husband's needs do not always come first. The woman must direct the intercourse, moving by herself for herself. The couple is taught that the clitoral orgasm is not separate, distinct, and inferior to the so-called "vaginal" orgasm. Coital orgasm is usually produced by direct and indirect clitoral stimulation, i.e., through the bumping and grinding movements of pelvic apposition and the inevitable tugging on the clitoral hood that occurs when the labia minora are depressed during thrusting (1). If this is not sufficient to produce orgasm, the technique of simultaneous clitoral stimulation during coitus is taught. Side-to-side and vaginal rear entry positions are taught because they allow for easy simultaneous clitoral stimulation and penile containment. If the woman is willing, she can learn to stimulate her clitoris during coitus, since she knows the most effective technique (25).

For Psychogenic Impotence. Psychogenic impotence is simply the inability to stay aroused during sex (30). Sensate focus is uniquely helpful in reassuring the couple that the symptom, regardless of its ultimate explanation, will disappear if the man can become and stay aroused. Loss of erection is translated into loss of arousal, which is explained by sudden anxiety or concentration lapses. The exercises focus on having the man relax and be caressed until he develops a lasting erection. The attainment of the first lasting erection decreases performance anxiety, which is manifested by loss of erection prior to or during penetration. For many men, penetration is the "true" test—the rest was merely foreplay. The persistence of this attitude indicates incomplete success. All men, however, experience increased worry at this stage. The confidence of the therapist, the partner's support, and the man's ability to concentrate on sensation during foreplay enable penetration, vaginal containment, and thrusting to orgasm.

For Female Primary Excitement Phase Dysfunction. Technically, the approach to the inability to obtain or maintain arousal is the same as the approach to impotence. The therapy, however, often turns out to be more complicated. Many of the women who are helped to overcome arousal problems do not seem to be capable of regularly achieving orgasm. This is not as frequent in impotent men. Also, it becomes apparent during sensate focus that many of these women suffer from a more basic problem of desire.

For Male and Female Desire Problems. Secondary desire problems are usually caused by physical illness, medications, depression, relationship deterioration, and other longstanding sexual dysfunctions. Attention to these more basic issues may resolve the problem.

Primary desire problems present therapists with the current major therapeutic enigma (9). While patients can be helped to concentrate on sensation and relax during sex, there is no set of instructions for transforming indifference into willingness or fear and antipathy into desire. A thorough, careful appreciation of the historical sources of resistance to the first set of sensate focus instructions may resolve the problem if it is psychogenic and not constitutional, i.e., acquired from past experience, rather than dictated by neuroendocrine organization. It is often necessary to switch from couple to individual psychotherapy.

Treatment Approaches for Individuals

Sex therapy is not a uniform treatment approach. Its techniques are variously applied by therapists with diverse professional training. Married couples with dysfunctions may be treated by one therapist or by opposite-sexed co-therapists. The therapy sessions may be scheduled daily for two weeks, weekly for a predetermined period, or weekly until a stable improvement is either achieved or recognized as not being possible. Therapy may also be conducted with groups of dysfunctional couples. Other couples may be treated with a marital therapy which does not include sensate focus. Such therapy is usually recommended to dysfunctional couples with seriously disturbed nonsexual relationships. Couples with relationship problems which seem to stem from the dysfunction are more likely to be treated with sex therapy.

There are special problems involved in treating unmarried dysfunctional individuals who have partners, i.e., the single, divorced, separated, widowed. Sex therapy with such couples often falters over the issue of commitment. The symptom-bearer may not be able to be completely honest, for fear of losing the partner. The partner may have a hidden motive for participating. One or both partners usually end up questioning the viability of the current relationship. Engaged couples, for example, may discover their marked ambivalence toward marriage during sex therapy.

Many unmarried dysfunctional individuals have no partners. There are currently three basic therapeutic options for them: 1. Sex therapy in a group of other same-sexed, dysfunctional individuals. Individuals are put through highly-structured educational group processes, e.g., groups of nonorgasmic women or premature ejaculators (32,33). The unique combination of support, education, role modeling, and competition may enable such endeavors to be effective. 2. Individual psychotherapy. The widespread publicity devoted to sex therapy has obscured the fact that traditional one-to-one therapies have helped many individuals overcome their problems. Early attempts to justify the growth of sex therapy usually mentioned the lack of evidence confirming the effectiveness of psychotherapy for sexual problems. This lack was contrasted with Masters and Johnson's impressive couple treatment results (2). Even today, however, there are no comparable data on the results of therapy with single individuals—with the possible exception of group therapy. 3. Sex therapy with a surrogate partner. This technique is not widely available and continues to be controversial for many reasons—not the least of which is the possibility that a man may be successful with a surrogate and still not be able to function with his own partner.

Experience with a variety of techniques has demonstrated that there is no single optimum approach to all individuals with any given sexual dysfunction. A decade ago, almost all symptom-bearers were referred for individual psychotherapy—often a long-term, expensive process with unpredictable results. Sex therapy also has certain strengths and limitations, which were revealed when the initial enthusiasm about the new approach was replaced by more experienced, critical evaluation. Decisions about suitable modes of therapy, i.e., sex therapy, individual psychotherapy, marital therapy, or none at all, remain matters of clinical judgment. These decisions would be simplified if one could state, for instance, that all married men with secondary psychologic impotence should be treated with sensate focus techniques. Unfortunately, treatment choice is not determined solely by the chief complaint. Some other factors are age, patient's psychological-mindedness, cause of the symptom, degree of support from wife, mental health, financial background, and subculture.

CONCLUDING REMARKS

Individuals with psychologic dysfunctions may be helped in a number of ways. The success of these therapeutic endeavors ultimately depends upon the causes of the symptoms. Although one can never be certain that all the influences have been ascertained and appreciated, it is possible to enable symptom removal with incomplete information. Sexual problems are often closely linked to other life problems. Thus, a sex therapist must know about broader emotional subjects; similarly, clinicians without specific training in sex therapy techniques may improve an individual's sexual functioning by dealing with other facets of the person. Although psychoanalysis was once considered the only viable clinical approach to sexual problems, it is not an ideal treatment for the majority of dysfunctional patients. Moreover, it has fostered erroneous concepts, e.g., only vaginal orgasm is normal; all sexual symptoms arise from unconscious conflict, and given only limited consideration to constitutional, organic, and interpersonal determinants of dysfunction. Despite some deficiencies, however, many basic psychoanalytic assumptions about psychogenic sexual symptoms are clinically verifiable. Symptoms do stem from underlying conflicts, some of which may be better understood by delving into an individual's past. After the first decade of experience with sex therapy, the study of sexual problems may be able to proceed along less ideologic lines and concentrate on illuminating the many remaining questions about sexual life.

REFERENCES

1. Masters WH, Johnson VE: *Human Sexual Response*. Boston, Little Brown & Co, 1966.
2. Masters WH, Johnson VE: *Human Sexual Inadequacy*. Boston, Little Brown & Co, 1970.
3. Frank E, Anderson C, Rubenstein D: Frequency of sexual dysfunction in "normal" couples. *N Engl J Med* 1978;299:111-115.
4. Levine SB, Yost MA Jr: Frequency of sexual dysfunction in a general gynecological clinic: An epidemiological approach. *Arch Sex Behav* 1976;5:229-238.
5. Martin C: Sexual activity in the aging male, in Money J, Musaph H (eds): *Handbook of Sexology*. Amsterdam, Excerpta Medical, 1977, pp 813-824.
6. Raboch J, Mellan J, Starka L: Klinefelter's syndrome: Sexual development and activity. *Arch Sex Behav* 1979;8:333-339.
7. Bentler PM, Reeler WH: Models of female orgasm. *Arch Sex Behav* 1979;8:405-423.
8. Kaplan HS: *The New Sex Therapy*. New York, Brunner/mazel, 1974.
9. Kaplan HS: Hypoactive sexual desire. *J Sex Marital Ther* 1977;3:3-9.
10. American Psychiatric Association Task Force on Nomenclature and Statistics: *DSM-III: Diagnostic Criteria Draft*. New York, American Psychiatric Association, 1978.
11. Levine SB: Marital sexual dysfunction: Introductory concepts. *Ann Intern Med* 1976; 84:448-453.
12. Vaillant GE: *Adaptation to Life*. Boston, Little Brown & Co, 1977.
13. Zohar J, Meiraz BM, Durst N: Factors influencing sexual activity after prostatectomy: A prospective study. *J Urol* 1976;116:332-334.
14. Bloch A, Maeder JP, Haissly JC: Sexual problems after myocardial infarction. *Am Heart J* 1975;90:536-537.
15. Wellisch DK, Jamison KR, Pasnau RO: Psychosocial aspects of mastectomy: II. The man's perspective. *Am J Psychiatry* 1978;135:543-546.
16. Fisher S: *The Female Orgasm*. New York, Basic Books Inc, 1973.
17. Munjack D, Cristol A, Goldstein A, et al.: Behavioral treatment of orgasmic dysfunction: A controlled study. *Br J Psychiatry* 1976;129:497-502.
18. Kilmann PR, Auerbach R: Treatments of premature ejaculation and psychogenic impotence: A critical review of the literature. *Arch Sex Behav* 1979;8:81-100.
19. Bieber I: The psychoanalytic treatment of sexual disorders. *J Sex Marital Ther* 1974;1:5-15.
20. Annon JS: *The Behavioral Treatment of Sexual Problems*. Honolulu, Enabling Systems Inc, 1974, vol 1.

21. Gagnon JH, Simon W: *Sexual Conduct: The Social Sources of Human Sexuality.* Chicago, Aldine Publishing Co, 1973.

22. Steinglass P: The conceptualization of marriage from a systems theory perspective, in Paolino TJ Jr, McCrady BS (eds): *Marriage and Marital Therapy.* New York, Brunner Mazel, 1978, pp 298–365.

23. Sluzki CE: Marital Therapy from a systems theory perspective, in Paolino TJ Jr, McCrady BS (eds): *Marriage and Marital Therapy.* New York, Brunner/Mazel, 1978, pp 366–394.

24. Wright J, Perreault R, Mathiew M: The treatment of sexual dysfunction. *Arch Gen Psychiatry* 1977;34:881–890.

25. Kaplan HS: *The Illustrated Manual of Sex Therapy.* New York, Quadrangel/ The New York Times Book Co, 1975.

26. Semans JH: Premature ejaculation: A new approach. *South Med J* 1956;49:353–357.

27. Silverstein J: *Sexual Enhancement for Women.* Arlington, MA, Jay Publishing Co, 1978.

28. LoPiccolo J, Lobitz WC: The role of masturbation in the treatment of orgasmic dysfunction. *Arch Sex Behav* 1972;2:163–171.

29. Hite S: *The Hite Report.* New York, Macmillan Publishing Co, 1976.

30. Levine SB: Marital sexual dysfunction: Erectile dysfunction. *Ann Intern Med* 1976; 85:342–350.

31. Levine SB, Agle D: The effectiveness of sex therapy for chronic secondary psychological impotence. *J Sex Marital Ther* 1978;4:235–258.

32. Barbach LG: Group treatment of preorgasmic women. *J Sex Marital Ther* 1974; 1:139–145.

33. Kaplan HS, Kohl RN, Pomeroy WB, *et al.:* Group treatment of premature ejaculation. *Arch Sex Behav* 1974;3:443–452.

Chapter 24

ADOLESCENT SEXUALITY
STEPHEN B. ZINN, M.D.

INTRODUCTION

Perpetuation of the species through sexual reproduction has always been a driving force behind human activity. During adolescence, sexual, aggressive, and cognitive motivations erupt with a momentum that is unequalled in any preceding or subsequent life stage.

From its earliest usage, the term "adolescence" has primarily referred to the biological changes initiated by puberty, which occur during the second decade of life. Beginning with the acquisition of secondary sexual characteristics, puberty continues for approximately two to three years. Puberty and its accompanying psychosexual adaptations are cross-cultural phenomena which invariably occur during the second decade. According to another definition, adolescence is a broad psychosocial concept, involving issues of emancipation and autonomy which may be highly age variable and culturally dependent. In some cultures and subcultures, for example, physical and emotional emancipation from the home do not occur until the late 20s or early 30s. Couples may marry and have children while continuing to live in the parental home under parental direction. The psychosocial tasks traditionally associated with adolescence may be prolonged, renegotiated, and sometimes never completed. The onset of puberty, however, makes it more difficult to postpone an individual's arrival at some resolution about their sexuality.

Achieving comfortable control and competence with sexuality is one of the primary tasks of adolescence. Core gender identity, i.e., sense of maleness or femaleness [1], is established by age 3; gender identity, i.e., sense of masculinity or femininity, is a continually developing part of the child's ego identity. The child's developing sexual identity can be traced along two separate continua: 1. core gender identity; 2. sexual orientation or the expression of heteroerotic or homoerotic behavior. Although a great deal of se development has already occurred, the adolescent must now come to terms with the psychophysiological implications and expressions of his or her sexual self. The adolescent must consolidate the increased recognition of sexual drive and management of erotic feelings into a comfortable, interpersonal and intrapsychic sexual orientation. Sexuality is not commonly thought of as something that needs to be mastered. However, like other developmental lines (2) or processes—such as the capacity to play, work, and relate to people—acquiring the capacity to express and feel comfortable with sexuality is a maturational task. The degree of mastery is partly dependent upon the successful intrapsychic integration of sexual and aggressive drives into a comfortable sexual identity. To master sexuality, one must achieve a sense of secure gender identity, discover comfortable erotic responsiveness, and learn how to use one's body pleasurably with others.

PRE-ADOLESCENT SEXUAL DEVELOPMENT

Human sexuality in the male embryo begins midway through the first trimester with the development of testes, which soon synthesize sex hormones, primarily androgens. The female embryo develops ovaries during the second trimester. Without the testicular hormonal stimulation of the first trimester, the embryo would develop along female lines. This may partly explain why males are more vulnerable to developmental errors than females. Although 140 males are conceived for every 100 girls, only 106 males are born for every 100 girls. Males are susceptible to a wide variety of childhood diseases, e.g., metabolic diseases; infantile autism; dyslexia; color blindness; stuttering. Early developmental differences favor girls with relatively more advanced social and verbal skills, and boys with more action-oriented behavior and relatively more advanced spatial-perceptual tasks (3).

There is a large body of descriptive literature detailing observations of children as their definitions of sexual selves unfold. A longitudinal study by Kogan and Moss (4) attempted to assess male and female behavior from birth through age 14. The study demonstrated that 2- and 3-year-old children gravitated toward strong sexual role characteristics in their play and daily activities. Sexual behaviors, coping patterns, and activity levels tended to persist throughout subsequent phases of childhood into adolescence. Boys who demonstrated early patterns of coping through passivity and lower levels of sexual activity had more sexual anxiety during early adolescence and beyond. Early active male coping mechanisms tended to be predictive of higher levels of sexual activity during adolescence and young adulthood. These predictive, action-oriented behaviors were less obvious in female sexual behaviors.

Most studies of early sexual development conclude that, within a given cultural context, a child who develops a comfortable sense of sexual self, which is neither too inhibiting nor too consumed with uncontrollable excitement, is more likely to have a self-fulfilling, healthy, adolescent sexual adjustment. This comfortable sexual definition of self is dependent upon the many variables of sexual expression within a given culture in a given historical context. For example, in the 1980s, as compared with the 1950s, there is much less societal repression of sexual mores; controlling sexual excitement is more difficult.

PUBERTY AND EARLY ADOLESCENT SEXUAL CONCERNS

Sexual maturation occurs along biological and psychosocial continua simultaneously. Pubescence, the transitional stage between the end of latency and the beginning of adolescence, marks the beginning of secondary sexual development. During this second surge of hormonal activity (the first surge is in utero), neurohormonal mechanisms initiate formation of the secondary sex characteristics. Although the process continues throughout adolescence, the most noticeable changes occur during the first 2–3 years.

Girls experience the onset of puberty between the ages of 10 and 13, two years before boys; the most active male pubertal changes occur between the ages of 12 and 15. The initial changes in girls are: pelvic widening; breast budding; skeletal growth; beginning of pubic hair. Menarche normally occurs between the ages of 10 and 16, with the highest incidence at age 13. After menarche, there are significant changes in body shape and mature pubic and axillary hair appear. In boys, puberty begins with growth in the size of the testicles, scrotum, and penis. Psychosocial and intrapsychic factors greatly influence the age of first seminal emissions. Most boys, however, have their first seminal emissions 1–2 years after the onset of puberty. Kinsey (5) reported that the large majority of boys experience orgasm within at least two years of puberty. The first seminal emission is followed by more pronounced penile growth, and the development of pubic and axillary hair. Facial hair develops last.

All early adolescents worry about whether the physiologic changes taking place in their bodies are normal. Girls worry about their breasts being too small or too big; boys worry about their penis size. Boys usually experience their first nocturnal emissions or wet dreams between the ages of 12½ and 14 (6). If unprepared, they may be ashamed of having "urinated" in bed, and fear being discovered and embarrassed by their parents. They may think something is abnormal about their genitals, or that their developing sexuality is "weird" or "perverted." Girls may also develop severe anxiety-producing fantasies around menarche—most involving guilt and a fear of bodily injury.

In addition to anxiety about normal pubertal changes, adolescents have sexual concerns about being physically different from their peers. They have an intense need ·for peer group acceptance. Physical comparisons between themselves and peers are greatest during early and late adolescence. The continuing conscience or superego development often causes them to be highly critical of themselves and their bodies. They also have a strong need to control their bodies and increasing sexual drives. Much of their anxiety can be alleviated by early education about pubertal changes. Some common adolescent problems are: delayed puberty; obesity; cryptochidism or undescended testicles (2-3% incidence at one year of age) (7); precocious sexual development; menstrual irregularities.

Pubertal boys and girls also undergo dramatic psychosocial changes. These changes are reflected in strong group behaviors, loyalties, and the evolution of intense same- and opposite-sex relationships. As the primary family attachments become less important, the adolescent begins the mastery of intimate relationships with peers and "role modeling" adults. Most typical of the early adolescent beginning intimate relationship is the "crush" of the junior high school years. Often brief in duration, highly intense, and ideological, the "crush" is the precursor of the "tender love" (8) or "going steady" of high school and mid-late adolescence. The adolescent resolves his or her sexual identity through these trial and error experiences.

MASTURBATION

Of all the common expressions of sexuality, masturbation has been subject to the most deeply-rooted societal misunderstanding and rigid moral judgments. As people have become more open about their sexual habits, some of the societal prohibitions against masturbation have lessened. Even so, almost all adolescents experience considerable guilt and shame about masturbation. Some guilt about masturbation and all other sexual practices is probably developmentally adaptive. The adolescent uses guilt as a mechanism for controlling sexual drives. Excessive guilt can, however, prevent the adolescent from attaining a comfortable sexual identity.

Masturbation is an important transitional practice in the development of mature sexuality. Conflicts about masturbation may reflect disturbances in sexual development. Kinsey, in 1948 (5), reported that 80% of boys and 20% of girls had masturbated to orgasm at some time during adolescence. One-third of all girls have masturbated to orgasm by the end of adolescence, although rarely before age 15 (9). More recent studies report a higher incidence of masturbation.

Sexual fantasies are an important part of adolescent masturbation. Boys' fantasies are usually explicit erotic visualizations, often stimulated by pictures and sex-oriented magazines. Girls tend to fantasize more about romantic love, involving courtship, kissing, and embracing. It is not uncommon for their fantasies to be completely dissociated from an awareness of their bodies. The adolescent girl's fantasies become more concretely sexual as she grows older. Adolescent girls are aroused by concrete sexual material.

Masturbation is an autoerotic activity which prepares the adolescent for competency in adult sexual relationships. For example, having a masturbatory orgasm alleviates the fear of orgasm. Non-masturbatory anorgasmic women are frightened of orgasm because they have never experienced it.

SEXUAL INTERCOURSE

Whether today's adolescents are more sexually active than those of previous generations is debatable. We do know, however, that today's adolescent is less likely than those in the preceding generation to have a first coital experience with a prostitute, be a virgin, have a "double standard" for males and females, or feel guilty about sexuality. Kinsey (5) reported that 30% of boys eighteen and under had had sexual intercourse. In 1969, Offer (10,11) did a study of 103 "typical" boys, selected from a total sample of 326 freshmen boys from two suburban high schools. He reported that 10% of the total had had sexual intercourse at least once during high school; 30% had had sexual intercourse by the end of their freshman year in college.

Sorenson (12) has thus far done the most complete survey of adolescent sexual behaviors and attitudes. His report sampled 2,042 randomly selected rural and suburban households within the continental United States. Twenty-two percent of the adolescent respondents (20% of all boys; 25% of all girls) denied having any sexual experience; of these, 75% said, "I've never had sex with a girl/boy because I'm not really ready for it." Sorensen further reports that 17% of all adolescents (14% of all boys; 19% of all girls) are sexual beginners, i.e., adolescents who have had some sexual experience, such as fondling or petting, but no sexual intercourse. Fifty-two percent of all adolescents in this survey reported having had sexual intercourse. The data, which show a surprisingly high incidence of sexual intercourse among adolescents, are probably very close to true incidence. A 1972 study on teenage pregnancy conducted by the President's Commission on Population Growth revealed that 46% of all adolescent girls had had sexual intercourse by the age of 19 (13).

Sorenson's data include many questions on attitudes toward sexual and emotional intimacy. Some of his data confirm the adolescent's striving for sexual and emotional intimacy, e.g., only 15% of all adolescents (24% of all boys; 6% of all girls) seek multiple sexual relationships, and have "no interest in a continuous or monogamous relationship with one sexual partner."

TABLE I
INTERCOURSE EXPERIENCE

	Yes	No	Total
BOYS			
All	59%	41%	100%
Age 13-15	44%	56%	100%
Age 16-19	72%	28%	100%
GIRLS			
All	45%	55%	100%
Age 13-15	30%	70%	100%
Age 16-19	57%	43%	100%
All Adolescents	52%	48%	100%

The fact that more adolescents engage in overt sexual practices does not necessarily mean that adolescents feel more comfortable with their developing sexuality. They still have the same doubts, conflicts about loss of physical and emotional control, and insecurities about sexual identity as those in preceding generations. All adolescent males worry about mastering premature ejaculation. Indeed, the increased trend toward sexual expression may greatly intensify the adolescent's conflicts. Many adolescents feel developmentally unprepared (in the psychic sense) for the situations in which they find themselves. A physician treating adolescents must, therefore, have a great deal of understanding, empathy, and knowledge.

PREGNANCY

Most adolescents fail to use contraception at some time. Sorenson (12) reported that neither partner used birth control for the first sexual intercourse in 55% of the cases; another 13% were not sure whether it had been used. More recently, Zelnik, Kim, and Kantner (14) have used life-table analysis to show that 10% of U.S. women have at least one pregnancy by age 17, 25% have at least one pregnancy by age 19.

There are over 400,000 illegitimate births annually. Over half of those mothers are adolescents. While the number of unwed births has increased, the adult female unwed birth rate has been leveling off; the adolescent rate has proportionally and steadily increased. Further evidence of widespread adolescent pregnancy is reflected in the abortion statistics from the early seventies. One-third of all abortions in the United States were performed on women 19 and under. Approximately 300,000 adolescents obtain abortions annually, and half of them are 17 years of age or younger (15).

Most adolescents are not aware of the advances and increased education in contraceptive techniques. Many, if not most, either misunderstand or deny their reproductive capacities. Many believe that a low frequency of intercourse will either deter or prevent the possibility of pregnancy. Some believe they won't become pregnant if they have sexual intercourse standing up. Many adolescents associate taking the pill with sexual promiscuity; others are afraid of its side effects. Some adolescents deny the possibility of becoming pregnant because they unconsciously want it to happen.

The need for complete service programs related to adolescent pregnancy cannot be overstated. First trimester abortion should be readily available within a community, and supportive counseling services for follow-up should be routine. Most adolescents associate the abortion with grief and mourning and need supportive aftercare. Physicians dealing with adolescent populations should give priority to general sexual and contraceptive education. Both partners need counseling when pregnancy occurs. Alleviating guilt about the pregnancy can prevent traumatic conflicts which might later affect sexual functioning and emotional life.

HOMOSEXUALITY

Strong same-sex emotional attachments are normal during early adolescence—usually in the form of dyadic friendships or group loyalties. These strong attachments are frequently influenced by the erotic manner in which the early adolescent experiences things. Touching, wrestling, patting each other, backrubs, and innocent caresses often become unconscious outlets for homoerotic feelings. These common, acceptable feelings can also lead to more overt, but isolated, homosexual behaviors. Homosexual experiences are more common among boys, usually in the form of mutual genital manipulation and/or masturbation; they sometimes include fellatio. Most surveys indicate that around 10% of adolescent males and 5% of adolescent females have at least one homosexual experience during early adolescence.

With the beginning of mid-adolescence (around 15 years of age), overt homosexual experience sharply decreases in favor of heterosexual attachments. True homosexuals begin to establish their identies at this time. Adolescent heterosexual, and especially homosexual, identity formation is flexible and unpredictable. In mid- and late-adolescence, members of both sexes need to be reassured that a few homosexual experiences do not make them homosexuals. Their anxiety can be greatly alleviated through reassurance and understanding.

REFERENCES

1. Stoller RS: *Sex and Gender: On the Development* of Masculinity and Feminity. New York, Science House, 1968.
2. Freud A: *Normality and Pathology in Childhood: Assessments in Development: The Writings of Anna Freud.* New York, International Universities Press, 1965, vol 6.
3. Chilman CS: *Adolescent Sexuality in a Changing American Society.* New York, John Wiley & Sons, 1983.
4. Kagan J, Moss HA: *Birth to Maturity.* New York, John Wiley & Sons Inc, 1962.
5. Kinsey AC, Pomeroy WB, Martin CE: *Sexual Behavior in the Human Male.* Philadelphia, WB Saunders, 1948.
6. Oliver G: *Clinical Sexuality,* ed 3. Philadelphia, JP Lippincott, 1974.
7. Malmquist CP: *Handbood of Adolescence.* New York, Jason Aronson, 1978.
8. Blos P: *On Adolescence.* New York, Free Press, 1962.
9. Jensen G: Adolescent Sexuality, in Saddock BJ, Kaplan H, Freedman A (eds): *The Sexual Experience.* Baltimore, Williams & Wilkins, 1976.
10. Offer D, Offer JL: Normal Adolescents Mature. *Seminars in Psychiatry* 1969;1:46–56.
11. Offer D, Offer JL: Growing Up: A Follow-Up Study of Normal Adolescents. *Seminars in Psychiatry* 1969;1.
12. Sorenson C: *Adolescent Sexuality in Contemporary America.* New York, World Publishing, 1973.
13. *U.S. Commission on Population Growth and the American Future.* Government Printing Office, 1972.
14. Zelnik M, Kim YJ, Kantner JF: Probabilities of Intercourse and Conception Among U.S. Teenage Women, *Family Planning Perspectives* 1979;11:177–183.
15. Fielding JE: Adolescent Pregnancy Revisited. *N Engl J Med* 1978;299:893–896.

Chapter 25

MALE SEXUAL DYSFUNCTION: PSYCHOGENIC IMPOTENCE

STEPHEN B. LEVINE, M.D.

Prior to 1970, most male sexual performance difficulties were considered impotence and assumed to be psychogenic. Since then, however, a careful classification system of specific dysfunctions has emerged (1), along with an awareness of organic contributants to erectile problems (2). Impotence per se is not a formal diagnosis. The DSM-III system distinguishes between psychosexual erectile failure due to a deficient drive and the incapacity to obtain or sustain excitement. This classification implies that the pathogeneses, treatments, or prognoses of these problems are essentially separate.

DSM-III distinctions clearly represent an important advance. Their application, however, is still problematic—not only because desire and excitement problems often coexist, but because organic factors may share in the pathogenesis. This chapter presents an overview of the psychogenic causes, and discusses a conservative approach to the differential diagnosis of organic and psychogenic erectile dysfunction.

DEFINITION AND EPIDEMIOLOGY

The inability to sustain an adequate erection for the duration of a desired sexual act is generally known as impotence. This definition is broad enough to include impotence among homosexuals, and to allow for considerable fluctuation in the degree of erectile turgidity during sexual behavior. Many men have a relative impotence, i.e., the degree of turgidity is compromised, but intercourse is possible. Clinically important nuances, such as the degree of turgidity, episodic nature of erectile failures, and distinctions between loss of desire and loss of erectile capacity, have not yet been reflected in the few relevant epidemiologic studies (3-8). These limitations may be causing an underestimation of the prevalence of potency problems. Regardless of methodologic flaws, existing data do, however, indicate that these problems

319

are quite common and increase dramatically with age (9,10). A baseline level of prevalence among young adults ranges from 0–3.5% (3,10,11). After age 45, however, there is a steady increase. The rate of increase accelerates even more after age 60. By age 70, 50% of men are, for all practical purposes, impotent. These guesstimates do not relate to etiology.

PATHOGENESIS OF PURE PSYCHOGENIC IMPOTENCE

Thorough discussion of the pathogenesis of psychogenic impotence is rare in the literature. Most papers focus on its recognition or its treatment. Etiology is usually summarized in terms of competing, seemingly mutually exclusive theories. Although there is a strong analytic tradition of assuming that oedipal dynamics underlie most impotence, few therapists who see many impotent men perceive the problem as having such a universal pathogenesis (12–16). Impotence, like other psychological symptoms, is overdetermined, i.e., it is the end product of temperamental, familial, affectual, cognitive, cultural, maturational, *and* biological influences. While each of the theoretical constructs which are often applied to the search for psychologic causality—psychodynamic (17); behavioral (18); cognitive (19); systems theory (20)—may provide an illuminating perspective, the questions which arise from their explanations are often unanswerable.

Performance anxiety is the modern explanation for the final common pathway to psychogenic impotence (21,22). After an episode of erectile failure, almost any man will become worried, if not preoccupied, about the state of subsequent erections. Performance anxiety can be severe enough to distract the man from the sensual stimuli that ordinarily enable and maintain excitement. The baffling questions about performance anxiety are: Why this man, at this time, with this particular symptom?

The practical clinician can articulate cogent answers to these questions, even though their ultimate validity may be difficult to ascertain. These answers often emerge from an initial evaluation for psychogenic impotence which considers the symptom from four perspectives: 1. Stage of the life cycle; 2. Quality and quantity of sexual desire; 3. Role of the partner; 4. Significance of past developmental experiences. Exploration and synthesis of these perspectives enables treatment appropriate to the pathogenesis.

Perspective One: At What Stage of Life Does the Symptom Appear?

It is useful to separate men with lifelong, or primary, impotence from those whose symptoms follow a long period of aproblematic sexual functioning (i.e., secondary impotence) (21). The causes of these two types of impotence, as well as the response to therapy, are usually quite discrete. Secondary psychologic impotence is far more prevalent than primary impotence. Simple conceptual models of the etiologies of these two types of impotence are presented below. It is important to realize that many psychogenic cases are complicated; a synthesis of concepts derived from both models is needed to adequately explain the symptom.

   1. Model for Secondary Impotence—Unrecognized Affects Stemming from New Life Circumstances

Occasional sexual failures are understandable when one considers the difficulty involved in achieving the three basic requirements of good sexual function, i.e., willingness to make love; capacity to relax; ability to concentrate on sensation (23). Strong feeling states, such as anger, guilt, shame, disgust, anxiety, and sadness, can induce a temporary unwillingness to make love, inability to relax, or preoccupation with other matters. Although the men are physically present, they are not always psychologically available for lovemaking. In addition, substance abuse may cause a physiologic inability to erect. The vast majority of erectile failures are followed by sexual encounters under better psychological and physiological conditions. The performance anxiety initially evoked by impotence fades away after one or more successful experiences.

Persistent impotence usually means that the initial failure was not due to an incident of minor personal significance. Curiously, these men often consider their dysfunctions inexplicable, despite recent major transitions in their lives, e.g., changes involving the quality of longstanding relationships, partners, or work. It is hard to avoid relating such problems to the widespread male belief that sex should be possible anytime, anywhere, with anybody. Secondary psychogenic impotence is a reminder that the penis is not a machine. The unrecognized affects that cause impotence are products of meaningful, personal life changes. Several such changes are illustrated in the following vignettes:

   Case #1: Hostile, Unreceptive Partner.

   A 50-year-old hardworking, religious, devoted father was married to a woman who prided herself on her worldliness and was contemptuous of his limitations. She had a series of affairs and was disinterested in having sexual contact with her husband. He did not seem to realize that his wife's blatant derision was relevant to his years of deteriorating potency.

   Case #2: Lingering Distrust of Women; Fear of Being Hurt Again.

   A mild-mannered air traffic controller claimed that his wife's decision to divorce him was a complete surprise. For six months after being "thrown out," he visited his children, worked, and drank heavily in his lonely apartment. His deep sense of loss and bitterness was gradually modified by an increasingly intimate relationship with the woman he eventually married. He was totally baffled by his erectile failure with his fiance.

Case #3: Inadequately Resolved Grief; Guilt Over Premature Intimacy.

Three months after his wife's death, a 58-year-old man began dating. He sought help for impotence after sexual failures with three partners. When asked if thoughts of his wife intruded upon him during sexual intimacies, he replied, "Never! My children have been very supportive of my dating. Logically, there is no reason for me not to date. Life must go on!" He then cried throughout his lengthy description of their many beautiful years of marriage and the horror of her slow, painful death. Leaving the interview, he said, "Maybe I did feel strange with other women."

Case #4: Displaced Anxiety Over Job Function.

A middle-aged man developed impotence the night after his boss urged him to assume a supervisory position. He was quite worried about his competence—"panicked, in fact"—because this position had previously been held only by engineers. He never related his worries about inadequacy in his new career role to his new sexual anxiety.

These men failed to appreciate the presence and significance of unpleasant affects during sexual intimacy. Case #1 was unable to face the reality of his painful position as a cuckold. Case #2 was unable to account for his tension whenever he engaged in sexual activity with a woman he loved. Case #3 almost succeeded in isolating the painful past from his new intimacies with other women. Case #4 tried to use sex for a respite from his mental preoccupation with job problems. Prior to entering their new life circumstances, none of these men had any erectile difficulties.

Any list of the psychological causes of secondary impotence could be extended to great length. Its exact contents are less important than the recognition of the patient's inability to deal with the affects (e.g., anxiety; anger; fear; guilt) behind the "causes"—e.g., marital deterioration; extramarital affair; job failure. These feelings may be avoided with defense mechanisms, but are ultimately expressed as performance anxiety.

2. *Model for Primary Psychogenic Impotence—Developmental Failure to Overcome Fear of Women*

First coital opportunities are typically accompanied by considerable anxiety. This anxiety is manifested as nervousness rather than a discrete fear, and detracts from the pleasure of this important rite of passage. Once coital success begins to dispel this nervousness, subsequent experiences can be more leisurely and pleasurable.

It is likely that clinicians only see a fraction of those who are initially impotent. Most impotent beginners achieve success in subsequent experiences with the same partners. Some, however, are so humiliated that they avoid intimacy for a long time. Those few who seek help are likely to present as young, panicky heterosexuals. The clinician's warmth, sympathy, and reassurance usually relieves their anxiety and enables them to try again. While such cases are gratifying to the clinician, they offer little insight into the sources of the anxiety.

Most men with longstanding primary impotence have other obvious psychiatric difficulties. An appreciation of these other difficulties places their sexual symptom in perspective. Associated disorders fall into five categories: Gender identity problems, e.g., transsexualism, transvestism; Perversions, e.g., sadism, pedophilia, masochism; Homosexuality, e.g., homoerotic male trying to be a heterosexual; Character neurosis, e.g., obsessive-compulsive disorder, passive-dependent character; Psychosis, e.g., schizophrenia or borderline disorders.

Case #5: Gender Identity Disorder.

A man who eventually had sex reassignment surgery was married for twenty years without having intercourse. After failing in his initial coital attempts, he was only rarely able to participate in mutual genital play; such activity was always accompanied by the fantasy that her body was his body. He had been secretly cross-dressing since early childhood, and often lapsed into a fantasy of being a girl. He had neither the desire nor the self-confidence necessary for intercourse.

Case #6: Masochistic Perversion.

A socially isolated, 63-year-old school teacher wanted to be put in touch with a sexual surrogate in order to have intercourse once before he died. His auto-erotic life was dominated by a spanking scenario. A few times a year he hired a prostitute. Pretending that he had been naughty, she would put him over her knees and spank him. He usually achieved orgasm with masturbation immediately afterward. He had never been able to maintain an erection for intercourse and had given up trying. He was too fearful and ashamed of himself to attempt any sexual intimacies with the few women he had ever dated.

Case #7: Ego-Dystonic Homosexuality.

A passive, effeminate musician and his devoted wife were referred for help in consummating their 16-year marriage. Their two children were adopted. Their mutual masturbatory sexual pattern caused them periodic distress. His weak desire for sex with his wife contrasted with his strong homoerotic interests. Although he had experienced these attractions since adolescence, he had not had any actual homosexual experiences. He fled from a religious order at age 20 when faced with an opportunity for homosexual behavior. For two years thereafter, constant anxiety prevented his going to school and work. He was embarrassed by his fear of being swallowed up in his wife's vagina.

Case #8: Character Neurosis.

A passive, obsessive-compulsive, heterosexual 28-year-old had been
unable to have intercourse with his wife of four years. Their verbal communication had dwindled considerably, and there had been no physical
contact for over three years. Prior to having cardiac surgery at age 8, the
patient had been chronically ill. He continued to be a quiet, socially isolated child. He dated only one girl. His future in-laws made their disappointment with their daughter's choice painfully obvious. Although he
petted eagerly prior to marriage, he claimed that religious beliefs prevented him from attempting intercourse. After the wedding, however, he
could not get excited with his wife.

Despite diverse etiologies, a defective sense of self generally precedes
primary impotence. It is a serious error to attribute doubts about masculinity
only to the initial sexual failure. The issues involved in the therapy of such
men are not usually as simple and discrete as those in cases of pure secondary
impotence. The success rates achieved with any approach to primary impotence are always much lower than those achieved with men who have had
a great deal of successful coital experience. Men with longstanding primary
impotence may achieve coital success (e.g., Case #8); more often than not,
however, both the patient and the therapist become concerned about matters
more basic than potency, e.g., identity; inability to form close relationships;
fear of loss of psychologic integrity through physical union with a woman;
pervasive passivity. Such men are basically frightened of women. The
sources of their fears are not readily accessible. Short-term therapies for impotent men with obvious psychiatric difficulties—especially those without
supportive partners—are not likely to enable *lasting* potency.

Some elemental fear of women is normal, even among potent young men.
Many men are unable to acknowledge this fear, and most cannot account
for it. This fear may derive from unconscious sources which are qualitatively
similar to those that cause impotence, e.g., fear of losing their separate masculine identity by merging with a woman; anger over real or imagined past
maternal injustices; guilt over past excitement and sexual desires for both parents; sense of inadequate masculinity stemming from limited paternal involvement. The vital differences, however, lie in the degrees of unconscious fear,
the fear-suppressing capacities, or the ability to be excited by their partners.

On rare occasions, a relatively normal young man seeks help for the persistent inability to achieve intercourse. Although this masculine heterosexual
without perverse tendencies may be socially at ease, successful in his work
sphere, and lacking in neurotic symptoms, an inexplicable anxiety prevents
him from having intercourse. The presence of such ego strengths generally
indicates that the focal problem will be quite amenable to treatment.

The first perspective can now be refocused: "What developmental task was in progress when the erectile problem began?" For most men, the answer involves dealing with a new life challenge; for some, however, the task was establishing an initial heterosexual relationship. The refocused perspective enables concepualization of the ultimate therapeutic task.

Perspective Two: Is Sexual Desire Inhibited, Deficient, Or Intact?

Despite their expressed desires for intercourse and their repeated coital attempts, many psychologically impotent men lack genuine sexual drive. What seems like sexual drive is only an expression of their wish to be capable of having coitus. As such, it should be considered cognitive desire and contrasted with somatically-experienced desire. The latter can be evaluated by asking about the presence of "horniness" and the length of time that elapses between perceived feelings about needing a sexual outlet (14). These questions usually enable the clinicial to make the useful distinction between cognitive and visceral desire.

DSM-III has separate diagnoses for men with deficient desire (desire inhibition) and those who have sexual drive but cannot maintain excitement (excitement inhibition) (15). Since excitement inhibitions are the most easily treated sexual dysfunctions, this distinction is quite important. Men with excitement inhibitions are trapped by their fears of sexual failure and vigilant preoccupation with their erections during lovemaking. When their pernicious performance anxiety stems from largely resolved psychological dilemmas, they can be significantly helped by simple interventions. The therapist needs to explain the origin and maintenance of the problem in a way that makes sense to the patient, i.e., label the original interfering affects and explain the destructive features of performance anxiety. The patient needs to be reassured that the symptom is neither rare nor permanent. Lovemaking without intercourse, i.e., sensate focus (21)—is usually prescribed. This procedure enables the man to relax, concentrate on sensation, and become aroused. Some patients report being cured by the following visit. It is far more common for the underlying psychological dilemma to be ongoing; in such cases, the therapeutic focus should be on its resolution. Once the dilemma is resolved, interventions aimed at excitement inhibitions can be employed.

Unfortunately, most psychologically impotent men cannot be rapidly and effectively treated because, in DSM-III terminology, they have "desire inhibitions." The differential diagnosis of "desire inhibitions" can be quite complicated. Desire *deficiency* states, such as those found among patients with unrecognized depressions, systemic illnesses, drug effects, and other biogenic low libido states, e.g., Klinefelter's, may be erroneously diagnosed as inhibitions. In patients with true inhibitions, the drive is present but deflected or hidden from the conscious self. Questions concerning masturbatory activity and imagery, dream imagery, nocturnal emissions, and sex with other partners are useful in recognizing the distinctions between drive deficiencies and true inhibitions. This decision is vital because therapy for a deficiency is quite different than that for an inhibition. This dilemma is especially common in physically normal older men with weakened libidos (9).

Although there is little knowledge about the physiologic basis for libido, a number of clinically useful phenomena have been observed. Viscerally experienced drive often disappears under the following conditions: preoccupation with life crises; grief; depression; partner unavailability due to illness, sexual disinterest, separation, or death; "falling out of love"; aging; psychosis. Easily-recognized inhibitions commonly occur as a result of fear of death or injury following physical illness (e.g., myocardial infarction or cardiac surgery); persistent erectile, ejaculatory, or partner dysfunction; suppressed anger at partner. Inhibitions which are more difficult to recognize can occur in men who: have a maternal transference to their sexual partners; enter into heterosexual relationships in an attempt to conceal gender identity disorders, paraphilias, homosexuality; demonstrate a characteristic inability to express anger.

The psychologic cause of the desire problem is, of course, the determining factor in its treatment. Problems stemming from either a deficiency or inhibition of drive do not respond to techniques which effectively alleviate excitement inhibition. Sensate focus exercises will not help men who have a cognitive desire for sex but lack any genuine sexual interest in their partners. The patient's attention needs to be focused on the underlying problem, rather than the sexual failure per se. Mental health professionals are quite familiar with such problems. The fact that sex therapists have been able to help these men indicates their competence in treating communication problems, interpersonal conflicts, and intrapsychic inhibition of affect expression. Both sex therapists and mental health professionals soon learn, however, that many desire problems cannot be resolved with current therapeutic techniques (24).

Perspective Three: The Partner as Victim—Partner as Saboteur Spectrum

When a woman maintains a warm, receptive, supportive attitude prior to and during her partner's impotence, she may be viewed as a victim of his intrapsychic conflicts and performance anxiety. Many partners deal with their new sexual deprivation and narcissistic worries in a non-critical, unpressured interpersonal manner. In such relationships, impotence is a product of intrapsychic dynamics, e.g., previous unresolved marital entanglements; unconscious maternal cathexes.

When a partner deliberately or inadvertently, consciously or unconsciously functions as saboteur, the etiology and therapy of the problem are very different. Although the impotence in such relationships is associated with male intrapsychic conflict, it is more accurately assessed as a response to intuitively experienced partner unreceptivity. Conjoint therapy employing sensate focus exercises can quickly unmask the saboteur. When potency begins to return, the woman ceases to cooperate, develops a new symptom, or launches a vitriolic attack on her partner. The various motives behind such sabotage must be understood and resolved before a viable, sexually and emotionally gratifying relationship can be established.

Evaluation of the wives of psychogenically impotent men is almost always helpful. The wife-victim of a man with secondary impotence may know more about the problem than does her husband; the wife-saboteur reveals her critical attitudes and conflicted motives in her discussions with the clinician. Some wives begin as victims. They inadvertently become saboteurs in response to their anger at the man's withdrawal. Probably the most common treatment mistake with secondarily impotent married men is the failure to appreciate the current interpersonal milieu. The man's conflicts, however neurotically expressed in the past, never previously prevented intercourse.

Perspective Four: Significance of the Unconscious Processes

Unconscious processes are probably involved in every case of psychogenic impotence. Even in cases with obvious precipitants, symptoms may be attributed to both the immediate antecedents and the unconscious conflicts and affects they provoke. For example, guilt over being unfaithful to his hopelessly demented wife caused a very proper, 60-year-old man to become impotent. However, much of his new sexual anxiety was generated by his experiences coping with his mother's promiscuity when he was 12.

Treatment planning is largely dependent upon the answers to two questions about unconscious determinants:

1. Are unmastered developmental processes the most significant contributants to an individual's vulnerability to impotence? Certain patterns of erectile dysfunction indicate a serious vulnerability to sexual failure: persistent primary impotence; only potent with derogated women; frequent, recurring impotence throughout adulthood; potency only occurs when the needs of the partner are ignored. (The latter three are sometimes classified imprecisely as "situational" impotence.) Treatments aimed at mastery of the remote focus responsible for the man's constriction are usually indicated. Unless the partner is especially supportive and intuitive, her involvement in therapy ceases once the underlying vulnerability is diagnosed.

2. Are the significant unconscious determinants accessible to exploration? Kaplan has categorized the sources of unconscious anxiety which produce inhibited desire and excitement into three levels (24). Mild sources include performance anxiety, guilt over sexual activity and pleasure, overconcern with the partner's pleasure, and response to partner dysfunction. These problems are often quickly resolved with conjoint or individual therapies. Mid level sources include angry inhibitions due to interpersonal conflict and fears of success and intimacy. Deeper sources include severe relationship problems, castration anxiety associated with oedipal conflicts or preoedipal pathologic introjects. Many mid level, and most deep, problems do not generally respond to brief and/or conjoint approaches; the results achieved with classic analytic therapies are also frequently disappointing.

The issue of accessibility is not limited to the depth of the underlying problem; the nature of the man's defensive structure is also involved. Those who employ primitive or immature defensive patterns complicate any therapeutic endeavor. A very passive factory worker who had been unable to consummate his 8-year marriage also suffered from almost complete amnesia about his childhood. His emotional poverty and repression provide a striking contrast to Case #8, the meek, obsessive-compulsive who was at least capable of recalling and discussing his life. He achieved lasting potency in four months of weekly conjoint therapy. The amnesic man seems incapable of even thinking about his present or past problems.

Accessibility of the underlying problem is also a function of the therapist's proficiency in, and willingness to use, various therapeutic techniques. Based on the experience of sex therapists of various theoretical orientations, it is apparently possible to restore or enable potency without resolving all of the patient's character and developmental problems. Considerable empirical evidence suggests that a variety of approaches may help impotent patients as long as the problem is carefully diagnosed (25-27). It is just as important for clinicians to recognize deeply rooted intrapsychic problems which require intensive individual therapy as it is to recognize those which can be handled with any number of briefer approaches.

In summary, clinicians should not look for a single method to treat psychogenic impotence. The concept of a specific treatment for a specific symptom is too simple. Impotence is a symptom, not a disease. Etiology *is* important to treatment results. The reports of new behavioral, cognitive, and dynamic treatment approaches have generally been favorable—but somewhat misleading. Unfavorable results are not usually reported. Regardless of the stated treatment paradigm, the process of therapy is more than technique; it is often a continual reappraisal of etiology. Treatment results extend beyond numerical summaries (28). The DSM-III division of psychogenic impotence into two categories only touches the surface of the etiologic issue. It is, however, a start.

Clinical Recognition of the Psychogenicity of Impotence

Soon after Masters and Johnson revealed the encouraging results of their therapeutic efforts, clinicians began to suspect that many "psychogenic" symptoms were actually due to unrecognized organic or mixed organo-psychologic problems (29). Since the new therapies failed to help at least one-third of patients (21,25,26), and many others were unable to sustain their initial improvements (30), further research was obviously needed. The improvement of the penile prosthesis was an important stimulus to the detection of organic factors. Since it is now possible to surgically restore coital capacity to men with irreversible organic impotence, the clinician is under greater pressure to make a correct diagnosis. The sleep laboratory has provided an objective means for distinguishing organic from pure psychologic impotence; it does not pinpoint specific causes (31,32). Other diagnostic methods have elucidated the pathogeneses of different causal factors. Atonic bladder, diagnosed by cystometric examination, is highly correlated with diabetic neuropathic impotence (33); radioimmunoassay has added hyperprolactinemia to the list of irreversible endocrine causes (34,35); penile blood flow and pressure measurements provide important diagnostic clues to vasculogenic impotence (2,36). Sympathetic blocking agents are now widely recognized as a source of impaired potency (37). Approximately half of men in their seventies have significant erectile impairments, many of which are idiopathic. Many men may be affected much earlier by the undefined process that produces the desire and excitement problems of aging (38,39).

These important recent developments have escalated the difficulties of clinicians who try to thoroughly evaluate complaints of impotence. Observations in sleep laboratories have questioned the validity of the sexual history as a guide to etiology, e.g., nocturnal tumescence observed in men with "organic" histories; absence of tumescence in men with "psychogenic" histories. Two observations need to be considered before further denigrating the interview as a diagnostic tool. First, the extent of the error involved in a careful clinical approach has not been documented. Second, nocturnal tumescence monitoring is not always valid; nor is the diagnostic interpretation of the results always clear-cut (31,40,41). Sleep studies must monitor both penile circumference and rigidity. Home monitoring studies are no longer considered valuable, since they do not measure nocturnal penile rigidity (42–44). Even if initial laboratory evaluation can be proven vastly superior to careful clinical evaluation, the lack of sleep laboratory facilities will still force the clinician to carry the burden of differential diagnosis.

Although there is strong disagreement (43,44), sleep studies are best reserved for those with uncertain diagnoses and those contemplating surgery.

Some impotent men can be easily diagnosed as psychogenic during the initial history. Prompt recognition of these clear-cut cases obviates the need for expensive diagnostic medical procedures and facilitates the provision of appropriate therapeutic services.

Pure psychogenic impotence is simply a deficiency of the affect state of arousal. The man's neural, hormonal, and hemodynamic mediators of erection are intact; he doesn't have the required erections because he cannot generate or maintain the necessary emotion. Clear-cut psychogenic cases are characterized by:

1. A selective pattern of erectile function since the onset of the problem, i.e., lasting, turgid erections under some circumstances. For example: an erection can be obtained during masturbation, but not with the partner; consistent potency with one partner but not another; erection is maintained throughout prolonged foreplay, but turgidity is lost immediately prior to or following intromission; turgid middle-of-the-night and morning erections, but none with any partner. The alternation between full potency and impairment is only a clear-cut indication of psychogenicity if: a. it cannot be linked to episodic drug abuse or medication use; b. the potency episodes are characterized by fully turgid, not just barely adequate erections.

2. Onset of dysfunction after a significant personal event, e.g., loss of a job; argument; being jilted; infidelity; discovery of infertility.

3. Evidence of sexual drive. For diagnostic purposes, it is reassuring to hear that a man feels "horny" episodically. It indicates that his brain mechanisms for spontaneous arousal are intact.

Many middle-aged and older men with psychogenic impotence appear to have an organic pattern of erectile dysfunction. Their weakened libido masks the selective pattern of potency that is the hallmark of psychogenicity. They indicate that their erectile impairment is constant under all circumstances, i.e., with their partner, nocturnal and morning erections, masturbation, other partners. Such a history in a younger man is usually indicative of organic impairment. In middle-aged and older populations, however, the absence of an understandable impotence-inducing life change is another useful criterion of organic impotence. When libido is deficient and the pattern of erectile dysfunction is not clearly psychogenic, the clinician must sort through all the usual organic and psychologic causes of libido impairment.

The work-up of men who do not demonstrate the three characteristics of clear-cut psychogenic impotence must be based on clinical judgment. The clinician must always carefully search for a recent important change in the man's mood, family relationships, or work sphere. If a personally significant upheaval has occurred prior to the potency disorder, it is reasonable to delay a sophisticated organic work-up. The essential psychogenicity of the problem may sometimes be recognized by a brief return of good potency after the initial consultation or therapeutic intervention.

Conclusion

Less than a decade ago, the proper diagnostic question was, "Is the impotence organic or psychogenic?" Today this oversimplified question has been replaced with, "What are the organic and psychogenic contributants to this man's (couple's) erectile insufficiency?" The broad etiologic schema of impotence includes: pure organic causes, due to medications, disease processes, and surgery; pure psychogenic causes, due to developmental or interpersonal sources; mixed organic-psychologic causes, due to a basic organic defect that causes the patient to react with disabling performance anxiety, or an organic cause coexisting with an unrelated intrapsychic or interpersonal disturbance. The mental health professional dealing with impotence needs to be familiar with the diagnosis of recognized organic contributants, in addition to having a considerable sophistication about the diverse dilemmas which may undermine the capacity to engage in intercourse.

REFERENCES

1. American Psychiatric Association Task Force on Nomenclature and Statistics: *Diagnostic and Statistical Manual of Mental Disorders* (DSM-III), ed 3. Washington, DC, American Psychiatric Association, 1980.
2. Wagner G, Green R: *Impotence: Physiological, Psychological, Surgical Diagnosis and Treatment.* New York, Plenum Press, 1981.
3. Kinsey AC, Pomeroy WB, Martin CE: *Sexual Behavior in the Human Male.* Philadelphia, WB Saunders, 1948.
4. Finkle AL, Moyers AB, Tobenkin MI, *et al.:* Sexual potency in aging males. *JAMA* 1959;170:1391–1393.
5. Bower CM, Cross RR, Lloyd FA: Sexual function and urologic disease in the elderly male. *J Am Geriatr Soc* 1963;11:647–652.
6. Martin CE: Marital and sexual factors in relation to age, disease, and longevity, in Wirt RD, Winokur G, Rolf M (eds): *Life History Research in Psychopathology.* Minneapolis, University of Minnesota Press, 1975, vol 4.
7. Pfeiffer E, Verwoedt A, Davis GC: Sexual behavior in middle life. *Am J Psychiatry* 1972;126:1262–1267.
8. Pfeiffer E, Davis GC: Determinants of sexual behavior in middle and old age. *J Am Geriatr Soc* 1972;20:151–158.
9. Martin CE: Factors affecting sexual functioning in 60 to 79-year-old married males. *Arch Sex Behav* 1981;10:399–420.
10. Lester E, Grant AJ, Woodruff FJ: Impotence in diabetic and nondiabetic hospital outpatients. *Br Med J* 1980;281:354–355.

11. Jensen SJ: Diabetic sexual function: A comparative study of 160 insulin-treated diabetic men and women and age matched controls. *Arch Sex Behav* 1981;10:493-504.

12. Kolodny RC, Masters WH, Johnson VE: *Textbook of Sexual Medicine.* Boston, Little Brown & Co, 1979.

13. Kaplan HS: *The New Sex Therapy.* New York, Brunner/Mazel, 1974.

14. Munjack DJ, Oziel J, Kanno PH, *et al.:* Psychological characteristics of males with secondary erectile failure. *Arch Sex Behav* 1981;10:123-132.

15. Derogatis LR, Meyer JK: A psychologic profile of the sexual dysfunctions. *Arch Sex Behav* 1979;8:201-224.

16. Stekel W: *Sexual Impotence in the Male.* New York, Liveright Publishing Corp, 1927, vol 2.

17. Freud S: On the universal tendency to debasement in the sphere of love (1912), in Strachy J (ed): *The Complete Psychological Works of Sigmund Freud,* st'd ed. London, Hogarth Press, 1957, vol 11, pp 177-190.

18. LoPiccolo J, LoPiccolo L (eds): *Handbook of Sex Therapy.* New York, Plenum Press, 1978.

19. Gagnon JH, Rosen RC, Lieblum SR: Cognitive and social aspects of sexual dysfunction: Sexual scripts in sex therapy. *J Sex Marital Ther* 1982;8:44-56.

20. Cole CM, Blaheney PE: The myth of the symptomatic vs. asymptomatic partner in conjoint treatment of sexual dysfunction. *J Sex Marital Ther* 1979;5:79-89.

21. Masters WH, Johnson VE: *Human Sexual Inadequacy.* Boston, Little Brown & Co, 1970.

22. Quadland MC: Private self consciousness, attribution of responsibility, perfectionistic thinking and secondary erectile dysfunction. *J Sex Marital There* 1980;6:47-55.

23. Levine SB: Marital sexual dysfunction: Introductory concepts. *Ann Intern Med* 1976; 84:448-453.

24. Kaplan HS: *Disorders of Sexual Desire.* New York, Simon & Schuster, 1979.

25. Wright J, Perrault R, Mathiew M: The treatment of sexual dysfunction. *Arch Gen Psychiatry* 1977;34:881-890.

26. Kilman PR, Auerback R: Treatments of premature ejaculation and psychogenic impotence: A critical review of the literature. *Arch Sex Behav* 1979;8:81-100.

27. Karacan I: The treatment of erectile dysfunction. *Directions in Psychiatry* 1: Lesson 13, 1981.

28. Levine SB: Conceptual suggestions for outcome research in sex therapy. *J Sex Marital Ther* 1980;6:102-108.

29. Schumacher S, Lloyd DW: Physiological and psychological factors in impotence. *J Sex Res* 1981;17:40-53.

30. Levine SB, Agle D: The effectiveness of sex therapy for chronic secondary psychological impotence. *J Sex Marital Ther* 1978;4:235-258.

31. Fisher C, Schiavi R, *et al.:* Evaluation of nocturnal penile tumescence in differential diagnosis of sexual impotence: A quantitative study. *Arch Gen Psychiatry* 1979; 36:431-437.

32. Karacan I, Saks PJ, Williams RL: The role of the sleep laboratory in the diagnosis and treatment of impotence, in Williams RL, Karacan I (eds): *Sleep Disorder Diagnosis and Treatment.* New York, Wiley, 1978.

33. Ellenberg M: Impotence in diabetes: The neurologic factor. *Ann Intern Med* 1971; 75:213-219.

34. Spark RF, White RA, Connolly PB: Impotence is not always psychogenic: New insights into the hypothalamic-pituitary-gonadal axis. *JAMA* 1980;243:750-755.

35. Franks S, Jacobs HS, Martin N, *et al.:* Hyperprolactinemia and impotence. *Clin Endocrinol* 1978;8:277-287.

36. Wagner G, Metz P: Vascular impotence. *J Sex Marital Ther* 1980;6:223-233.

37. Segraves RT: Pharmacological agents causing sexual dysfunction. *J Sex Marital Ther* 1977;3:157-176.
38. Edwards AE, Husted JR: Penile sensitivity, age and sexual behavior. *J Clin Psychiatry* 1976;32:697-700.
39. Solnick RL, Birren JE: age and male erectile responsiveness. *Arch Sex Behav* 1977; 6:1-9.
40. Marshall P, Senedge D, Delva N: The role of nocturnal penile tumescence in differentiating between organic and psychogenic impotence: The first stage of validation. *Arch Sex Behav* 1981;10:1-10.
41. Allen RP: Erectile impotence: Objective diagnosis from sleep-related erections. Guest Editorial. *J Urol* 1981;126:353.
42. Wein AJ, Fishkin R, Carpiniello VL, *et al.:* Expansion without significant rigidity during nocturnal penile tumescence testing: A potential source of misinterpretation. *J Urol* 1982;126:343-344.
43. Marshall P, Morales A, Surridge D: Unreliability of nocturnal penile tumescence recording and MMPI profiles in assessment of impotence. *Urol* 1981;17:136-139.
44. Karacan I: Nocturnal penile tumescence as a biologic marker in assessing erectile dysfunction. *Psychosomatics* 1982;23:349-360.
45. Schmidt HS, Wise HA: Significance of impaired penile tumescence and associated polysomnographic abnormalities in the impotent patient. *J Urol* 1981;126:348-351.

Chapter 26

FEMALE SEXUAL DYSFUNCTION
MIRIAM ROSENTHAL, M.D.

INTRODUCTION

Despite the tremendous increase in our biologic and psychologic knowledge, female sexuality remains less well understood than male sexuality. Viewed from the traditional male perspective, only immoral women expected to derive pleasure from sexual interactions. Many women were so inhibited by their cultures that they lived through courtship, marriage, childbearing, and menopause without ever experiencing sexual arousal or orgasm.

Due to recent sociocultural changes, women are now more likely to be active participants in their sexual lives. The growth of industrial societies and the population explosion have changed children from economic assets to liabilities. Changing roles, widely disseminated new sexual knowledge, and birth control technology have revolutionized sexual relationships. A female born in 1900 had a life expectancy of 48 years; the current life expectancy is 77. Family structures are also changing. Only 17% of American families consist of a full-time homemaker mother, a bread-winning father, and dependent children. In 28% of homes with children, both parents work. There are no children in one-third of American families.

This chapter is an introduction to the complex issues of female sexuality, including dysfunctions and some therapeutic approaches.

DEVELOPMENTAL ISSUES

It is important to remember that adult sexual behaviors are influenced by constitutional, biological, and psychological factors which begin in prenatal life. Although it is modified throughout the life cycle, the ability to sustain intimate relationships has its roots in the earliest infant-parent bonds. The wish to recreate the pleasure caused by a loving parent's touch is the earliest impetus for touching the genitals. Genital self-touching in the first 2 years of life enables exploration and definition of bodily boundaries. Later, families may regard the toddler's interest in pleasurable genital sensations with disgust, shame, and censure. Latency age girls often masturbate with clitoral stimulation via indirect rhythmic activities, such as jumping rope, bicycling, dancing, running water over their genitals, pressing their thighs together, or directly rubbing the clitoris. Prepubertal girls are probably often aware of vaginal sensations, and experience their bodies as sources of pleasure. Some girls may displace their genital manipulation by playing with their hair, ears, or mouths. The onset of menses helps to more clearly define a girl's internal reproductive organs and establish the monthly rhythm of her adult reproductive years. Cultural myths of uncleanliness, loss of bodily control, and dirtiness make it difficult for many girls to consider menstruation a source of pride. The attitudes of surrounding adults make a very significant difference. As a rehearsal for adult sexuality, adolescent masturbation is accompanied by fantasies expressing deep sexual longings. (See N. Friday, *My Secret Garden* [1] for an excellent description of women's sexual fantasies.) Fantasy has an important role in development.

Girls often begin genital sexual activity with a partner because they wish to preserve a relationship. Experimentation with male and female partners occurs in adolescence. First intercourse for girls is often painful, and rarely results in orgasm. In 1976, more than half of 19-year-old American females had had intercourse.

FEMALE SEXUAL DYSFUNCTIONS

Although the classification of female sexual dysfunctions has been summarized in the preceding sections, a reminder is in order. Masters and Johnson's description of the 4 phases of sexual physiology implies that there is a smooth continuum from desire to excitement to plateau to orgasm to resolution. There are really 3 distinct phases: *desire;* with its cortical component; general *vasocongestion,* to produce lubrication (under control of parasympathetic autonomic nervous system); reflex *muscular contractions* of organs, which are under sympathetic nervous system control. Each of these components differs in its vulnerability to physical trauma, illness, drugs, aging, partner problems, and intrapsychic difficulties; each may respond to different treatment approaches. A careful history and physical is essential to clarify the problem and treat it accordingly. Most of these dysfunctions apply to women with lesbian or heterosexual orientations. (*Causes* of sexual dysfunctions have been summarized in the preceding sections.) (2,3)

CLINICAL CONSIDERATIONS

Some of the most common female sexual complaints are: 1. "I don't want sex. I'm not interested." 2. "I don't have orgasm." 3. "It hurts when I have sex" (3).

Inhibited Sexual Desire—"I don't want sex. I'm not interested."

Inhibited sexual desire is probably the most common of all female sexual complaints. The problem may be primary, i.e., lifelong, or secondary, i.e., developing after a period of normal functioning. Its presence does not imply a lack of physiologic response; arousal and orgasm are possible in the face of very little desire. Many women with primary inhibited sexual desire (ISD) have never consciously masturbated, come from severely inhibited backgrounds, or have been sexually traumatized in childhood or adolescence. They may avoid social relationships to avoid sex. Sexual repression is strong, and is associated with unpleasant emotions. Some of these women will tolerate sex because they need to be close to another human being. Treatment consists of simultaneous psychotherapy and behavioral methods, to help make them more comfortable with their bodies and lessen their inhibitions.

Secondary inhibited sexual desire often develops after partner difficulties which cause anger, physical or emotional traumas, illness, drugs, surgery, and, frequently, depression. A careful history is essential, and should include recent life changes, losses, and medical and drug histories. Female desire does vary with the menstrual cycle, and there is some evidence of an increase around the time of ovulation (4). Desire problems related to concerns about pregnancy may decrease with the use of good, reliable contraception. Desire may increase after menopause when fertility is no longer a worry; conversely, it may decrease when sex is no longer associated with procreation. There is a wide variation in sexual appetites, some of which is certainly biologically determined. It is important to look for changes in sexual patterns, which arise when partners have considerably different levels of desire. Treatment involves determining and resolving the cause of the problem (5).

Sexual Phobias

Women with very specific fears of sex develop patterns of avoidance. These fears are not related to sexual failure. The thought of sex arouses panic and anxiety. These individuals may avoid any reference to sex in jokes, movies, or books. They may become socially isolated. Treatment consists of education, support, psychotherapy, and behavioral techniques, which may be used in conjunction with antipanic medications, such as imipramine (6).

Orgasmic Problems—"I don't have orgasm. I don't have the right kind of orgasm. I have to fake orgasm."

Orgasmic problems are very common. About 8–10% of adult women in the United States have never been orgasmic, another 10% can only achieve orgasm with fantasy (7). Most women fall somewhere in between the two extremes, demonstrating a variety of responses. Women with primary orgasmic problems have never experienced orgasm in any situation, even after prolonged, effective sexual stimulation. Those with secondary orgasmic problems have had periods of normal functioning. In both primary and secondary cases, the women may lubricate easily, enjoy lovemaking, and feel satisfaction. Somehow they get "stuck" in the plateau phase of the sexual response cycle. Some women are not really sure if they have reached orgasm; others regularly "fake" orgasm in order to please their partners. A number of women are orgasmic with clitoral stimulation, but not during intercourse. For others, the presence of the penis, a strong erotic stimulus, is necessary for orgasm.

Orgasm is a reflex triggered by afferent impulses from the clitoris, nipples, other body parts, and the cortex. The efferent fibers cause contractions of the perivaginal musculature. The uterus and other body parts may also contract. Like other reflexes, orgasm can be inhibited by many things, such as distractions, fears, and anger at the partner. Orgasm is not a passive process.

The woman with primary orgasmic dysfunction is likely to have some very basic fears about sexuality and relationships. She may fear losing control, urinating, getting pregnant, or giving herself pleasure. She may experience performance anxiety, and may or may not be sexually inhibited in general. Not having a trusted partner is sometimes a factor.

Theories which labelled vaginal orgasms mature and clitoral orgasms immature have hopefully been laid to rest. There are innumerable orgasmic variations. The goal of any treatment is to help the individual achieve her first orgasm, if she has never had one, or to reestablish orgasmic achievement if it has ceased. Although every woman is physiologically capable of having an orgasm, the orgasm mania of our current cultural climate sometimes makes its achievement more difficult for some women. Pressure may also come from partners who insist that a woman's lack of orgasm is due to the male partner's failure.

Treatment is aimed at enhancing sensory stimulation and extinguishing the woman's involuntary over-control. The therapist's first task is to make certain that the woman has had sufficient clitoral stimulation and is able to communicate her needs to her partner. She needs to know that it is all right to be sexual. Sometimes these educational techniques are enough to overcome the problem. Barbach's book, *For Yourself,* has been very helpful to many women (8).

A woman with primary orgasmic dysfunction needs to learn what it feels like to have an orgasm. She may have to disregard her obsessive thoughts and distractions, and focus on the erotic thoughts and premonitory feelings which directly precede orgasm. The use of fantasy can be very helpful. Women with very religious backgrounds may find the idea of erotic fantasy, i.e., thinking of other partners and being overcome by a loving partner, more guilt-provoking than sex itself. Self-stimulation is often recommended as a means of learning what feels good and helps the woman become sexually aroused. The long-standing prohibition against masturbation in her value system may be difficult to overcome. She may prefer to masturbate in privacy, rather than with a partner. Some women have marked success with a vibrator, at first alone and then, possibly with the partner. In addition to mastering the physical aspects of achieving orgasm, women need to understand and discuss their fears. Many patients find it helpful to join a women's group. Besides discussing educational issues, members are assigned specific sexual tasks, such as masturbation. Tasks are performed in privacy, and responses are later shared with the group members. They may also be able to share fantasies and give one another support.

Transferring orgasmic achievement to a partner situation is the final step in most treatment situations. Heterosexual women are encouraged to heighten arousal before penetration. They learn that the greatest clitoral stimulation comes from the indirect friction of the hood being pulled back and forth over this organ. Each woman needs to learn the most effective means of increasing her own pleasure, e.g., active thrusting and use of pelvic and thigh musculature; avoidance of distracting thoughts; free use of erotic and exciting fantasies. Lastly, a beloved, trusted partner is a big help. The prognosis is very good (5,9).

Pain With Sex—"It hurts when I have sex."
Pain during a sexual interaction can be especially destructive. Even when the actual pain is gone, its memory may remain and interfere with pleasure. Some women may assume that sex will be painful because they associate menstruation and childbirth with pain; these woman may have no background of trauma or major inhibitions. A careful history and physical exam is essential. The following Table lists the physical reasons for dyspareunia. It is also important to look for psychological contributants.

Treatment for each of the above conditions is very specific. While treating the physical problems, the psychological aspects, especially the effects on sexuality, should also be assessed. It is often important to see both the partner and the patient.

Vaginismus is the painful reflex spasm of the perivaginal and thigh adductor muscles which occurs in anticipation of any vaginal penetration. It oc-

TABLE I
SOME PHYSICAL REASONS FOR DYSPAREUNIA (9)

Vaginal Opening:

hymen—rare
tender episiotomy scar
aging—with decreased elasticity
labia—Bartholin gland abscess
other lesions

Clitoris

irritations
infections

Vagina

infections
sensitivity reactions
atrophic reactions
decreased lubrication

Uterus, Tubes, Ovaries

endometriosis
pelvic inflammatory disease
ectopic pregnancy
numerous others

curs most often in young, inexperienced women from strict homes. Some patients may have been subjected to rape or incest as children or adults. Severe pain secondary to trauma or medical procedures in the vaginal area may sometimes cause the problem. Insufficient lubrication from lack of arousal or sexual phobias may also cause pain with intercourse and vaginismus.

Vaginismus must be diagnosed by history and physical exam. Gynecologists often institute a program of gradual vaginal dilitation, using dilators, the woman's finger, or the partner's finger; not all women respond to this prescription. Some may have more serious problems which require psychotherapy. It is not unusual for a woman who has overcome her difficulty to find that her partner has developed erectile problems. This finding supports the belief that sexual problems are rarely limited to one partner.

FEMALE SEXUAL DYSFUNCTION IN SPECIFIC SITUATIONS

Sex and the Adolescent

Recent statistical analysis indicates that premarital intercourse is increasing among teenagers of all races and ethnic origins. Most sexual encounters occur at the home of one partner, and there is a seasonal rise in the summer. Although contraceptive use is increasing, it does not begin with the onset of intercourse. Between 1971 and 1976, the pill and IUD's have become more popular; the use of condoms, douches, and withdrawal as contraceptive methods has declined. The adverse publicity about medical side effects of the pill and IUD's, along with renewed support for the use of the diaphragm, may change this trend in the 1980s. Adolescent sexuality is a mixture of experimentation, performance anxiety, strong biological desires, and fear of pregnancy. The physician can play a very significant role in a young woman's sexual education (10–12).

Sex and Pregnancy

Numerous factors affect couples' sexuality during pregnancy: physiological, endocrine, and body image changes; concerns about feeling sexually desirable; conflicting roles of wife and career woman; partner attitudes about the pregnancy; patient's reaction to the pregnancy; anticipated changes in the family system. Despite increased or decreased libido, most women want more physical closeness during pregnancy. Libido generally declines during the first trimester. This period is characterized by nausea, considerable fatigue, possible ambivalence about the pregnancy, and a general turning inward as the woman begins to adapt to the growing fetus inside her. Increased pelvic vascularity in the second trimester may lead to increased desire and orgasmic capability.

There is considerable variation in the third trimester, when the awkwardness of the large abdomen may make sex uncomfortable. Unless there is a history of miscarriage or bleeding, it is generally believed that sex can continue until term. Obstetricians who are concerned about infection and premature labor may ask the couple to abstain in the last few weeks. Non-coital forms of sexual interactions can help. Blowing air into the vagina is contraindicated during pregnancy, since it may cause air emboli. Since orgasm causes the uterus to contract, women with histories of miscarriages should avoid it in the last few weeks. It is very important that the physician talk to the couple about sex during the pregnancy. Otherwise it may be a source of trouble and ignorance at a time when the partners should be growing closer (13–16).

Sex and Gynecological Surgery

Ten percent of all adult women in the United States have had hysterectomies. In 1975, 725,000 hysterectomies and 471,000 oophorectomies were performed on women under 45 years of age. Several factors determine the effects of the operation on the woman's sexual functioning: 1. age at the time of hysterectomy; 2. type of surgical procedure; 3. the woman's physical history; 4. reactions to the procedures; 5. woman's environmental supports. Some women have decreased libido after hysterectomy even if the ovaries are not removed. While physicians used to tell their patients this was all psychological, there is evidence to support the role of physical factors. Many women find the sensation of the penis pushing against the cervix extremely pleasurable. The uterus may contract during orgasm. The ovary is a source of androgens which, in the form of testosterone, may enhance libido. Discussing these changes with a patient may help her with post-operative sexual functioning. It is important to include the partner in these discussions. Many males believe that a hysterectomy leaves their partner with an empty cavity from labia to umbilicus. Management therefore consists of pre- and post-operative educational counseling. Knowledge of the patient's pre-operative sexual functioning is a prerequisite for post-operative counseling. Hormone replacement may sometimes be necessary, and sensate focus exercises can help to enhance total body pleasure (17-19).

Sexual Dysfunctions Following Rape and Incest

The incidence of sexual dysfunctions following rape and/or incest is estimated to be about 70%. Rape victims often go through a rape trauma syndrome characterized by a number of emotional changes, including fears, nightmares, and depression. They may experience a variety of anxiety and panic reactions to any sexual stimuli, dyspareunia, and problems with desire, arousal, orgasm, and sexual satisfaction. The enormous variety of reactions necessitates an individualized approach. Psychological and physical assessments should be followed by appropriate psychotherapy and support (20).

Sex and Abortion

In general, there are no major psychological sequelae to abortion. The association of sexuality and the loss of a child may, however, affect a woman's sexual functioning. A thorough history will clarify this situation and enable the initiation of appropriate psychotherapy.

Sex and Infertility

Infertility, a major problem for many couples today, has a great impact upon each partner's sexual functioning. Sexuality is most affected at 3 times during the experience: 1. when the diagnosis is first made; 2. during the infertility work-up; 3. when the couple is told that there is little or no hope for their having a child of their own. Sexual desire may diminish as sex becomes very goal-oriented—i.e., the physician directs the couple to have sex at certain times of the month, using certain positions, to maximize the possibility of pregnancy. Pleasure is sometimes diminished by temperature-taking to determine the times of ovulation. Arousal becomes difficult during the most fertile times of the month. The man's inability to achieve an erection at the time of the wife's ovulation is referred to as "this is the night syndrome." Couples are frequently unable to discuss these problems with their doctors for fear of seeming uncooperative or not really desirous of pregnancy. The depression which accompanies the appearance of the menstrual period each month also inhibits sexuality. Partners often feel blame and guilt, which interferes with their sexual interactions. Sexual dysfunctions also contribute to infertility, e.g., vaginismus; retarded ejaculation; erectile problems. If they become severe, dealing with the sexual dysfunctions may take precedence over completing the infertility work-up. Standard approaches should be used in treating these dysfunctions; the therapist should, however, be aware of the current stresses caused by the medical situation.

CONCLUSION

The advantages to the new openness about sexuality are tempered by the pressures on many women to "measure up" to their often incorrect conceptions of the current sexual norms. By becoming actively involved in, and deriving pleasure from, their sexual lives, women reap the greatest benefits of this new attitude. The physician's role is to educate, understand, and be knowledgeable about diagnoses, treatments, and referrals to sex therapists.

REFERENCES

1. Friday N: *My Secret Garden*. New York, Pocket Books, 1974.
2. Levine SB, Rosenthal MB: Marital sexual dysfunction: Female dysfunction. *Ann Intern Med* 1977;86:588-597.
3. Masters WH, Johnson VE: *Human Sexual Inadequacy* Boston, Little Brown & Co, 1970.
4. Adams DB, Gold A, Burt AD: Rise in female-initiated sexual activity at ovulation and its suppression by oral contraceptives. *N Engl J Med* 1978;299:1145-1150.
5. Kaplan H: *The New Sex Therapy*. New York, Brunner/Mazel, 1974.
6. Kaplan HS, Fyer A, Novick A: The treatment of sexual phobias: The combined use of antipanic medication and sex therapy. *J Sex Marital Ther* 1982;8:29-43.
7. Kuriansky JB, Sharpe L, O'Conner D: The treatment of anorgasmia. Long term effectiveness of a short term behavioral group therapy. *J Sex Marital Ther* 1982;8:29-43.
8. Barbach LG: *For Yourself. The Fulfillment of Female Sexuality*. New York, Doubleday & Co, 1975.
9. Wabrek A, Wabrek CJ: Dyspareunia. *J Sex Marital Ther* 1975;1:3.
10. Miller WB: Sexual and contraceptive behavior in young unmarried women. *Primary Care* 1976;3:327-453.
11. Rosenthal MB: Sexual counseling and interviewing of adolescents. *Primary Care* 1977;2:
12. Zelnik M, Kantner JF: Sexual and contraceptive experience of young, unmarried women in the United States, 1976 and 1971. *Fam Plann Perspect* 1977;9:55-71.
13. Lief H: Sexual desire and responsivity during pregnancy. *Med Aspects Hum Sex* 1977; :56-57.

14. Perkins R: Sexual behavior and response in relation to complications of pregnancy. *Am J Obstet Gynecol* 1979;134:498-505.
15. Solberg DA, Butler J, Wagner N: Sexual behavior in pregnancy. *N Engl J Med* 1973; 288:1096-1103.
16. Tolor A, DiGrazia PV: Sexual attitudes and behavior patterns during and following pregnancy. *Arch Sex Behav* 1976;5:539-551.
17. Amias AG: Sexual life after gynecologic operations. *Br Med J* 1975;2:608-609.
18. Dennerstein L, Wood C, Burrows G: Sexual dysfunction following hysterectomy. *Aust Fam Physician* 1977;6:92-96.
19. Zussman L, Zussman S, Sunley R, *et al.:* Sexual response after hysterectomy-oophorectomy: Recent studies and reconsideration of psychogenesis. *Am J Obstet Gynecol* 1981; 140:725-729.
20. Becker JV, Skinner LJ, Abel G, *et al.:* Incidence and types of sexual dysfunctions in rape and incest victims. *J Sex Marital Ther* 1982;8:65-74.

Chapter 27

VICTIM RESPONSE TO RAPE AND VIOLENCE
PHILLIP J. RESNICK, M.D.

We live in a violent society. A white man in the United States has one chance in 186 of being a murder victim during his lifetime; the odds increase to one in 29 for a black man. Each year an American has more than three chances in one hundred of being the victim of a violent crime (1). Victims of physical assault or rape often require psychological support. Physicians should be sensitive to victims' immediate needs, and be familiar with the common psychological sequelae of such attacks.

VICTIM RESPONSE TO VIOLENCE

Most people respond to a personal attack of sudden, unexpected violence with momentary shock and disbelief. This is often followed by a frozen, frightened response, which may be analogous to the tonic immobility seen in animals when they are victims of predators. Statements such as, "My body felt paralyzed," or "My body went absolutely stiff" are quite common among rape victims (2). Victims usually react to a life-threatening situation with submission, compliance, or other ingratiating behavior. The fear may be so profound that the victim concludes that all hope for survival depends upon appeasing the criminal.

Ingratiating behavior by the victim may lead others to the false conclusion that the victim caused or participated in the criminal act. Victims are later likely to play down such behavior because of shame or guilt (3). Other victims respond to their fright with anger; they may scream, strike their assailant with a purse, or say, "Get the hell away, or I'll call the police." Some criminals back down, but the majority beat the victim into compliance. One robbery victim said to a criminal, "I'll never forget your face;" she was shot in the head and permanently blinded. Attempts to cling to the criminal or make him feel guilty are likely to be ineffective, and may, in fact, cause more assaultive behavior.

Men and women respond differently to being victims. Policemen and combat soldiers readily submit to superior force without loss of self-respect. Female victims, on the other hand, tend to express shame and outrage over having submitted. Women feel they submitted to the criminal; most men feel they submitted to the gun, rather than the man holding it. Violent criminals who have been victims report that they readily submit without protest. They acknowledge their fear—for example, one criminal stated, "I'd be scared of a midget with a gun." Men and women differ in their attitudes toward their responses, rather than their actual behavior. Women often feel ashamed or stupid, and seem to expect more from themselves than men. When men are boys, they learn that submission to a stronger force allows them to fight another day. Women frequently fantasize further harm from the criminal, whereas men are more likely to fantasize revenge.

Terror may induce a psychological regression which reduces the victim to a child-like clinging. Such behavior is analagous to a child who buries his head in his mother's skirts when she is angry with him. Anger is suppressed to avoid any further provocation, which could cause additional punishment.

Society has a strange attitude toward victims of violence (4). The innocent or accidental nature of the victim's involvement is difficult to accept. Friends may aggressively question victims about their reasons for placing themselves in a position to be attacked. Such questioning is prompted by people's need to find rational explanations for violent crimes. We feel less vulnerable and helpless if we can believe that the victim contributed to the crime in some way. We can then reassure ourselves that we would never be that careless or "stupid."

Being a victim of violence can be compared to experiencing a sudden and unexpected loss. There may be loss of money, physical well-being, and self-respect—because of viewing compliant behavior with shame. Victims often lose their belief that society will protect them from harm. Being the victim of an unsympathetic society after a crime may cause the victim to view the world as an even more hostile place.

Victims of violence, including rape, often suffer a post-traumatic stress disorder, as delineated in DSM-III (5). The attack is a stressor that would evoke significant symptoms of distress in almost anyone. The characteristic symptoms include: reexperiencing the traumatic event; numbing of responses; a variety of autonomic, dysphoric, or cognitive symptoms. Victims commonly have recurrent, intrusive recollections and dreams of the assault. The numbing of responsiveness to the world, which usually begins shortly after the trauma, may be manifested by diminished interest in activities, feelings of detachment from others, and constricted affect. Victims also commonly demonstrate hyperalertness, an exaggerated startle response, sleep disturbances, and concentration difficulties. They are likely to avoid activities which arouse recollections of the assault. Symptoms are intensified by events which resemble or symbolize the attack. If a second victim was killed or seriously injured, the other victim may feel guilty for having survived.

VICTIM RESPONSE TO RAPE

Short of homicide, rape is the ultimate violation of the self. It involves the invasion of one's innermost private space, as well as the loss of autonomy and control (6). It is dehumanizing to be forced to participate in what otherwise would be an intimate and loving act. It is the person's self, not an orifice, that has been invaded. The core meaning of rape is the same for a virgin, a housewife, a lesbian, and a prostitute. Most women are never totally free of the fear of rape (6). Under current conditions, a conservative estimate is that 20–30 percent of girls now twelve years old will suffer violent sexual attacks during their lifetimes (7).

Since the late 1960s, the women's movement in the United States has been successful in changing a number of attitudes about rape. Several state laws have been changed to: 1. eliminate the possibility of bringing up the victim's past sexual behavior during rape trials; 2. provide an attorney to protect the victim's rights during trials. Although some improvement has been made in the conviction rate, rape is still one of the most difficult crimes to successfully prosecute.

In spite of better public education about rape, certain myths still persist. The first myth is, "Nice girls don't get raped, and bad girls shouldn't complain." This sexist statement retains the use of the word "girls" instead of "women." Unfortunately, even victims often believe this myth. Because they blame themselves, they need help recognizing that they are truly *victims*. The second myth is that victims cannot be raped unless they want to be. This is patently ridiculous in view of the fact that some rapists threaten their victims with guns or knives. It tends to perpetuate the idea that women are safe unless they choose to submit to the situation. A final myth is that proper women should tolerate considerable brutality as evidence that they did not consent to sexual relations. No one suggests that a robbery victim undergo a beating before giving up a wallet. The persistence of these myths contributes to the difficulty in convincing juries to convict rapists.

It is estimated that at least 50 percent of rape victims do not report the crime to the police—either out of fear of additional assault by the rapist or embarrassment. Some victims, especially single women, fear being publicly accused of active participation. Changes of public attitudes in the last decade, and the passage of laws to protect victims have reduced this problem. Also, victims commonly believe that the rapist will not be convicted anyway. It is true that few rapists are brought to trial, and only a minority are convicted. Out of 1085 arrests for rape in New York City in 1970, there were only 18 convictions (8). Rape Crisis Centers in major cities now play an important role in assisting victims, whether or not they report the rape to the police.

The "rape trauma syndrome" was first described by Burgess and Holmstrom (9) in 1974, prior to the DSM-III description of post-traumatic stress disorder. Today, the rape trauma syndrome is best conceptualized as a variant of post-traumatic stress disorder. The victim's life-style is completely disrupted by the rape. The physical, emotional, and behavioral stress reactions characteristic of the syndrome result from the victim's confrontation with a life-threatening event.

Physical reactions include general feelings of body soreness, and sleep and eating pattern disturbances. Fear is the primary emotional reaction—fear of physical injury, mutilation, and death. Additional feelings range from humiliation, degradation, guilt, shame, and embarrassment to self-blame, anger, and revenge (10). The victim continually tries to block out thoughts of the assault, although she is continually haunted by memories. In trying to find some way to undo what happened, the victim may ruminate over how she might have escaped from the assailant.

The acute phase of the rape trauma syndrome is manifested by momentary shock, similar to that experienced by any victim of sudden violent assault. The victim's overt reaction may be expressive, in which case sobbing occurs, or controlled, in which case feelings are masked. The immediate overt response is not a reliable indicator of the amount of the victim's psychological distress. In the intermediate phase, there is a pseudoadjustment and work is resumed. The victim may experience guilt over exercising "poor judgment," whether she did so or not.

Victims are particularly upset by the humiliation of the rape experience. There is no more clear way of demonstrating power over another than by using sex to humiliate the other person. This is evident in prisons where men regularly use homosexual behavior to exercise power over other inmates. Whether or not humiliation is the conscious intention of the rapist, it is experienced by all victims. Women are very reluctant to talk about humiliating behaviors during their rape, besides forced intercourse or fellatio. In one study, 47 of 63 rapes showed fairly clear evidence of intent to humiliate (11).

There are various long-term changes in rape victims' life-styles. Some women limit their activities to those that are work or school-related. Others respond to the rape by staying home, and only venturing out of the house with a friend. Victims commonly seek support from family members who were not normally seen on a daily basis. This often means travelling to some other city for a brief stay with parents. Many victims move to a new residence, or at least request new, unlisted telephone numbers.

Recurrent dreams and nightmares commonly occur during both the acute and long-term phases of the rape trauma syndrome. One type of nightmare involves the victim's failure to escape from circumstances similar to those of the actual rape. In later dreams, the victims themselves may commit acts of violence, such as killing or stabbing the rapist or others.

Phobias are likely to develop in relation to the specific circumstances of the rape. Victims may become fearful of being alone on the street or at home. Victims may show a global fear of everyone, or just men who resemble the assailant. A fear of sex and sexual dysfunction often occur after rape. The reaction, sensitivity, and patience of the victim's sexual partner may have a major effect upon her long-term sexual adjustment.

The following case illustrates many common responses of rape victims:

> Miss A, a 19-year-old, white waitress, and her roommate, Miss B, were raped in their first floor apartment. Miss A had some prior problems with her self-image. When she was 16 years old, she visited a psychiatrist several times because of depression. One year after graduating from high school, she moved out of her parents' home to live with Miss B.
>
> Miss A was awakened at 4:30 a.m. by a large black man, holding his hand over her mouth and a switchblade knife over her heart. He instructed her not to scream. Miss A's initial reaction was disbelief and numbness. The intruder told her that he would not hurt her if she gave him her money. Her immediate fear was of being killed. Her hands were tied behind her back, and a sock was tied around her mouth as a gag. The rapist went into the other bedroom and tied up Miss B, who slept in the nude. He then forced Miss A to show him where the money was kept.
>
> Miss A was "in shock" and was surprised that she did not "pass out." She felt certain that she was going to die. She cried a good deal, whereas Miss B was overtly angry and called the rapist names. For example, she called him a "mother-fucking bastard." He said, "What did you call me?" Miss A replied, "She said you were a very nice robber." When the rapist was in her roommate's room, Miss A managed to free her hands; however, she was too fearful to try to escape. She pleaded with the rapist to go, and "asked him a hundred times," "Are you going to kill us?" The whole series of events took about one hour.
>
> The intruder asked if there was any more money. Miss A replied, "No." He said, "If you don't come up with another $10.00, someone is going to get fucked." Miss A then felt her hopes of getting away safely "fall apart." The rapist dragged Miss B to the floor, and held his knife to her chest. He said, "Are you going to fuck me?" He pressed the knife to her chest until she agreed.
>
> Miss A was screaming for him to stop. The rapist tried to quiet her while he raped her roommate. He had trouble maintaining a full erection, but did penetrate Miss B without reaching a climax. He then tried

to have vaginal intercourse with Miss A, but did not fully penetrate her. After two tries with each victim, he realized that he would not be successful. He then demanded that they both kneel and give him a "blow job." He forced one after the other to perform fellatio. Miss A gagged almost continually. She reports that he smelled terrible. He did not reach a climax by this method either.

After forcing both women into the shower, the rapist left. Once they realized he was gone, they went out into the corridor and banged on the doors of all their neighbors. They were taken to the hospital by the police. Miss A was afraid that she would "flip out," or "go insane." She continued to feel "scared and paranoid." She wondered how she could ever lead a normal life again. She was quite concerned that no man could ever love her because she was "damaged goods."

Miss A agreed to sleep in her apartment the next night only if a police lieutenant stayed with her for protection. Her thoughts were "racing" and she was fearful she would "freak out." She felt unable to sleep in her bedroom, and fared no better on the couch. She was afraid of being left alone for even a short time. Her biggest fear was that the rapist would return and kill her.

She handled her emotional distress by talking a great deal with her roommate; they talked of nothing else for two weeks. After a temporary stay with her parents, Miss A moved into the third floor of an apartment building that had a security officer on duty all night. Nonetheless, she put a slide bolt, dead bolt, chain lock, and bells on her door.

She felt she could never move into a home because an intruder could gain entrance to the first floor. Each time she comes into her apartment, she checks the closets to be sure that no one is hiding there. She remains very concerned about being unable to hear someone coming in.

She developed a "tremendous awareness" of crime after the rape. She takes extreme precautions because she feels so vulnerable. Since she was raped in her own home, she does not feel safe anywhere. Prior to the rape, she did not believe that such a thing could happen to her. She used to feel that people were basically good. Now she is uneasy with all strangers. Although she is less afraid with men she knows, she feels unable to fully trust anybody. In her work as a waitress, she is sometimes rude to a male customer to make it absolutely clear that she is not sexually available.

She initially had nightmares every night in which she was tied up and helpless. In one dream, several men surrounded her bed and planned to kill her. She has daydreams of revenge against the rapist. She would like him to be castrated, and to "look in his eyes in the light of day and tell him that he'll fry in hell if the police don't get him."

After having sexual relations, the rape comes into her mind. She concentrates on the warmth and caring of her current relationship to differentiate it from the rape experience.

Miss A showed the following common responses to her rape. She was immobilized by fear. Her concern about being killed was far more important than the sexual violation. She demonstrated an expressive initial reaction, in contrast to her roommate, who was overtly more calm, except for her outbursts of anger. After the rape, she was anxious about being alone because she feared the rapist would return to kill her. She had an immediate need to move out of her apartment. The particular circumstances of her rape made her extremely sensitive to being able to hear warning signs of a future assault. She exhibited a sleep disturbance, recurring nightmares, a sense of vulnerability, difficulty trusting men, and extreme concern about security in her new apartment. She was able to mentally separate the rape experience from a caring sexual relationship more quickly than most rape victims.

Miss B sustained fewer symptoms subsequent to the rape. This may have been due to greater maturity, more self-esteem, or her less ingratiating behavior during the rape.

Follow-up studies of rape victims: Follow-up studies demonstrate more serious long-term sequelae than clinicians originally suspected. Nadelson *et al.* (12) found that victims experienced the following persistent symptoms 12–30 months after the rape: suspicion of others (75%); restricted activities (60%); fear of being alone (60%); sexual difficulties (50%); sleep troubles including nightmares (25%); decreased concentration (25%). Although three-fourths of those in Burgess and Holstrom's study (13) felt recovered four to six years later, one-half felt that it took years. Ellis *et al.* (14) compared 27 adult victims who had been raped three years earlier to nonvictim controls. The victims were more depressed, got less enjoyment from their daily lives, and were more tense and fatigued. Depressions following the assault were so severe that 50% reported having suicidal thoughts. Twelve victims had discussed the rape with virtually no one, a factor which they felt contributed to guilt, isolation, and depression. Victims of sudden assault by complete strangers had more persistent problems of depression and more phobias; they were also more likely to report persistent avoidance of dating.

The following statement from a rape victim conveys the ongoing anguish. "In some ways, rape is never erased. Years later, even the word 'rape' or the shadow of a familiar face can cause unexpected pain. The raped woman often cannot bear to be touched. Isolation is her condition. Touched, she knows she cannot feel; touched, she remains untouched. She is incarcerated in Hades. Her mother is outside and cannot hear her." (15)

Men respond to the rape of their wives, girlfriends, or daughters with anger at both the attacker and at the victim—for being "compliant." They may become overprotective, partly from guilt over failing to protect their loved one (16). Sometimes a man feels his masculinity threatened by an attack on "his" woman. Feelings of helplessness are engendered. During wars, the victors have traditionally raped the women of the conquered nation in front of their men, to symbolically violate their property rights. Occasionally, a man insists upon having sex with his wife shortly after a rape, to reassert his "property rights." Husbands may be less able to offer emotional support to their wives because of concerns about "used merchandise." The idea of sharing a woman with the rapist may also create homosexual conflicts in some men. The husband's failure to offer support may cause the victim to feel betrayed by both the male rapist and her male protector, thereby contributing to her diminished trust in men.

Treatment of the Victim: Treatment of victims of sudden, unexpected violence should be aimed at reducing target symptoms and preventing chronic disability. The therapist should inquire about the victim's experience and feelings in detail. Going over the event in a non-judgmental manner may help to desensitize memories. Having the victim return to routine activities as soon as possible is likely to reduce long-term emotional disability. Progressive desensitization may be used to treat specific phobic symptoms. Minor tranquilizers should be used judiciously to decrease symptoms of anxiety.

Medical treatment for rape victims should be offered for two purposes: 1. treatment of physical injury, venereal disease prophylaxis, pregnancy testing, and emotional support; 2. collection of evidence for the rapist's possible prosecution. Physicians should listen to the rape experience in a manner that supports and validates the victim's feelings. The victim should be encouraged to express these feelings in her own way.

The phrasing of questions about the rapist's behavior is very important— particularly if any activities other than "straight" vaginal intercourse were included—for example, fellatio, cunnilingus, or anal intercourse. Women may feel especially humiliated by such experiences. The doctor should avoid phrases which suggest ordinary intercourse or lovemaking; nor should one infer that the victim took any initiative. For example, avoid such phrases as, "Did you put your mouth on his penis?" Questions of this sort may increase the victim's feelings of guilt or shame. Instead, one might ask, "Did the rapist put his penis in your mouth?" The latter phrase transfers responsibility for the action to the rapist.

The victim may be shocked to discover the range of people's reactions to her rape. She can be prepared for this situation by learning about people's needs to make unsympathetic responses. It may be extremely helpful for the victim to select a good friend or loved one as a confidant. Although the doctor may feel angry toward unsympathetic or accusatory members of the victim's family, it is important for them to be able to "ventilate" their feelings and calm down.

The woman should be allowed to talk about the incident and attempt to determine what she did "wrong"—i.e., should have done differently. She may need to review the event a number of times before she can accept the fact that the rapist is responsible for its occurrence. Discussing some of the general mythology about rape—such as women being responsible for male sexuality—may be helpful.

The victim's fears, which are likely to be particularly strong if the rapist threatened further harm, should also be discussed. Suggesting various methods of protection may increase her awareness of choice, give her a stronger sense of control, and reduce her fear.

Since a significant portion of women still do not report rapes, clinicians should be alert for the "silent-rape reaction" (17). Because they have blocked their feelings and reactions, such women carry a tremendous psychological burden. Avoidance of sexual relationships, or the sudden onset of phobic reactions, should alert the clinician to the possibility of unreported rape. Direct questioning about any attempted assaults may release considerable unresolved feeling.

It is difficult to convey the overwhelming fear and vulnerability felt by a rape victim. The following "Rape Poem" by Marge Piercy (18) does it well:

> There is no difference between being raped
> and being pushed down a flight of cement steps
> except that the wounds also bleed inside.
>
> There is no difference between being raped
> and being run over by a truck
> except that afterward men ask if you enjoyed it.
>
> There is no difference between being raped
> and being bit on the ankle by a rattlesnake
> except that people ask if your skirt was short
> and why you were out alone anyhow.
>
> There is no difference between being raped
> and going head first through a windshield
> except that afterward you are afraid
> not of cars
> but half the human race.
>
> The rapist is your boyfriend's brother.
> He sits beside you in the movies eating popcorn.
> Rape fattens on the fantasies of the normal male
> like a maggot in garbage.
>
> Fear of rape is a cold wind blowing
> all of the time on a woman's hunched back.
> Never to stroll alone on a sand road through pine woods,

never to climb a trail across a bald
without that aluminum in the mouth
when I see a man climbing toward me.

Never to open the door to a knock
without that razor just grazing the throat.
The fear of the dark side of hedges,
the back seat of the car, the empty house
rattling keys like a snake's warning.
The fear of the smiling man
in whose pocket is a knife.
The fear of the serious man
in whose fist is locked hatred.

All it takes to cast a rapist to be able to see your body
as jackhammer, as blowtorch, as adding-machine-gun.
All it takes is hating that body
your own, your self, your muscle that softens to flab.

All it takes is to push what you hate,
what you fear onto the soft alien flesh.
To bucket out invincible as a tank
armored with treads without senses
to possess and punish in one act,
to rip up pleasure, to murder those who dare
live in the leafy flesh open to love.*

*From *Living in the Open,* by Marge Piercy. Copyright 1976 by Marge Piercy. Reprinted by permission of Alfred A. Knopf, Inc.

REFERENCES

1. *Victims of Crime.* NCJ-79615, Bureau of Justice Statistics Bulletin, November, 1981.
2. Gallup GG, Suarez SD: Tonic immobility as a response to rape in humans. *Psychological Record* 1979;29:315-320.
3. Symonds M: Victims of senseless violence. *Psychiat Worldview* 1977;1:1-3.
4. Symonds M: Victims of violence: Psychological effects and aftereffects. *Am J Psychoanal* 1975;35:19-26.
5. American Psychiatric Association Committee on Nomenclature and Statistics: *Diagnostic and Statistical Manual of Mental Disorders,* ed 3. Washington, DC, American Psychiatric Association, 1980.
6. Hilberman E: *The Rape Victim.* Washington, DC, The American Psychiatric Association, 1976.
7. Johnson AG: On the prevalence of rape in the United States. Signs: *J Women in Culture and Society* 1980;6:136-146.
8. Cooke KH: Results of corroboration and requirements in New York City. *Yale L J* 1972;81:12-21.
9. Burgess AW, Holmstrom LL: Rape trauma syndrome. *Am J Psychiatry* 1974;131:981-986.

10. Notman MT, Nadelson CC: The rape victim: Psychodynamic considerations. *Am J Psychiatry* 1976;133:408–413.
11. Marshall W: Inferring humiliation as motivation in sexual offenses. *Treatment for Sexual Aggressives News* 5:1–3.
12. Nadelson CC, Notman MT, Zackson H, *et al.*: A follow-up study of rape victims. *Am J Psychiatry* 1982;139:1266–1270.
13. Burgess AW, Holmstrom LL: Recovery from rape and prior life stress. *Res Nurs Health* 1978;1:165–174.
14. Ellis EM, Atkeson BM, Calhoun KS: An assessment of long-term reaction to rape. *J Abnormal Psychology* 1981;90:263–266.
15. Metzger D: It is always the woman who is raped. *Am J Psychiatry* 1976;133:405–408.
16. Nadelson CC, Notman MT: Psychological responses to rape. *Psychiatric Opinion* 1977; 14:13–18.
17. Burgess AW, Holmstrom LL: *Rape: Victims of Crisis.* Bowie, Maryland, Robert J Brady Co, 1974, pp 3–50.
18. Piercy M: *Living in the Open.* New York, Alfred Knopf, 1976.

Chapter 28

SEXUALITY AND AGING
STEPHEN B. LEVINE, M.D.

INTRODUCTION

Sexual desire and behavior normally continue throughout the entire life cycle. Most people, however, erroneously assume that sexual desire and behavior are attributes of youth. Young adults who may be able to acknowledge that their parents have a sex life usually cannot seriously discuss such a possibility in relation to their grandparents. (These same people may only recently have realized that sex was a part of their parents' lives.)

Old age provides many people with a convenient excuse to cut down on or discontinue sexual practices if they have found sex unfulfilling or troublesome. Partner loss through death, illness, or divorce is also a primary cause of the decline in sexual behavior among the aging, especially women. Our culture is so strongly imbued with the myth that old age is barren of sexual desire and behavior that those who are interested in sex often feel embarrassed or abnormal. Many men become so afraid of losing their potency as they approach 50 that their anxiety may actually serve as a self-fulfilling prophecy. When dealing with clinical problems in the elderly, it is important for the physician to understand that sexual expression is possible throughout the life cycle (1-4).

MALES

General Considerations

The first problem is one of definition. When does old age begin? When do changes become apparent? The biological forces, structures, and functions involved with sexual expression evolve slowly. It is possible that some men never undergo any significant alteration of their sexual apparatus. It is assumed here, however, that, beginning with the sixth decade, men are likely to notice some physiological changes.

The Changes

Erectile Response. The erection which used to occur in seconds may now require several minutes. The turgidity may not be as great as before, even when an erection occurs in this early stage of arousal. Men who are unaware of the normality of the phenomenon may mistakenly conclude that they are impotent.

Pre-ejaculatory Emission. The few drops from the Cowper's gland which commonly appear shortly before ejaculation may be reduced in volume or disappear entirely.

Ease of Ejaculation. The older man has a distinct advantage over the younger man, who typically has more difficulty delaying ejaculation. An older man's ejaculatory control allows him to prolong intercourse, often providing his partner with great pleasure. The same gradual physiological change that enables ejaculatory control is the basis for the occasional inability to ejaculate noted by many men in their sixties.

Ejaculation Inevitability. The two- to four-second period prior to expulsion of semen is associated with intense pleasure, due to the contractions of the internal sexual apparatus; it may occasionally be prolonged if the prostate develops a spastic contraction, but is usually decreased. Ejaculatory inevitability may disappear entirely if the preceding intercourse was prolonged or exciting, and followed a long period of abstinence. A low level of circulating testosterone may also eliminate this initial stage of ejaculation (1).

Force. The force of ejaculation, which can be great in young men, is often reduced considerably. Semen may ooze out instead of being propelled.

Volume. Volume of ejaculation is often reduced. Despite the reductions in ejaculatory volume and force, the experience of the orgasm may still bring great pleasure and release.

Resolution. Detumescence in older men can be extremely rapid, just a few seconds. The refractory period may increase to the point where re-erection is not possible for twenty-four hours—even if ejaculation has not occurred.

Overview

The capacities for sexual feeling and expression, unless limited by severe illness, depression, or social restriction, continue far into old age. These changes do not occur at the same time for all men and are often only intermittently present. It is vital for men to understand the normality of these changes in order to maintain their self-esteem.

A Syndrome of Testicular Insufficiency?

The existence of a male climacteric has long been debated. Diminished sexual responses in some men reflect diminished testosterone secretion and can be improved with supplements. Symptoms of testosterone deficiency include: painful orgasm, despite a normal prostate gland; constant presence of one-stage ejaculation with reduced volume under little or no pressure. Testosterone should be administered intramuscularly because of poor oral absorption. Most of the functional decrements in aging men are not due to testosterone deficiency; if there is a documented deficiency, intramuscular testosterone is the treatment of choice.

The Female Who Fails to Understand: A Pernicious Trap

A female's lack of intuitive or factual awareness of the aging man's sexual patterns may play a significant role in the premature cessation of sexual relations. The man's erectile slowness may be erroneously considered indicative of a lack of love. The reduction in his demand for ejaculation may make some females feel they are not doing their duty. A female's determination to induce ejaculation may decrease the man's desire to participate at all. The man, and not his partner, should have the privilege of choosing whether and when to ejaculate.

FEMALES

General Considerations

The end of menstruation marks the end of a woman's reproductive capacity, not her sexual life. This loss of the capacity to bear children may induce a significant grief response in some women, causing sexual desire to lessen or disappear. This is a form of mourning, and is usually temporary. Given an adequate sexual adjustment prior to menopause, there is no reason to expect sexual life to decline immediately thereafter. In fact, some women report increased sexual desire and responsiveness when freed from the possibility of pregnancy.

Aging does, however, affect sexual anatomy, physiology, and psychology. The sexual apparatus gradually loses its capacity, as do other organ systems. Many of the sexual organ changes caused by aging are either reversible or delayable through treatment with exogenous estrogens. An active, regular sexual life with an interesting, interested partner, however, is far more important than exogenous estrogen in insuring a continuation of sexual pleasure, responsiveness, and orgasm.

The Changes with Age and Estrogen Deficiency

Delay in Vaginal Lubrication. Lubrication in a young woman may occur within thirty seconds of sexual arousal; it may take as long as five minutes in older women. This delay in lubrication is thought to be due to the thinning of the vaginal barrel. The rugae atrophy with increasing age and change from a rich, dark purple color to pink. Older women who have frequent intercourse have no delay in lubrication, in spite of atrophic changes in the vagina.

Decrease in Vaginal Lubrication. When lubrication does occur, its volume may no longer be as copious or consistently adequate as before.

Reduction in Vaginal Expansion. There is a slowing of, and a reduction in, the involuntary expansion of vaginal length and diameter. This is partly due to a loss of tissue elasticity. It is also related to the reduction of uterine elevation which, in younger women, produces a tenting effect on the inner vagina. The vagina will still expand with high levels of excitement, but not as much as in premenopausal days.

Loss of Reduction of Labia Minora "Sex Skin" Color Change. In younger women, the change in the color of the labia minora is a reliable indicator of impending orgasm. This color change is greatly reduced in older women.

Loss of "Invitation to Intercourse." The labia majora widen and flatten out on the perineum in younger women during the plateau stage of excitement. In older women, the loss of elasticity results in the labia majora hanging at the vaginal outlet.

Clitoral Changes. There may be some slight late postmenopausal reduction in the size of the clitoris. More often, however, there is an atrophy of the clitoral hood and the mons veneris fat pad. Despite this change, the clitoris in older women elevates and flattens on the anterior border of the symphysis with sexual excitement, as it does in younger women.

Orgasm Shortening. The number of rhythmic contractions of the orgasmic platform decreases from 12 to 4 or 5, shortening the duration of the orgasm. Older women may continue to be multiply orgasmic.

Uterine Orgasmic Responses:

1. As in younger women, the uterus may rhythmically contract in waves that pass from the fundus to the lower segment. This occurs only once or twice in older women.
2. There may, however, be a spastic contraction of the uterus which produces pain. The pain may be severe, and located in the lower abdominal region, vagina, and legs. This painful orgasmic response is an indication of a need for estrogens.

Resolution. Vasocongestion and myotonia disappear in a matter of seconds rather than minutes.

Practical Problems

Dyspareunia. The atrophy of the vaginal barrel causes a loss of the natural cushion to the force of penile thrusting. The loss can result in pain and bladder or urethral irritation. The urge to urinate immediately following intercourse is a tip-off. If intercourse is unusually prolonged, or repeated without a day's rest, the atrophic dry vagina is liable to crack and cause pain.

Irritation of the Clitoris. Clitoral stimulation remains an effective means of arousal in older women. Pain or irritation may replace excitement, however, if a too-direct approach is employed. This increased susceptibility to clitoral irritation is probably due to the loss of mons fat tissue and atrophy of the clitoral hood. Estrogen may reverse this problem.

Some decrement of sexual desire may result from an estrogen deficiency, although this is not a major factor in most cases.

Increased Frequency of Masturbation. Because of the higher male death rate and the increasing prevalence of potency problems, many women masturbate occasionally for relief of their sexual tensions. Although this is a normal phenomenon, it may produce a great deal of guilt; physicians will occasionally be indirectly questioned about it.

The Role of the Physician

Many older people feel it is unnatural or perverted to have sexual relations. When they were young the discussion of sexual topics was very inhibited; consequently, their sexual value systems are quite restrictive. There are a large number of remarriages within the geriatric population, and sexual concerns are universal. Physicians can encourage such basic activities as intercourse and masturbation. With couples whose intercourse is limited, physicians can also emphasize the fact that sex is not restricted to coitus.

HELPFUL GENERAL IDEAS

The following quotation is taken from Robert N. Butler's "Psychiatry and the Elderly: An Overview":

> There is also a developmental potential in sexuality. Sex in young people tends to be urgent and explosive, involved largely with physical pleasure and/or the conception of children. This "first language of sex" is biological and instinctive. It often becomes a way of asserting independence, strength, prowess, and power in the process of discovering one's abilities to be sexually desirable and sexually effective. The first language of sex has been much discussed and written about because it lends itself to study—one can measure physical response, frequency of contact, forms of outlet, sexual positions, and physical skills in lovemaking. There is, however, a second language of sex, which is largely learned rather than instinctive and is often vastly underdeveloped because it depends on the ability to recognize and share feelings in words and actions and to achieve a mutual tenderness and thoughtfulness. In its richest form, the second language becomes highly creative and imaginative, with bountiful possibilities for enough new emotional experiences to last a lifetime. Yet it is an art that must be developed slowly and painstakingly through years of experience in giving and receiving. This sec-

ond language expresses the developmental potential of sexuality and needs further study from the life cycle perspective (5).

The richness of Dr. Butler's concept becomes apparent when one contrasts the lack of sexual contact in those couples whose sexual lives have a first language signature ("Foreplay is preparation for intercourse; I can't do the 'job' anymore.") with the continued sexual activity in those that have a second language signature ("We love to caress and have orgasms. Sometimes I'm harder than others. We make do with what we have."). Many people do not realize that orgasm without erection is possible. The physician can often educate the man, woman, or couple about the importance of psychological nurturance through sex. It is vital, however, that the physician view sex as more than penile-vaginal union.

Sexuality in the older years is often a matter of autoeroticism. A recent study (6) revealed that 60% of single people over 60 masturbate regularly. Over 90% of subjects between 60 and 95 expressed a strong interest in sex. Many considered sex a crucial part of their lives; it provides them with a general sense of well-being and a good feeling about themselves. Physicians should take care not to impugn the autoerotic or partner sexual activities of celibate or married older persons; rather, they should support and encourage their continuation.

REFERENCES

1. Masters WH, Johnson VE: *Human Sexual Inadequacy.* Boston, Little Brown & Co, 1970, pp 316-350.
2. Rubin I: *Sexual Life After Sixty.* New York, Basic Books, 1965.
3. Pfeiffer E, Davis GD: Determinants of sexual behavior in middle and old age. *J Am Geriatr Soc* 1972;151:151-158.
4. Busse E, Pfeiffer E: *Behavior and Adaptation in Late Life.* Boston, Little Brown & Co, 1969.
5. Butler RN: Psychiatry and the elderly: An overview. *Am J Psychiatry* 1975;132:893-900.
6. Starr B, Weiner MB: *The Starr-Weiner Report on Sex and Sexuality in the Mature Years.* New York, Stein & Day, 1981.

Chapter 29

PHYSICAL ILLNESS AND SEXUAL FUNCTION
STANLEY E. ALTHOF, Ph.D.

GOALS

1. To acquaint students with the effects of physical illnesses and treatments on sexual functioning.
2. To impart knowledge about the prevention and treatment of sexual dysfunctions associated with physical illness.

OVERVIEW

Various mechanisms can interfere with sexual functioning:

Illness—Diseases may impair desire, arousal (potency), orgasm, satisfaction, and fertility via chromosomal, hormonal, neural, or vascular damage —e.g., Klinefelter's syndrome, hypogonadism, spinal cord injury, diabetes, LeRiche Syndrome.

Surgical treatment—Surgery may compromise neural integrity. For example, men who have had bilateral sympathectomies can no longer ejaculate. Women report decreased genital sensation after surgery on the distal aorta.

Pharmacological treatment—Via various pathways, medications can preclude desire, excitement, orgasm, and fertility. In addition, certain drugs can lead to erectile and ejaculatory disturbances (phenothiazines; antihypertensive agents).

Psychological reaction to illness and/or treatment—A serious disease and its treatment may assault a patient's self-esteem, self-worth, and sense of attractiveness. Persistent negative affects associated with being ill, e.g., anxiety/fear (about abandonment, further loss of function, death); depression; anger; guilt; shame, may compromise sexual function. The manner in which each individual copes with illness and treatment varies according to personality organization. Thus, one cannot predict how any one person will react to any illness/treatment. Most physical illnesses affect sexual life. ᵃᵗ

361

least temporarily. In many situations, however, illness and treatment should not result in profound, chronic sexual dysfunctions. Awareness of alternative treatment regimens and advice concerning sexual practices can often alleviate and minimize the sexual sequelae.

The most important means of minimizing sexual sequelae is open, frank discussion with patients and partners of both their premorbid sexual lives and the potential consequences of any illness and/or treatment. Even a brief discussion lets the patient know that it is all right to raise sexual concerns and future problems, which may or may not be related to their physical condition. Open communication is often hindered by physicians' discomfort about discussing sexuality and lack of information about sexual functioning.

SPECIFIC ILLNESSES AND TREATMENTS

Myocardial Infarction

The widespread fear of sudden death during sexual intercourse is often parodied in expressions such as, "He died in the saddle," or "He went out smiling." This fear is based on the belief that sexual intercourse/orgasm causes significant increases in the heart and respiratory rates, blood pressure, and oxygen consumption. Unfortunately, the initial research into the physiologic cost of sexual activity perpetuated this myth.

Masters and Johnson (1) compared the physiological responses to sexual intercourse of young, healthy, recently married men and older married men with sexual problems. The data were recorded in a laboratory situation. Orgasm produced profound changes in blood pressure, heart, and respiratory rates in both groups. Hellerstein and Friedman's (2,3) findings at University Hospitals of Cleveland were more encouraging. By continuously monitoring the ECG's of a group of middle-aged, middle-class, married men over a 24–48 hour period, they were able to measure maximal and average heart rates, and estimate the equivalent oxygen cost and blood pressure increases during sexual activity. They concluded that, "The physiological cost (of sexual activity) is certainly modest with maximal heart rate response averaging less than 120 beats per minute and lasting for 10–15 seconds at most. The equivalent oxygen cost is similar to that of climbing a flight of stairs, walking briskly, or performing ordinary tasks in any occupation" (2,3). After consistent, independent replication, Hellerstein and Friedman's work is now widely accepted as the standard for the physiological cost of intercourse/orgasm. The discrepancies between Masters and Johnson's initial studies and Hellerstein and Friedman's results are due to methodological problems of sample bias and the conditions under which the measurements were gathered.

After examining more than 5,000 cases of sudden death over a four-year period, Uneo (4) reported the death rate (30 out of 5,559) from coital coronaries to be 0.6%. The vast majority of men who experienced "coital coronaries" were involved in extramarital affairs. These men are said to be at greater risk for coronaries because of circumstances associated with extramarital activity: increased alcohol and food intake; unfamiliar circumstances; excitement of being with a new partner.

DeSilva and Lown's (5) report on sudden death states that while coronary artery disease is often the underlying pathological condition, hemodynamic stresses are rarely implicated as causal factors in deaths. These authors suggest that neural activity resulting in cardiac arrhythmia may play a causal role in sudden death. Derogatis (6), therefore, cautions clinicians against being too complacent about the effects of sexual activity after MI. He hypothesizes that sexual activity results in intense sympathetic nervous system activity, leading to fatal arrhythmias. At present while Derogatis' hypothesis is thought provoking, there are no hard data linking sexual activity and sudden death. Resumption of sexual activity after an uncomplicated myocardial infarction is generally considered relatively safe and psychologically beneficial to the recuperative process.

The reported effects of MI's on mens' sexual lives are not so encouraging. Post-MI patients demonstrate prolonged, significant decreases in desire and sexual activity levels; estimates range from 43-75% decreased frequency in activity levels. They also develop various sexual dysfunctions (premature ejaculation—37%; retarded ejaculation—54%; erectile problems—64%) (7-13). Although beta blocking agents and diuretics are known to cause sexual dysfunction in some individuals, studies have failed to reveal any statistically significant correlation between medications and sexual functioning (9,10).

MI's predispose men to moderate levels of depression and anxiety (14), accompanied by irritability, exhaustion, boredom, feelings of hopelessness, and psychophysiological pain, i.e., pain not due to any organic condition. Patients' wives experienced moderate depression, anxiety, and guilt about their roles in these illnesses (15). A 28% to 58% incidence of post-MI marital conflicts and dissatisfaction has also been reported.

Men have been the primary targets of investigation in studies of heart disease and sexuality; women have largely been ignored. There appears to be a tacit assumption that the effects of MI on male sexuality can be generalized to female sexuality. This assumption needs further study and clarification.

Intervention. Physicians should take a history of the patient's pre-illness level of sexual functioning. Specific questions include frequency of activity, levels of desire, arousal, and orgasmic capacity, and levels of satisfaction, as well as any previous sexual dysfunction of the patient or partner. Since the energy requirements for coitus are known, the patient's physiologic capability to engage in intercourse can be tested with stress tests and/or bicycle ergometry. Any remaining doubts may be resolved by having patients engage in intercourse while hooked up to a Holter monitor. Patients who fail to meet the minimum physiological requirements should be clearly told to avoid intercourse. It is, however, equally important to discuss alternative outlets with both the patient and partner, i.e., touching, kissing, holding. A carefully designated exercise program may help increase the patient's physiologic capability. The physician should be alert to signs of depression, anxiety, irritability, marital discord, and psychophysiological pain.

If there are no medical contraindications, the patient and partner should be specifically told that they may resume their pre-illness level of sexual activity. They should be reassured that intercourse will not harm the patient. Patients should be told that it is normal to experience some anxiety upon resumption of sexual activity. They should also be instructed to avoid positions that increase isometric exertion (missionary position coupled with strenuous pelvic thrusting) and counterphobic sexual behaviors, such as being hypersexual. Physicians should be aware that many cardiac medications have sexual side effects. Anti-angina and anti-anxiety agents may be useful in the transition back to regular sexual function.

Short-term group counseling sessions are useful in helping patients work through their post-MI concerns, e.g., sudden death; recurrence of MI; ability to return to work; financial security; resumption of sexual activity (9,16). Leaders provide education about: drug regimens and possible side effects; the physiologic cost of sexual activity; suggestions regarding sexual techniques; management of chest pain; benefits of exercise and diet programs. Supportive psychotherapy is aimed at bolstering the patient's self-esteem and decreasing despair/depression. Some of these group meetings are open to patients' partners who need help with their feelings about the patient's illness/recuperation.

Diabetes Mellitus

Impotence, inhibited sexual desire, and retrograde ejaculation are the three male sexual dysfunctions caused by diabetes mellitus (17). Diabetic men in every age group have a higher prevalence of impotence than non-diabetic men (18,19). Aging is directly related to the increased frequency of erectile dysfunctions; estimates of impotence range from 29% of men under 30 to 40–73% of men in their 60s (19). The development of the impotence is gradual, and may be the first clue to the onset of diabetes. Erectile dysfunction does not appear to be related to metabolic control, severity, and duration of the illness (20). The pathogenesis of diabetic impotence is presently unknown, but is thought to involve interactions among various neural and vascular mechanisms.

An estimated 2% of diabetic men suffer from retrograde ejaculation, a condition in which the ejaculate is propelled backward into the bladder, rather than anterograde out of the urethra (21): The internal vesical sphincter's failure to close completely, as a result of the impaired sympathetic innervation, causes this phenomenon. Infertility is one consequence of retrograde ejaculation.

The relationship between diabetes and female sexual dysfunction is unclear. Kolodny (21) reported that diabetic women may develop orgasmic difficulties. In contrast, Ellenberg (22) and Jensen (17) report that, as a group, diabetic women have no greater incidence of anorgasmia than non-diabetic women.

Imagine what it's like to be invited to dinner at a friend's house or professional banquet and to be unable to eat what is served. How does it feel to always carry syringes, needles, insulin, urine testing paper, and candy around with you? Think what it's like to wonder if you've taken too much or too little insulin each time you feel tired or lightheaded. Is it possible that you might lose consciousness or even have convulsions? What will happen when you tell your employer that you're diabetic? These are only a few of the possible daily anxieties of diabetics.

The diagnosis of diabetes may result in a wide range of psychological reactions. A diabetic may experience chronic to moderate depression which focuses on a defective body image and sense of self-worth. The illness may magnify and exacerbate a negative self-image in an individual whose self-esteem has already been impaired. Some people consider the illness a punishment for sin.

"Control" is a key word for diabetics—control of diet, medication, and life-style. Yet, paradoxically, many diabetics consider their bodies "out-of-control." This idea may stem from the fact that their emotions and even sexual impulses also seem to be "out-of-control." Some people react to the regulation, restriction, and control of their lives by denying their illness and expressing their rebellion by overeating; others over-restrict their life-styles.

Anticipatory dread of the physical consequences of diabetes may lead to development of sexual dysfunctions. For instance, the male diabetic's fear of impotence may engender sufficient performance anxiety to render him psychologically impotent. Each sexual encounter is fraught with the fear of losing the erection. Women's realistic and exaggerated fears of pregnancy and congenital birth defects may lead to impairments of desire, arousal, and orgasmic capacity. Also, the diabetic's increased susceptibility to infection may lead to acute and chronic urinary tract and vaginal infections; these result in physical pain, psychological discomfort, and sexual dysfunction.

Intervention. The physician should routinely inquire about the diabetic male patient's erectile capacity and overall sexual functioning. Such questioning reveals the physician's concern about the patient's sexual life. The etiology of any reported potency problems should be ascertained. It is important to remember that not all impotence in diabetic men has an organic etiology. If psychogenic factors appear prominent, the patient should be referred to a mental health professional for further evaluation. If an organic diagnosis is confirmed, it should be acknowledged; the following alternatives should then be emphasized:

1. There are means other than intercourse of obtaining sexual gratification. The patient can thus continue to give and derive sexual pleasure.
2. The partner can be taught the "stuffing technique," i.e., flaccid penis is inserted into the vagina.
3. The patient can wear an external prosthetic device to enable intromission.
4. The patient can have a permanent prosthetic device surgically implanted.
5. The patient and partner can discontinue sexual activities.
6. Patients with retrograde ejaculation may need information about artificial insemination.

Female patients should also be encouraged to discuss their sexual concerns. Physicians should watch for signs of depression and psychophysiologic symptoms.

Mastectomy

The emotional suffering associated with mastectomy far outweighs the physical pain (23). At best, the loss of one or both breasts leads to profound psychological disturbances characterized by: depression; anxiety; alterations in body image, sense of femininity, and self-esteem; sexual dysfunctions. The cancer and traumatic treatment provoke many logical and illogical thoughts and feelings regarding:

1. *Health:* Will she die? Is she contagious? Will the cancer spread? Will she be in great pain? Will she deteriorate to a mere shadow of her former self?
2. *Sense of self:* Our culture glorifies breast consciousness and health. How will the loss of this organ affect the woman's self-esteem, feelings of self-worth, and femininity? Will she still feel feminine, attractive, alluring, and desirable? Or will she feel mutilated, disfigured, deformed, and only half a woman?
3. *Relationships with others:* How will they react? Will they stare at her? How can she tell others what she is experiencing? The woman's partner will have to cope with his reactions to the cancer/surgery. Partner reactions include: guilt for somehow having caused this misfortune; anger; fear; depression over the loss of the breast and the possible loss of the partner; helplessness; possible disgust; conflicts between the desire to demonstrate caring, love, and affection, and the fear of psychologically and/or physically harming the patient. Psychological rip-

ples are likely to be experienced by other family members, e.g., the effects on her teenage daughter's sense of femininity/sexuality/health. Will mom die?

The vast majority of women undergoing mastectomy make good emotional adjustments (24). While the overall outlook is positive, significant numbers of post-mastectomy women report: sexual problems; suicidal ideation; increased tranquilizer and alcohol use; a feeling that their femininity has been compromised (24-28). The period between the discovery of the mass and surgery is reported to be the most stressful. Unfortunately, this is not a time when patients are routinely provided with counseling or support. The other stressful times are immediately and two months post-surgery (24).

Women's major concerns focus on body image, attractiveness, self-esteem, and feared loss of love and affection from significant others. Fear of death or recurrence of illness is given a surprisingly low priority. Most women experience, at least temporarily, a mild to moderate regression. This temporary regressive shift leads to increased dependency and heightens the importance of being accepted by others at this stage in the rehabilitation process (27,28). Even at two years post-mastectomy, 20-30% of women report sexual difficulties; decreased frequency and orgasmic problems are the most common (25). The women usually wait for their partners to "make the first moves;" the partners may fear being rebuffed or hurting the patients. Forty percent of husbands report sleep disturbances, nightmares, and decreased concentration at work (29). Because they often feel left out of the decision-making process, many men experience themselves as impotent.

Young women with few support systems, whose pre-mastectomy emotional functioning was already somewhat compromised, are at risk for poor post-mastectomy outcomes. Younger women tend to have more trouble coping with the psychological and sexual sequelae of mastectomy (26).

An excerpt from Betty Rollins' book, *First You Cry,* poignantly describes her reactions to lovemaking after mastectomy (30).

> We made love that night . . . he needed it, I endured it. There was one part I couldn't endure; I couldn't endure his touching my one breast . . . it wasn't his fault. He touched me to be nice, I know, or maybe he wanted to, but when he cupped his hand and gently held me there, I screamed. I couldn't help it. Feeling his hand on that breast reminded me too much of the other one, the dead twin . . .
>
> I did not worry that my husband would no longer find me attractive. He found me attractive. He wanted me. The crazy thing was, I did not want him. He still found me attractive, all right, but I did not. I no longer found me attractive. I was damaged goods and I knew it . . . . I was mutilated, a deformed person. If you feel deformed it's hard to be sexy.

Intervention. The emotional pain can be lessened if physicians understand the anxieties associated with different phases of the mastectomy experience. Women experience the greatest distress after the lump has been discovered and prior to surgery. At this same time, men, who are left out of the decision-making process, experience themselves as helpless. Physicians who recognize the pre-mastectomy anxieties (fear of death; fear of surgery; questions about how much tissue will be removed) will begin to demonstrate their willingness to discuss the patient's feelings and offer support and reassurance. If appropriate, physicians may invite the partner for conjoint counseling sessions; this serves to lessen his sense of impotence and get his input regarding possible surgical options.

After surgery, physicians should routinely inquire about the patient's level of depression and possible suicidal ideation. The generous offer of support can help patients mourn their losses. As the women begin to feel better, they become more concerned about being accepted by others. The staff's comments or suggestions tend to reinforce femininity and heighten patients' self-esteem, e.g., comments about appearance; suggestions about wearing make-up, nightgowns, etc. Physicians should intervene promptly if the partner's distress is indicated by a lack of visitation. Some therapists recommend desensitization programs to lessen partners' anxiety about observing the surgical results. Others advocate having the partner assist in changing dressings.

The patient and partner are encouraged to openly discuss their feelings prior to discharge. To promote psychological healing and assist the couple in returning to their prior marital equilibrium, the physician should encourage them to be sexual. The physician should reassure the patient and partner that sexual activity will not be harmful. He should suggest sexual positions that protect the surgical site and lessen the woman's feeling of being overexposed, i.e., missionary position; lateral rear entry.

At follow-up visits, doctors should inquire about health-related problems and social/sexual difficulties. Questions should focus on: alcohol and tranquilizer usage; level of depression; sexual dysfunctions; concerns about prosthetic devices, cosmetic difficulties, and clothes.

Many hospitals have instituted routine counseling programs for mastectomy patients and their families. There are also a number of ongoing self-help groups. These individual and group counseling sessions try to give the patient and family support, practical advice, and assistance in working through the cycle of denial, depression, anger, and resolution. These programs encourage patients to frankly discuss fears about their illness, as well as changes in perception of body image, femininity, and self-worth. Group members give suggestions about clothing and information on prosthetic devices. Discussions of typical sexual anxieties help allay fears about resuming sexual activity. These programs also help the partner and family adjust to the patient's illness and surgery.

REFERENCES

1. Masters WH, Johnson VE: *Human Sexual Response*. Boston, Little Brown & Co, 1966.
2. Hellerstein HK, Friedman EH: Sexual activity and the post-coronary patient. *Med Aspects Hum Sex* 1969;3:70-96.
3. Hellerstein HK, Friedman EH: Sexual activity and the post-coronary patient. *Arch Intern Med* 1970;125:987-999.
4. Uneo M: The so-called coition death. *Japanese Journal of Legal Medicine* 1963;17: 333-337.
5. DeSilva RA, Lown B: Ventricular premature beats, stress and sudden death. *Psychosomatics* 1978;19:649-661.
6. Derogatis LR, King KM: The coital coronary: A reassessment of the concept. *Arch Sex Behav* 1981;10:325-335.
7. Bloch A, Marder JP, Haissly JC: Sexual problems after myocardial infarction. *Am Heart J* 1975;90:536-537.
9. Horgan JH, Craig AJ: Resumption of sexual activity after myocardial infarction. *Ir Med J* 1978;71:540-542.
9. Mann S, Yates JE, Raftery EB: The effects of myocardial infarction on sexual activity. *Journal of Cardiac Rehabilitation* 1981;1:187-194.
10. Mehta J, Krop H: The effect of myocardial infarction on sexual functioning. *Sexuality and Disability* 1979;2:115-121.
11. Papadopoulos C: A survey of social activity after myocardial infarction. *Cardiovascular Medicine* 1978;3:821-826.
12. Tuttle WB, Cook WL, Fitch E: Sexual behavior in post-myocardial infarction patients. *Am J Cardiol* 1964;13:140.
13. Wabrek AJ, Burchell RC: Male sexual dysfunction associated with coronary heart disease. *Arch Sex Behav* 1980;9:69-75.
14. Wishnie HA, Hackett TP, Cassem NH: Psychological hazards of convalescence following myocardial infarction. *JAMA* 1971;215:1292-1296.
15. Skelton M, Dominian J: Psychological stress in wives of patients with myocardial infarction. *Br Med J* 1973;2:101-103.
16. Adsett CA, Bruhn JC: Short-term group psychotherapy for post-myocardial infarction patients and their wives. *Can Med Assoc J* 1968;99:577-584.
17. Jensen SB: Diabetic sexual dysfunction: A comparative study of 160 insulin treated men and women and an age-matched control group. *Arch Sex Behav* 1981;10:493-504.
18. Levine SB: Sexual problems in the diabetic, in Bleiccher SJ, Brodoff B (eds): *Diabetes Mellitus and Obesity*. Baltimore, Williams & Wilkins, 1982.
19. Schiavi R: Sexuality and medical illness: Diabetes mellitus, in Green R (ed): *Human Sexuality, A Health Practitioners Text*, ed 2. Baltimore, Williams & Wilkins, 1979.
20. Rubin A, Babbott D: Impotence and diabetes mellitus. *JAMA* 1958;168:498-500.
21. Kolodny RC, Masters WH, Johnson VE: *Textbook of Sexual Medicine*. Boston, Little Brown & Co, 1979.
22. Ellenberg M: Sexual aspects of the female diabetic. *Mt. Sinai J Med* 1977;44:495-500.
23. Erwin CV: Psychological adjustment to mastectomy. *Med Aspects Hum Sex* 1973;7: 42-65.

24. Jamison KR, Wellisch DK, Pasnau RO: Psychological aspects of mastectomy: I. The woman's perspective. *Am J Psychiatry* 1978;135:432-436.
25. Amberger H, Henningsen B, Fey K: Rehabilitation after radical mastectomy, in Lewison EF, Montague ACW, Stowecifer GR (eds): *Breast Cancer*. New York, Alan R Liss Inc, 1977, pp 543-544.
26. Lyon JS: Management of psychological problems in breast cancer, in Stoll BA (ed): *Breast Cancer Management—Early and Late*. Chicago, William Heieman Medical Books, 1977.
27. Witkin MH: Sex therapy and mastectomy. *J Sex Marital Ther* 1975;1:290-303.
28. Witkin MH: Psychosexual counseling of the mastectomy patient. *J Sex Marital Ther* 1978;4:20-28.
29. Wellisch DK, Jamison KR, Pasnau RO: Psychological aspects of mastectomy: II. The man's perspective. *Am J Psychiatry* 1978;135:543-546.
30. Rollins B: *First You Cry*. Philadelphia, JP Lippincott, 1976.

Chapter 30

GENDER IDENTITY DEVELOPMENT
LESLIE M. LOTHSTEIN, Ph.D.

At the moment of delivery (or as determined by amniocentesis), all eyes focus upon the structure of the child's genitals. Once a sexual determination is made (sometimes with great difficulty in children with intersexual or hermaphroditic disorders, cf. Money and Ehrhardt [1]), the child is provided with its first identity theme—that is, whether it is a boy or a girl. The child's second identity theme is its name, which typically confirms its sex. Subsequently, the child's gender identity is profoundly shaped by the sex of rearing. In most instances, parents raise children according to their anatomical sex. The process for communicating gender roles and shaping gender identity involves a complex intergenerational and cultural signalling and message system, in which communications about the child's sex and gender serve to organize and stabilize the child's nascent gender-self system. Children typically evolve normal core male or female gender identities (2). Indeed, even by the end of the first year of life, children evidence the rudiments of an appropriate gender-self system (cf. Stoller, however, who states that all children exhibit *primary femininity*) (3). It must be realized that "masculinity" and "femininity" are value laden terms which depict (for our society) highly stereotypical and caricatured male or female gender behaviors and roles.

There are also children whose parents rear them contrary to their anatomical sexes. These children are typically gender dysphoric, experiencing gender confusion and diffusion throughout their lives. Some of these children may assume cross-gender identifications, acting like, and wishing to become, members of the opposite sex. Once they enter school, these children are often singled out and stigmatized as sissies or tomboys (though most tomboys and many sissies do not have severe gender confusion). While many of these gender dysphoric children become homosexuals, others may become transvestites or transsexuals. In addition to their gender dysphoria, these children may also evidence severe emotional pathology in non-gender-related areas of their lives; including serious developmental defects and a pathological organization of their self systems.

371

This chapter addresses the fact that a substantial number of children and adults manifest severe gender identity disturbances which warrant psychological and, possibly, medical interventions. While there is considerable historical, mythological, and literary evidence (4) of gender identity and role disorders being "un mal ancien" and not of recent origin, *psychosexual disorders* were not considered worthy of psychological attention until the publication of the third edition of the American Psychiatric Association's *Diagnostic and Statistical Manual* (DSM-III, 1980) (5). These disorders include: Transsexualism; Gender Identity Disorder of Childhood; Atypical Gender Identity Disorder.

Throughout this chapter, I shall use the terms "gender" and "sex" in very specific ways. The term "gender" is a psychological term which refers to a male or female's subjective feelings of masculinity (maleness) and femininity (femaleness), respectively. The term "sex" (as in *sexual identity*) shall always refer to one's chromosomal or genetic sex, or to one's secondary sexual characteristics.

PREVALENCE, INCIDENCE, SEX RATIO

Because of the problems involved in obtaining reliable data, the findings on prevalence, incidence, and sex ratio of gender identity disorders must be viewed cautiously. While DSM-III reports that the prevalence of gender identity disorders is 'rare,' the authors made no effort to report statistics. A number of worldwide reports suggest, however, that the prevalence of adult gender identity disorders ranges from 1/37,000 to 1/100,000 for males, and from 1/103,000 to 1/400,000 for females (6,7). Reker *et al.* (8) stated that the incidence of gender identity disorders for children was similar to that of adults (about 1/100,000), and that a child clinician in private practice would see about one seriously disturbed gender identity patient every 5 years.

Over the last two decades, a number of studies on the sex ratio of transsexualism revealed that the ratio is approaching 1:1; the results from various countries vary from as high as 10:1 (males to females) to 1.5:1. Despite the difficulty in obtaining reliable prevalence, incidence, and sex ratio data, it is clear that increasing numbers of patients are applying for psychological and medical help with their gender identity disorders. Any statistics on the prevalence and incidence of transsexualism are, therefore, bound to be, at best, conservative estimates of what appears to be a growing phenomenon. Indeed, the Harry Benjamin Gender Dysphoria Association (a research and clinical forum for practitioners engaged in treating individuals with gender identity disturbances) suggested that 3000–6000 adults have been hormonally and surgically revised, and 30,000–60,000 persons worldwide have been identified as transsexuals and requested sex reassignment surgery (SRS) (9). Over the last decade, the ratio of women to men has clearly approached parity.

DIFFERENTIAL DIAGNOSIS

The clinician evaluating a person with a gender identity disorder is faced with the initial problem of making a differential diagnosis between a functional and an organic disorder (that is, whether the patient's gender dysphoria is of a purely psychosexual nature or is rooted in an identifiable chromosomal or biochemical disorder). Secondarily, the clinician must distinguish between a primary psychosexual gender identity disorder and one which is caused by another serious psychological disorder (e.g., a personality disturbance, schizophrenia, etc.) or an acquired organic condition (e.g., temporal lobe epilepsy, result of cerebral trauma).

Transsexualism, the most severe of the gender identity disorders, was first named by Cauldwell (10) and clinically described by Benjamin (11). It is a profound disorder of the self system (12), in which the individual believes that s/he is trapped in the wrong body. According to DSM-III (5), the diagnosis of transsexualism can only be made if certain descriptive criteria are met: 1. the individual expresses a "sense of discomfort and inappropriateness about (their) anatomic sex;" 2. they wish to be rid of (their) genitals and to live as a member of the other sex;" 3. their disorder "has been continuous (not limited to periods of stress) for at least two years;" 4. there is no evidence of "physical intersex or genetic abnormality;" 5. the condition is "not due to another mental disorder, such as Schizophrenia."

Individuals diagnosed as transsexual are not typically delusional about their sexual status. They fully comprehend their biological status, but *wish* to become members of the opposite sex through surgery. Hence, the majority of transsexuals are not viewed as psychotic. If, however, a self-diagnosed transsexual entertains a delusion of sex change and sexual metamorphosis, the clinician should immediately suspect a primary disorder of schizophrenia or an organic condition, with the gender identity disturbance being of secondary importance.

There are also a number of individuals who may cross-dress and impersonate members of the opposite sex and gender, without wishing to change their sexes. Their cross-gender behavior must be differentiated from transsexualism. For example, transvestites, as opposed to transsexuals, do not have a primary gender dysphoria per se, as they do not reject their sexual status and do not wish to adopt cross-gender identities (13). The typical transvestite is a heterosexual male who is married and has children, though a number of women have also recently been identified as transvestites. These individuals are compulsively driven to cross-dress—initially for sexual excitement and gratification (masturbation), and later for the "self soothing" feelings that accompany cross-dressing. In either case, wearing the clothes of the opposite sex has an anxiety-reducing function. Transvestites do *not* want to get rid of their genitals and live in cross-gender roles. They usually cross-dress in private, though there are some transvestites who are compulsively driven to expose themselves in public. Once the masturbatory act is completed, the transvestite usually takes off the female/male clothing. In the majority of instances, the precipitant of a male transvestite's episodes is the experience of intense castration anxiety (14). By wearing female clothing, the transvestite feels symbolically identified, and partially fused, with his mother. The acts of cross-dressing and masturbation serve to reduce his castration anxiety and reinforce his masculinity.

Like the transvestite, the effeminate homosexual or butch dyke who cross-dresses does *not* want to become a member of the opposite sex. These individuals are comfortable with their sexual anatomy and do *not* want to change their sexes. They do *not* have primary gender identity disorders. They may adopt cross-gender roles for many purposes: sex role comfort; personality style; anxiety maintenance; sexual solicitation; arousal. There are also a number of secondary gender identity and role disorders which need to be distinguished from primary gender identity disorders, i.e., conditions in which gender identity and role are impaired secondarily to another major psychological disorder. These conditions may include: borderline personality disorder; identity disorder of adolescence; fetishism; sexual sadism and masochism; exhibitionism; toxic psychosis associated with drug abuse (e.g., amphetamines), in which sexual repressions are lifted; male and female impersonation; delusions of sex change and genital hallucinosis associated with schizophrenia.

Severe gender identity disorders in children need to be treated separately from adult disorders (8,15). These disorders are characterized by a child's hatred of, and disgust with, his sexual anatomy. The child either denies that s/he has the sexual anatomy which is congruent with their biological sex, or wishes to have the sexual anatomy of the opposite sex. These children also have a need to wear clothes and engage in activities and roles which are traditionally associated with the opposite sex. According to DSM-III (5), these disorders involve a "profound disturbance of the normal sense of maleness or femaleness" and are not to be confused with the "rejection of stereotypical sex role behavior as, for example, in 'tomboyishness' in girls or 'sissyish' behavior in boys."

THE EVALUATION OF SEVERE GENDER IDENTITY DISORDERS

All individuals who identify themselves as transsexuals should be given comprehensive medical and psychological evaluations. After ruling out an intersexual or genetic disorder. the clinician must still entertain the possibility that the patient may have an as yet undisclosed biological substratum to their gender disorder. In patients with possible organic conditions, a complete neurological work-up (including a neuropsychological assessment) may be indicated. If the clinician suspects the possibility of a neurohormonal disorder, the patient should be referred to a physician with some specialty training in endocrinology. Additionally, many self-labelled transsexuals who have been taking illicitly-obtained hormones may not reveal that information; thus, they may then be diagnosed as having a naturally occurring physiological condition. For example, some female-to-male transsexuals,in a few published studies,claimed to have spontaneous virilization; they were secretly administering androgens, which caused their hirsutism. Some of these patients were mistakenly diagnosed as having Stein-Leventhal syndrome. A well-trained physician should be able to differentially diagnose these various conditions and clarify many aspects of the patient's gender dysphoria. In addition, a comprehensive evaluation should include the following: complete objective and projective psychological testing; interviews with family members, close friends, and spouses or partners; and intensive interviews with the patient over a period of at least one year. The need to interview family members and friends is based on the finding that transsexual patients tend to falsify their social histories and lie about their conditions (16) in order to obtain surgery. The patient's problems are often similar to those in Munchhausen's syndrome.

The evaluation of a child gender identity disturbance requires an extensive social and medical history. The clinician should inquire about the child's pre- and post-natal development and ascertain whether the mother took any medications during pregnancy. Constructing a family genogram (17) can also provide important information about the intergenerational family dynamics, and how the targeted child was 'chosen' to act out the family's gender conflicts. All of the members of the child's immediate family should be involved in the evaluation procedure, although they do not have to be interviewed as a group. The clinician should be prepared to consult with the child's school counselor and teachers, since that is the milieu in which most behavioral difficulties, social harassment, and stigmatization occur.

ETIOLOGY OF SEVERE GENDER IDENTITY DISORDERS

Severe gender identity disorders which do not have apparent biological bases (i.e., are unrelated to chromosomal disorders and genetic abnormalities) can be explained by either physiological or psychological theories. Physiological theories have focused on the possible roles of cerebral pathology (18–20), prenatal hormones and neurohormonal disorders (1), enzyme defects (21), toxic effects of drugs (22), and effects of H-Y antigens (23,24) on cross-gender behavior. These theories are intriguing and often compelling because they provide a common sense explanation for the patient's complaints about being in the wrong body; there is, however, no crucial test for any of the hypotheses. Ehrhardt and Meyer-Bahlburg's (25) literature summary suggested that prenatal hormones may play a role in human psychosexual differentiation; however, "the development of gender identity seems to depend largely on the sex of rearing."

Psychological theories which explain male and female gender identity disorders (specifically transsexualism) have been quite diverse. Most researchers have focused on an explanation for male transsexualism, viewing female transsexualism as a qualitatively different disorder. Stoller (2,26), the most prolific writer in the field, viewed transsexualism as a psychological disorder evolving within the structure of family dynamics. He suggested, however, that two divergent theories were needed to explain male and female transsexualism. Male transsexualism (a rare disorder which Stoller viewed as only including a small number of males who actually applied for SRS) evolved out of a "blissful symbiosis" with the mother, an empty, bisexual, depressed woman with profound gender conflicts. The transsexual-to-be son evolved a female gender identity in a nonconflictual way, via a mechanism akin to imprinting (27,28) [1]. However, for female transsexuals, Stoller regarded the mechanisms of conflict, defense, and trauma as central to the etiology of their gender identity conflict.

Other theories (29) have viewed transsexualism as a defense against homosexuality; a perversion; the result of a thought disorder; a disorder of orality; a pregenital disorder related to intense separation anxiety and abandonment depression; a defense against annihilation anxiety [2]; the result of a developmental arrest; a variant of borderline schizophrenic pathology [3]; a disorder of the sense of self, a narcississtic disorder [4]; and a variant of paranoid psychosis.

In contrast to the psychiatric view of transsexualism as an illness, some sociologists and sexologists have viewed it simply as an alternative life style; the fact that it was resisted by society, makes it an iatrogenic disorder. Such a view is clinically untenable. The so-called transsexual life style is highly obligatory, not something which can be freely chosen. The transsexual is actually driven by his/her emotional pathology to act out his/her gender distress, which often reaches suicidal proportions.

My research with over 200 self-labelled transsexuals (about 150 men and 50 women who requested SRS) suggests that severe gender identity pathology evolves within the family matrix, and can only be explained in the context of the family dynamics. The typical self-labelled transsexual is born into a family with considerable gender confusion, but possibly no other family member who is designated as a transsexual. The transsexual's family is characterized by sexual chaos (e.g., incest and sexual exploitation of the patient by various family members) and violent behaviors, in most cases directed against the future transsexual. The patient's transsexualism evolves through a complex family communication process, in which the parents constantly express displeasure with their child's body, secondary sexual characteristics, and emerging psychosexual traits of masculinity or femininity. Throughout early childhood, the parents consistently assault and try to thwart the development of their child's core gender identity.

As a consequence of being raised in a chaotic family, the transsexual is unable to evolve stable ego mechanisms and functions and establish a cohesive self system. As a group, transsexuals evidence profound developmental arrests, intense separation anxieties and abandonment depressions, a broad range of affective disturbances, impaired ego functioning, nonspecific ego weaknesses, primitive and pathologically organized defense mechanisms, and typically borderline and narcissistic personality disturbances. Many of these patients also exhibit a variety of cognitive defects (especially a disturbance in symbol formation) and reveal a subtle thought disturbance; no more than 15% of all transsexuals are schizophrenic.

Research (12) suggests that severe gender identity disorders are psychologically "organized" sometime between 18 and 36 months of age. During this time, the child is attempting to stabilize his/her gender self-system; establish self and object constancy; and structuralize a core gender identity. The child is also developing semi-symbolic forms of reasoning; becoming aware of the anatomical distinctions between the sexes; experiencing an early genital phase; having a pre-oedipal castration reaction; beginning to progressively differentiate his/her body image and schema; revealing "an upsurge in object-loss anxiety, negativism, and an increased hostile dependence on the mother" from whom s/he needs to separate (during the so-called rapprochement period of separation-individuation); and developing a nuclear self-system. All of these developments and achievements are influenced by each child's unique environmental variables—that is, overall physical attractiveness; health; intelligence level; stability of ego functioning; birth of a new sibling; evidence of abandonments, separations, losses, changes, and death in the family; effects of other caretakers and peers; unpredictable environmental impingements which may significantly alter the child's reality. The birth of the genderal self and the establishment of gender-self constancy occurs in the second half of the second year of life, prior to the establishment of a core gender identity.

Rather than developing a core gender identity, transsexuals develop gender diffusion and confusion; their gender-self representations oscillate between "all good" opposite gender representations and "all bad" same gender representations. Consequently, these individuals come to hate anything associated with their developing body image and gender. Having predominantly borderline personality organizations, these individuals are constantly in search of some life goal which will make them feel "whole." As a result of advances in surgical technology, they have, unfortunately, come to look upon SRS as the source of their "wholeness." These individuals essentially lack a cohesive self-system. By matching their bodies to their minds through SRS, thereby resolving the split in their self-systems, they believe they will become "whole" people. The attempted reparation of structural defects in their ego and self-systems by surgery is a solution which is bound to fail.

THE TREATMENT OF GENDER IDENTITY DISORDERS

Once transsexualism is viewed as a disorder of the self-system, the clinician realizes that the *primary* treatment of choice is some form of long-term, intensive psychodynamically-oriented or ego supportive psychotherapy (30). The tactics and techniques for involving these difficult to treat patients in such a psychotherapy have been described in detail (12,31,32). The goals of any psychotherapy must be tailored to the patient's needs. The therapist must never limit treatment goals to the patient's readjustment to his/her original gender role. Therapy should be focused on viable goals, in terms of sexual preference, gender role, and identity (29). Approaching the treatment situation with preconceived, value-laden options will only preclude psychotherapy and make SRS a more viable option.

There will always be a small number of patients who will benefit from SRS, mostly because they have lived and worked so long in cross-gender roles; it is impossible, however, to identify these patients *a priori*. Moreover, there is increasing evidence, even from its proponents, that SRS may not be the treatment of choice for self-labelled and diagnosed transsexuals (33). Additionally, SRS is still an experimental treatment with results which are quite primitive.

From a socio-legal perspective, the law has protected transsexual surgeons from mayhem [5]. However, it has failed to consider the means of integrating post-surgical transsexuals into society as productive, satisfied, individuals (34). The fact that the law recognizes SRS as the *only* way to treat transsexuals, and insurance companies will pay for SRS but not psychotherapy, actually handicaps patients seeking relief from their transsexual anguish. The existence and spurious success claims of SRS have created a number of legal, social, family, community, religious, ethical, and bioethical dilemmas which cannot be solely addressed and answered by the medical-surgical community. These complex problems need to be addressed by interdisciplinary groups of individuals who are cognizant of the transsexuals' psychological defects and the availability of newer psychotherapeutic techniques for treating their condition.

One fact does stand out. When children present with severe gender identity and role pathologies (not to be confused with tomboyism and sissyness), the primary physician (usually the pediatrician) should *not* advise the parents that they will outgrow their condition. Without psychological intervention, a child's severe gender problems will develop into a full-blown gender identity or role disorder. All children with severe gender disorders should be referred for psychological treatment; their parents should be referred for counseling or psychotherapy. Every effort should be made to treat these problems psychologically. This is especially important with the adolescent patient, for whom a premature diagnosis of transsexualism may close the door to rehabilitative psychotherapy (15).

As clinicians learn more about transsexualism and other severe gender identity disorders, they will, hopefully, be able to empathically relate to the seriousness of gender pathologies and acquire the conceptual tools necessary for formulating adequate evaluation and treatment programs.

NOTES

1. *Imprinting* is an etiological term referring to an animal's instinctual development of an indelible attachment to its parent or surrogate. The term was first used clinically by Money *et al.* (Imprinting and the establishment of gender role. *Arch Neurol Psychiatry* 1957;77: 333–336), and elaborated by Lichtenstein in a 1961 article (cf. reference 27), which suggested that the mother used imprinting to provide her child with an identity. In 1968 and 1975, Stoller (cf. references 2,26) used the term "imprinting" in contrast to the psychoanalytic term "conflict." He suggested that the female identity of these male transsexuals was imprinted—that is, learned in a nonconflictual way as a result of a symbiotic attachment to mother.

2. *Annihilation anxiety* refers to an individual's fear of going crazy, becoming fragmented, falling apart, of dissociating. Often contrasted with "castration anxiety," it is viewed as a more primitive type of anxiety related to basic feelings of bodily and self disintegration; this type of fear is often seen in schizophrenics. Annihilation anxiety is, in fact, often synonymous with a diagnosed primitive mental condition such as schizophrenia.

3. *Borderline schizophrenic pathology* refers to a mental condition which falls somewhere between a severe neurosis and a schizophrenic disorder, although closer to schizophrenia. It is often used synonymously with the following terms: borderline schizophrenia; borderline states.

4. *Narcissistic disorder* refers to Kohut's concept of the development and elaboration of issues such as perfectionism, grandiosity, exhibitionism, omnipotence, admiration, greatness, and idealization, which relate to the cohesiveness of the self *(The Restoration of the Self.* New York, International Universities Press, 1977). To the extent that these issues are not integrated into an individual's self-system, s/he will have a narcissistic disorder. Moreover, his/her self-esteem, goals, ambitions, achievements, and assertiveness will also be impaired. A narcissistic disorder implies a severe and primitive developmental disturbance, involving developmental arrest, loss of self cohesion, and a structural defect of the self-system.

5. The term *mayhem* is used in an historical, legal sense, referring to "maiming statutes" in English law. These were initially instituted to protect individuals from losing limbs necessary to fight. Under English common law, it was a felony to inflict such an injury. According to Webster's *Third International Dictionary* (P. Grove (ed), Merriam Co, Springfield, Mass, 1966), "mayhem" is defined as "the malicious and permanent crippling, mutilation, or disfiguring of another, constituting a grave felony under modern statutes but in some jurisdictions requiring a specific intent, as distinguished from general malice.

REFERENCES

1. Money J, Ehrhardt A: *Man and Woman Boy and Girl.* Baltimore, Johns Hopkins Press, 1972.
2. Stoller R: *Sex and Gender.* New York, Science House, 1968.
3. Stoller R: Primary femininity. *J Am Psychoanal Assoc* 1976;24:59–78.
4. Green R: *Sexual Identity Conflicts in Children and Adults.* New York, Basic Books, 1974.
5. American Psychiatric Association Task Force on Nomenclature and Statistics: *Diagnostic and Statistical Manual of Mental Disorders,* ed 3. Washington, DC, American Psychiatric Association, 1980.
6. Ross M, Walinder J, Lundstrom B, *et al.:* Cross cultural approaches to transsexualism, a comparison between Sweden and Australia. *Acta Psychiatr Scand* 1981;63:75–82.
7. Walinder J: Incidence and sex ration of transsexualism in Sweden. *Br J Psychiatry* 1971;119:195–196.
8. Rekers G, Bentler P, Rosen A, *et al.:* Child gender disturbances: A clinical rationale for intervention. *Psychotherapy: Theory, Research and Practice* 1977;14:2–11.
9. Walker P, Berger J, Green R, *et al.: Standards of Care: The Hormonal and Surgical Sex Reassignment of Gender Dysphoric Persons.* Mimeo, distributed by the Harry Benjamin International Gender Dysphoria Association, c/o Paul Walker, Ph.D., 1952 Union Street, San Francisco, California, 94123.
10. Cauldwell D: Psychopathia transsexualis. *Sexology* 1949;16:274–280.
11. Benjamin H: *The Transsexual Phenomenon.* New York, Julian Press, 1966.
12. Lothstein L: *Female-to-Male Transsexualism.* London, Routledge & Kegan Paul, 1983.
13. Segal M: Transvestism as an impulse and a defense. *Int J Psychoanal* 1965;46:209–217.
14. Bak R, Stuart W: Fetishism, transvestism, and voyeurism: A psychoanalytic approach, in Arieti S, Brody E (eds): *American Handbook of Psychiatry.* New York, Grune & Stratton, 1970, vol 3.
15. Lothstein L: The adolescent gender dysphoric patient: An approach to treatment and management. *J Pediatr Psychol* 1980;5:93–109.
16. Walker P: Factitious presentations of 'transsexualism'—35 cases, in *Abstracts and Proceedings of the 7th International Gender Dysphoria Association.* Lake Tahoe, Nevada, 1981.
17. Guerin P, Fogarty TF: The family therapist's own family. *Int J Psychiatry* 1972;10:6–22.
18. Blumer D: Transsexualism; sexual dysfunction and temporal lobe disorders, in Green R, Money J (eds): *Transsexualism and Sex Reassignment.* Baltimore, Johns Hopkins Press, 1969.
19. Hoenig J, Torr J: EEG abnormalities and transsexualism. *Br J Psychiatry* 1979;134:293–300.
20. Spate Z: Zum abteil des limschen systems in her Pathogenese des Transvestismus. *Psychiatrie, Neurologie, und Medizinische Psychologie* 1970;22:209–217.

21. Stoller R: A contribution to the study of gender identity. Follow-up. *Int J Psychoanal* 1979;60:433–441.
22. Lothstein L: Amphetamine abuse and transsexualism. *J Nerv Ment Dis* 1982;170:568–571.
23. Eicher W, Spoljar M, Cleve H, *et al.:* H-Y antigen in trans-sexuality. *Lancet II,* No. 8152, pp 1137–1138, November, 1979.
24. Pfafflin F: H-Y antigen in transsexualism, in *Abstracts and Proceedings of the 7th International Gender Dysphoria Symposium.* Lake Tahoe, Nevada, 1981.
25. Ehrhardt A, Meyer-Bahlburt H: Effects of prenatal sex hormones on gender related behavior. *Science* 1981;211:1312–1317.
26. Stoller R: *Sex and Gender.* New York, Jason Aronson, 1975, vol 2.
27. Lichtenstein H: Identity and sexuality. *J Am Psychoanal Assoc* 1961;9:179–260.
28. Money J, Hampson J, Hampson J: Imprinting and the establishment of gender role. *Arch Neurol Psychiatry* 1957;77:333–336.
29. Lothstein L: Psychodynamics and sociodynamics of gender dysphoric states. *Am J Psychother* 1979;33:214–238.
30. Lothstein L: Psychotherapy with patients with gender dysphoria syndromes. *Bull Menninger Clin* 1977;41:563–582.
31. Lothstein L: Countertransference reactions to gender dysphoric patients: Implications for psychotherapy. *Psychotherapy: Theory, Research, and Practice.* 1977;14:21–31.
32. Lothstein L, Levine S: Expressive psychotherapy with gender dysphoric patients. *Arch Gen Psychiatry* 1981;38:924–929.
33. Lothstein L: Sex reassignment surgery: Historical, bioethical, and theoretical issues. *Am J Psychiatry* 1982;139:417–426.
34. Walz B: Transsexuals and the law. *J Contemporary Law* 1979;5:181–214.

Chapter 31

HOMOSEXUALITY
STEPHEN B. LEVINE, M.D.

INTRODUCTION

Why Study Homosexuality

1. There are millions of homosexuals in this country with special mental and physical health care needs.
2. It provides an opportunity to study the way societal laws and attitudes affect the psychological lives of minority group members.
3. It provides an opportunity to consider the ways in which cultural institutions—such as laws, restrictions, prejudice—result from forces originating in individual psychological development.
4. It illuminates the developmental processes of typical sexual orientation, i.e., heterosexuality.
5. It raises questions about the relationship between medical and societal values.
6. It is an introduction to the concept of gender identity.

The Problem—Prejudice

It is quite difficult to conduct an objective study of homosexuality. Most heterosexuals have had little personal experience with people they have recognized as being homosexuals. A primitive fear causes them to deride homosexuality and label it "pathological." Their thoughts about homosexuals tend to be unidimensional and stereotyped. Although most adults recognize individual styles of heterosexuality, they often think of homosexuality in strictly unitary terms. Homosexuals are: effeminate; passive; untrustworthy; child molesters; beauticians; dykes; masochistic; etc. The major characteristic that homosexual men and women have in common is an erotic preference for members of their own sex. In recent years, society has begun to abandon some of its stereotypes and recognize homosexuals as people with a wide range of personalities and sexual styles.

CLASSIFICATION AND DEFINITIONS

From Degeneracy to Perversion to ? Normality

In the nineteenth century, medical professionals considered homosexuality a degenerate disease of the nervous system—an hereditary taint. This was probably a medical translation of the predominant moral view of male homosexuals. Homosexuality embodied the exact opposite of the widely promulgated social ideal for sexual behavior, i.e., pleasureless sex for procreation, and was, therefore, degenerate.

In 1905, Freud dispelled the physical illness model and made it clear that homosexuality was an acquired psychological pattern. Homosexuality was thereafter grouped with other deviations in sexual development as a perversion (1). Other examples of "perverted" sexual preferences included: young children; the dead; men dressing in women's clothes; anal sexual play; public exhibition of the penis. Thus, although Freud's step represented a conceptual advance, the word "perversion" continued to connote moral displeasure, sin, and disapproval. Homosexuality came to be classified with other perversions as a personality disorder, i.e., a mental illness.

In 1974, the American Psychiatric Association responded to well-organized political pressure from gay organizations, homosexual psychiatrists, and political activists within APA by reviewing the status of homosexuality as a disease. It was concluded that homosexuality per se was not a mental illness. The task force didn't say it was normal—just that it wasn't necessarily abnormal (2). Those individuals who were unable to comfortably tolerate their sexual orientation were considered mentally ill. They are currently diagnosed as having "ego dystonic homosexuality" (3). Homosexuality is no longer classified as a perversion. The current euphemism is "deviation." This word reflects the increased tolerance for atypical sexual expression without the connotation of sin implied by "perversion."

What Is A Homosexual?

While for practical purposes people may be thought of as homosexual, there is no widely-accepted definition of the term. Sexual orientation (gender and other characteristics of attractive people) is not necessarily fixed in direction or intensity throughout the life cycle (4). The Kinsey Scale (5) was an attempt to objectify and rate the degree of a person's homosexuality. This scale is used in two ways: to rate purely subjective phenomena, such as arousal and fantasies, and to produce objective reports of sexual behavior with partners.

The Kinsey Scale

0   Exclusively heterosexual with no homosexuality
1   Predominantly heterosexual, only incidentally homosexual
2   Predominantly heterosexual, but more than incidentally homosexual
3   Equally heterosexual and homosexual
4   Predominantly homosexual, but more than incidentally heterosexual
5   Predominantly homosexual but incidentally heterosexual
6   Exclusively homosexual

Other Homosexual Phenomena

Any static classification of human sexuality quickly becomes extremely complicated. At some time in the lives of most people, there are some homoerotic thoughts, fantasies, curiosities, or wishes. Partner sexual behavior is not necessarily an indication of subjective sexual orientation. Some homosexual behavior can be attributed to the unavailability of members of the opposite sex; this common prison phenomenon is referred to as *"facultative"* homosexuality. Adults without previous significant homoerotic interests may briefly engage in homosexual behavior during periods of great emotional stress or intoxication. Such *"episodic"* homosexuality occurs throughout the life cycle. Some people with homoerotic fantasies are behaviorally asexual. Some homosexually active people may have relatively asexual fantasy lives. Therefore, the decision to label a person as "homosexual" is arbitrary. When this term is carefully used, it implies an unmistakable, persistent pattern of easy arousal and responsivity to members of the same sex.

Psychoanalysts use the term *"latent homosexuality"* to refer to the universal childhood experience of being attracted to members of the same sex (6). The inability to effectively repress these largely unconscious longings for closeness is sometimes thought responsible for some neurotic and psychotic symptoms. A more narrow usage of the term "latent homosexuality" is in reference to the consciously experienced plight of the homoerotic person who is either celibate or behaviorally heterosexual.

THE BIOLOGICAL BASIS FOR HOMOSEXUAL ORIENTATION, BEHAVIOR, AND INTEREST

The Basic Hypothesis

The assumption that biologic programming induces heterosexual interest and behavior is basic to most research into the etiology of atypical orientation. Male homosexual phenomena are assumed to represent a shift toward biologic femaleness, and vice versa. Thus, homosexual phenomena are considered manifestations of CNS pseudohermaphrodism. This hypothesis posits that homosexual and heterosexual brains are biologically different (7).

The Supportive Model

Some support is derived from animal models of sexual behavior. Androgen appears to be responsible for prenatal organization of male behavior in many animals. Typical rat mating behavior, for example, involves a definable pattern of mounting, intromission, and ejaculation; female mating behavior involves a downward arching of the back, referred to as lordosis. Lordosis in males and mounting behavior in females can be achieved by inducing an androgen deficiency in prenatal males, and giving androgens to prenatal females. The female cyclic and male tonic patterns of gonadotropin release can be similarly manipulated by prenatal androgens. In rats, then, there is evidence that fetal hormones program brains dimorphically, which in turn program post-natal behavior.

Extrapolating the rat model to the human results in the following hypothesis: if the prenatal androgen levels are sufficiently high, the preoptic anterior hypothalamic area will be organized; if the androgen level is low, for whatever reasons, the central medial nucleus, or the female center of the hypothalamic area, will predominate. An intermediate level of fetal androgenization would eventually result in bisexuality. The enormous jump from rat to human is in part reflected by the fact that rat mounting behavior is not the same phenomenon as human sexual orientation. The biologic hypothesis ignores the impressive fact that mating behavior can be affected by social learning—even in subhuman animals.

Possible Evidence from Humans

The Intersex Conditions. Human prenatal hormone disorders potentially provide some perspective on the pseudohermaphroditic brain hypothesis. Several studies of male 46 XY genotypes with complete androgen insensitivity or testicular feminization syndromes are relevant. These patients are reared as females because they have female external genitals. Ten such patients (8) were all sexually attracted to males. This seems to support the biologic hypothesis, but the social learning theory of gender development (gender identity and orientation follow the sex of rearing) is equally as explanatory. The consistency of the findings in many studies that sex of rearing is the crucial determinant of gender in intersexed patients (9) seemed to make it a basic principle. But recently, one of Money's cases, who was initially reported to have been successfully raised as a girl following accidental penile ablation at birth was revealed as being masculine, disturbed, and having trouble being a female at age 13 (10). The assumption that nurturing is more important than prenatal biological events is again being questioned.

Prenatal congenital adrenal hyperplasia causes the adrenals in genetic females to produce large amounts of androgens. Born with intersex genitalia, some of these genetic females are reared as males. If prenatal hormone theory is correct, these girls should have increased incidence of homosexuality. The preponderance of evidence is, however, that most girls with this syndrome are heterosexual, regardless of when treatment was instituted. Moreover, the vast majority of female homosexuals are endocrinologically normal, have regular menstrual patterns, and show no signs of virilization.

Much research has suggested that pre- and perinatal androgen levels affect aggression, rough-and-tumble play, and maternal behavior. It is interesting that childhood effeminacy is a predictor of homosexual orientation, and many male homosexuals exhibit various degrees of effeminacy. Experiments have shown the prenatal exposure of males to progestin or estrogens decreases the incidence of masculine behavior—thus linking effeminacy to prenatal hormonal level. It is also tempting to link the high incidence of childhood tomboyism in lesbians to high levels of prenatal androgen. Unfortunately, these phenomena can also be explained by social learning.

Hormonal Levels of Adult Homosexuals. A great many studies have focused on testosterone levels of adult male homosexuals (7). The vast majority of subjects have had normal testosterone levels. Significantly lower mean testosterone levels have only been found in 4 out of 22 studies. Three of these studies lacked good control groups, and a fourth was complicated by a high incidence of drug abuse. One study included a pair of monozygotic twins, who were discordant for sexual orientation but had equivalent normal levels. Elevated levels of testosterone among homosexuals have been demonstrated in two studies. Studies of gonadotropins have also failed to reveal any consistent, strong relationship between adult homosexuality and an abnormality in the hypothalamic pituitary gonadal axis.

The majority of female homosexuals appear to have normal testosterone-estrogen levels. However, androgen elevations have been found in a subgroup of approximately one-third (11,12). This is an interesting finding, although not a sufficient indication that high androgens cause homosexuality. In fact, it could mean exactly the opposite, i.e., that homosexuality induces the endocrine system to elevate androgen production.

In conclusion, there really is no compelling evidence to support the biologic theory of male or female homosexuality.

A Different Biologic Perspective

The previously mentioned studies are scientific, but limited by current technology. Personality theories cannot be scientifically tested and replicated in the same way. A child's temperament is genetic or biogenic in that it is ultimately a byproduct of the nervous system's organization. The neurophysiologic mechanism for determination of temperament is as yet unknown (13). It may be possible for certain temperamental or constitutional factors to predispose a child to experiences that will solidify homosexual orientation. For example, a very passive, inactive male child's preference for maternal closeness may cause the father to ignore his son because he is not "all boy." The son's continued rejection may lead to psychological and family dynamics that solidify the homosexual aspect of his character. Thus, orientation and behavior may ultimately depend upon the interaction of biologic and social forces that cannot be measured, but can be expressed in terms of temperament and goodness of fit between child and parents. If this interactive model, based on the convergence of multiple psychological and biological forces, is correct, the biologic theory of homosexual etiology is a colossal oversimplification.

PSYCHOLOGICAL FORCES WHICH MAY MOTIVATE MALE HOMOSEXUAL PREFERENCE

Politics and Science

Inquiry into the origins of homosexual preference will inevitably be viewed as more than a scientific venture. Its hypotheses will be drawn into the continuing moral and political debates about homosexuality. In fact, even the decision to undertake such an inquiry may arise from subtle moral and political assumptions. Homosexuals are the objects of social intolerance, which seeks to justify itself by discovering their biologic or social defects. Homosexual groups point out the methodologic limitations of the few available studies. These include: investigator bias that homosexuality is a pathology; failure to use nonpatient homosexuals; inertia about replication. In addition to being methodologically unsound, the studies are exploitative, i.e., they confirm the investigator's initial hypothesis that homosexuality is a curable mental illness. The psycho-politics of the 1970s did not permit discussions of cures for nondiseases. For those who view life as a continual process that integrates the present with the past, it is not possible to simply ignore hypotheses about the genesis of this developmental outcome. Homosexuality is studied because it exists and illuminates the process of typical development.

Two Descriptive Studies

The persistent psychological interest in, and responsiveness to, the same sex is determined, if not completely fixed, very early in life. Many homosexual men and women report that, "they have always been this way" (14). Such statements indicate that homosexuality probably develops prior to age 5. Human beings are not directly aware of the early life experiences that lead to sexual orientation.

Whitham administered questionnaires to 206 male homosexuals and controls looking for childhood indicators of male homosexuality (15). He found that ultimate male homosexuality was preceded by the following indicators: 1. interest in girl dolls; 2. cross-dressing; 3. preference for company of girls; 4. preference for company of older women rather than older men; 5. being regarded by other boys as a sissy; 6. sexual interest in other boys in childhood sex play. Whitham found that the greater the number of childhood indicators, the stronger the man's adult homosexual orientation.

In a subsequent study, Whitham demonstrated that these characteristics of the prehomosexual male child existed in three societies—United States, Guatemala, Brazil (16).

Most homosexual males are aware of their homoerotic preferences by age 14. Their sexuality is generally declared prior to that of heterosexuals. Saghir and Robins conceptualized three manifestations of sexual responsiveness (14):

Romantic emotional responses include dreams, fantasies, desire for nongenital contact, and an intensive wish for, or feeling of, closeness or affection. These responses were often platonic but did contain an admixture of genital desires.

The majority of male homosexuals became aware of their persistent and predominant responsiveness to males by late latency. Their heterosexual responsiveness was transient, occasional, poorly defined, and usually after age fourteen. The romantic responses of homosexuals tended to occur earlier than the romantic responses of heterosexuals.

Cognitional Rehearsals. Cognitional rehearsals are explicit sexual fantasies, i.e., mental responses to actual or imagined past or present olfactory, visual, tactile, or auditory stimuli. A small percentage of heterosexuals experience homosexual cognitional rehearsals, whereas almost all homosexuals have them prior to adolescence. Cognitional rehearsals with heterosexual content occur during adolescence in both hetero- and homosexuals.

Physical Sexual Arousal is pleasurable sensation from physical contact with or without erection or genital touching. Most experienced arousal prior to adolescence; only a small minority (2%) did not experience it until early adulthood. About one-third of heterosexual men reported homosexual arousal; for 90% it was transient and prior to age fourteen. About 40% of male homosexuals denied ever experiencing arousal from a female source. For heterosexuals, the earliest arousal comes from nongenital contact with a girl. For most homosexuals, the earliest arousal through physical contact involves genital contact with a male.

Composite View of the Prehomosexual Boy
Saghir and Robins found that two-thirds of 89 adult homosexual males evidenced sissiness prior to age 14. These boys showed persistent and multi-

faceted behaviors that made them the objects of ridicule from peers and family. The sissiness included: avoidance of other boys, boys' games, sports, and rough play; preference for playing with girls, dolls, performing domestic chores; social isolation. These children were often unhappy because of the teasing they received for being "girl-like" or a "mama's boy."

About a fourth of adult homosexuals report a consistent wish to belong to the opposite sex. Almost half of children with sissiness had the wish to become a girl. (Such data are the source of the hypothesis that homosexuality is the adult outcome of serious early life gender confusion, i.e., it is a gender identity disorder). Some of these children were motivated to repeatedly dress in girls' clothing when alone. The differences between homo- and heterosexuals in the prevalence of this reported behavior were not statistically significant, but the trend was impressive.

Masculine play patterns are preferred by most boys by age six to seven. The sissiness, i.e., the striking absence of these patterns, may be evident years before the awareness of erotic object preference.

This composite view does not apply to about one-third of adult homosexuals who gave no indication of being sissies. This suggests that there may be many paths to adult male homosexuality. Adult male homosexuals do not discuss the positive influences on their development of sexual preference. This may be due to the fact that homosexuality is solely a result of negative factors.

Bieber *et al.* (17) emphasize the fear of physical injury and excessive dependence on the mother prior to adolescence.

Several prospective studies (18,19) have confirmed these retrospective impressions that latent effeminacy is a forerunner of adolescent preferential homosexuality. One must remember that there are many degrees of "effeminacy," "sissiness," or discomfort with typical male latency behaviors.

Composite View of the Family that Produces a Homosexual Son —Bieber *et al.*'s Dynamic Study

1. Subsystems of Nuclear Family. One can speak of intrafamilial relations in several ways: the mother-child, father-child, mother-father, mother-father-child subsystems. Because of the constitutional and maturational differences between each child, and the character structure and maturation of each parent, each child in a family has a unique mother-father-child subsystem. The family is composed of a set of interlocking subsystems. Siblings do not necessarily share the same psychological environment.
2. The psychological environment of the homosexual son is thought to be critically different from that of other siblings.
3. The typical mother has been characterized as *Close, Binding, Intimate.* Sixty-nine percent of mothers in their study produced an intimate close-

ness that interfered with their prehomosexual son's masculine development by:

a. Overstimulating via seductiveness or sexual intimacy;
b. Teaching that masculine sexuality was aggressive, brutal, and unacceptable;
c. Restricting peer group relationships. Spirited boys were often referred to as roughnecks. They pushed this son into adult, rather than peer, relationships. They singled this son out as special, encouraging a competition that the siblings could not win.
d. Interfering with independence by preempting decision-making, showing excessive concern for safety, and encouraging social isolation;
e. Interfering with the father-son relationship by showing open preference for the son, by pitting father and son against each other, and by including the son in parental arguments or in the bedroom.

The other 31% of mothers studied were rejecting-minimizing-hostile, detached, or controlling-domineering. No homosexual was judged to have a nonpathological mother, in contrast to a heterosexual control group in which the mothers were viewed as less pathological.

4. Seventy-five percent of the fathers in the study were classified as detached. But even among the others, there was not one who was felt to relate warmly to his son. These fathers interfered with masculine development by:

a. Providing no male warmth. If the child became aware of this lack he often felt rejected. If he was unable to verbalize the lack of interest or affection, he might always sense a vague hunger for something unidentified. This suggests that part of the homosexual orientation is a search for what was lacking in the early father-son relationship.
b. Spending little time with these sons;
c. Failing to provide a model for identification;
d. Failing to protect the son from the mother's destructive qualities;
e. Open hostility.

The outstanding attitude of son to father in this study was hatred and fear. In addition, Bieber et al. suggest that if a father is not detached from his son, the son will not become homosexual (17).

5. Some criticisms of this composite family data (20):

a. These data were based upon patients in psychoanalysis and may not pertain to homosexuals who do not seek out therapy. This is a very important conceptual criticism, although diverse studies including nonpatients show similar patterns. Saghir and Robins found most of their homosexual group described their fathers as indifferent and uninvolved (particularly with the homosexual son).

b. These data emphasize the role of the parents, leaving out the inherent contributions of the son—i.e., constitutional components.
c. Not all homosexuals report poor relationships with their fathers.
d. The pattern of a dominant, seductive, over-controlling mother and a passive, indifferent, hostile father is hardly specific to homosexuality. Similar family backgrounds are reported for diverse adult and child pathologies. This criticism may not be so much an argument against the cause of homosexuality as it is an impressive clue to what children require for the development of smoothly functioning heterosexual character structures.

Psychological Motivation for a Homosexual Object Choice: A Cautious Summary

The motivation for homosexual object choice has not been thoroughly studied prospectively. It seems clear that childhood gender confusion predisposes to recurring adolescent and adult homoerotic interests. Gender identity and role confusion reflect either the child's failure to accept his designation as a "boy" or his prolonged uncertainty about his identity. These difficulties with the formation of the sense of self are initially greatly influenced by parent-child relationships. The resultant gender ambiguity soon begins to be a force unto itself in the family's life. To oversimplify this set of forces, male homosexuality may result from excessive maternal closeness or insufficient parental love in the first two years, or later developmental problems after the rudiments of a masculine sense of self have been established.

MALE HOMOSEXUAL BEHAVIOR

The Sexual Behavior of Overt Homosexuals (14)

Masturbation. It has been repeatedly observed that, beginning with preadolescence, larger numbers of homosexuals than heterosexuals masturbate, and with greater frequency. Masturbation continues in spite of partner outlets. This may reflect a stronger biologic sex drive. It may also be an indication that homosexuals derive a psychological satisfaction through masturbation that cannot be obtained through other sexual outlets.

Mutual Masturbation. Ninety-three percent of homosexuals and 23% of heterosexuals had this type of experience by middle adolescence.

Fellatio. Ninety-nine percent of homosexuals and 3% of heterosexuals engaged in male-to-male oral-genital contact. About 25% of homosexuals began this prior to age 14.

Anal Intercourse. Ninety-three percent of homosexuals engaged in anal intercourse at some time in their lives, 8% prior to age 14. No heterosexuals reported this experience.

Object Anal Insertion. Nine percent of homosexuals reported the occasional insertion of penis-shaped objects in the rectum for masturbation.

Heterosexual Intercourse. About half of the homosexual men have had heterosexual intercourse—in contrast to about two-thirds of the single heterosexual controls. About half of each group first had intercourse during adolescence. Only 5% of those homosexuals who tried intercourse were impotent, but none reported being emotionally satisfied with heterosexual intercourse. They were either emotionally or sexually indifferent, derived slight pleasure, or felt somewhat clumsy and inadequate. Fear of women was specifically reported by only 3% of homosexuals. (This is in stark contrast to Bieber *et al.* [16] and wide clinical experience in which fear of women is assumed.)

Insertee-Insertor

A homosexual used to be classified as "masculine" if he inserted his penis, and "feminine" if he received the penis during intercourse. After data became available, it became apparent that it does not make sense to classify homosexual acts according to active and passive roles. One can actively seek a passive role, or passively perform an active role, in anal intercourse. The distinctions have even less meaning with regard to fellatio. Too much emphasis on who is active and who is passive limits one's understanding of what is actually taking place.

The one who inserts his penis into another's orifice can be designated the "insertor;" the "owner" of the orifice, the "insertee." In Saghir and Robins' study, 36% of homosexuals adopted an insertee role for at least one year after age 15; 12% adopted an insertor role; 52% interchanged sex roles and considered themselves as neither insertees nor insertors. Sixty percent of the men who were insertees considered themselves feminine or neuter. Twenty-two percent of the insertors considered themselves feminine.

Social Structure and Homosexual Behavior

"Coming out" is a term which refers to three related phenomena: recognition of self as homosexual; entrance into the homosexual community; public declaration of homosexuality. With regard to the second level:

a. Most homosexuals who come out do so prior to age 30, many before age 21.

b. Coming out is not necessarily pleasant. The sense of belonging and relief it provides to individuals who have long felt isolated, different or "queer" may replace the guilt and shame associated with deviance.

"Cruising" is the process of picking up a partner of the same sex. In early adolescence partners tend to be found among friends at school. In later adolescence, the public parks, washrooms, book stores, and particular streets expand access. As the homosexual becomes older, a wider variety of opportunities opens up, including bars, certain larger cities, movie houses, and organizations. Added opportunities for sexual liaisons are provided by homophile organizations, although they do not exist solely for this purpose. Many homosexual men find cruising quite objectionable.

Promiscuity. Many homosexual men have significant periods during their adolescence or adulthood in which they have numerous sexual encounters without a relationship. There is no minimum level for defining promiscuity, but most homosexual men feel they are or have been promiscuous. The number of their partners may be astoundingly high. Homosexual men are not invariably promiscuous throughout their lives.

Prostitution. Homosexual prostitution is more common than heterosexual prostitution. Five percent of the homosexual men interviewed by Saghir and Robins prostituted for at least one month, most for over one year. Male prostitutes tend to be under 25.

Group Sex. More homosexuals than heterosexuals have had sex with three or more persons.

CONSEQUENCES OF A HOMOEROTIC PATTERN

The Basic Decision—Can I Accept This?

A variety of illusions can be used to prevent recognition of one's homosexual desires. Eventually rationalizations such as "I just haven't met the right girl," "I'll grow out of it," or "I do it just for kicks" no longer work, and the issue of self-acceptance must be confronted.

There are numerous ways of not accepting one's homosexuality. One can become relatively asexual, substitute numerous activities, busy oneself with career or recreation, and live a primarily autoerotic life. One can escape into heterosexuality—dating, engaging in sexual relations, marrying, and raising a family. Occasionally individuals who cannot accept their homosexual inclinations seek out professional help.

Accepting oneself as homosexual requires dealing with the internalized attitude of society toward homosexuality. This is no easy task, since homosexuals are commonly regarded as queer, inferior, ludicrous, perverted, sick. Homosexuals are a despised and harassed minority; joining them, even mentally, may cause a considerable struggle. When one can recognize and accept his homosexuality without anxiety, depression, or hypochondriasis, he must deal with the problem of disclosure. Despite increased sexual permissiveness, self disclosure is done at great risk, and is a rare and relatively recent phenomenon. Indirect forms of public disclosure include working and living in homosexual communities and choosing careers associated with homosexuals. Many develop a double life, maintaining a facade of heterosexuality by day and a retreat into a homosexual subculture by night.

Even those who have come out at all three levels (self-recognition, in gay community, to the world in general) may have considerable private pain about being homosexual. It is particularly difficult to discuss one's homosexuality directly with one's parents—even though it seems the parents already know. Telling the father is probably the most difficult aspect. (*Consenting Adults* [21], a novel by Laura Hobson, deals with this subject sensitively.)

Delay is the most common response to the issue of self-acceptance; it is not so difficult to understand, considering the significance of the decision. External problems associated with a disclosure of homosexuality include: a change in location; career shift; rejection by family and friends. Internal problems involving the internalized values of one's family, religion, and dominant culture may be even more formidable. Perhaps as many as one-third of homosexuals never reach a comfortable stage of self-acceptance.

Some individuals do find the right girl after a period of homosexuality, or are able to find unconscious outlets for these inclinations before many of these consequences and dilemmas have to be consciously faced.

Lasting Love Relationships

The majority of homosexuals seek and find relationships with men characterized by strong affectual bonds. The physical relations include kissing, fondling, tender nongenital sex, and genital contact. They fall in love, live together, and function as a social unit in the homosexual subculture. While some of these "marriages" may last over a decade, most do not last longer than three years. The chances of any given male homosexual relationship lasting for a lifetime are very slim. Jealousies, infidelity, and decreasing interest in sex plague these relationships.

Special Difficulties

1. *Blackmail.* Men living double lives are vulnerable to homosexual blackmailers. Victims may not seek recourse through police channels because they fear disclosure. In addition, many homosexuals are assaulted and robbed by their sexual partners.
2. *Police Harassment.* The majority of arrests of homosexuals are made for solicitation or loitering in public places. Entrapment is the method used. A young policeman in plain clothes may entice a homosexual into genital contact and then serve as a witness when his nearby partner arrests the unsuspecting person. This practice, and the periodic raids of gay bars, are

disappearing due to the increased political power of homosexual organizations.

3. *Armed Forces Discrimination.* Homosexuality is currently sufficient cause for a discharge with less than honorable status.

4. *Job Security Risk.* Security clearances for important government offices are not given to recognized homosexuals, apparently because they are thought to be vulnerable to blackmail. Homosexuality can serve as an excuse for dismissal to hide radically different motives. Points 2, 3, 4 emphasize the fact that the civil rights of homosexuals are compromised by society.

5. *Medically Viewed as Sick or Perverse.* Homosexuals do become ill, but their physicians rarely know of their homosexuality. Physicians' embarrassment about taking a sexual history may interfere with the detection of venereal disease, highly prevalent among promiscuous homosexuals. Several serious new illnesses discovered among homosexuals reemphasize the need for physicians to become comfortable and skillful in dealing with the sexual lives of this minority. Articulate members of homophile organizations point out that society's intolerant, prejudiced views about homosexuality are the source of the homosexual sickness. They feel that mental health cannot be achieved by helping a homosexual adjust to a maladjusted society. Quoting Franklin Kameny, "Psychiatry is totally irrelevant to the problems of homosexuals in a hostile society. At the very least psychiatry and psychiatrists are ignored; more often they are attacked as the 'enemy incarnate'—and with considerable justification. Psychiatrists have been discredited and dethroned as sources of wisdom, knowledge, and authority . . . Having defaulted in areas in which they could assist us, and having shown themselves totally insensitive to the consequences of the theories which they irresponsibly promulgate, psychiatrists are felt to have nothing whatever of value to offer us and are thought to be doing us very real harm."

Saghir and Robins and Bell and Weinberg have found, however, that most of their homosexual samples felt that psychiatric care was effective and beneficial. Male homosexuals are commonly seen by psychiatrists for the same types of problems seen in heterosexuals—i.e., depression; neurotic symptoms; difficulties in relationships.

The Mental Health of Male Homosexuals

In 1978, Bell and Weinberg published a major sociological survey of male and female homosexuality in San Francisco (22). While their sample is not representative of all homosexuals (Nobody knows what sample would be representative.), its size and the fact that it included black and white, male and female homosexuals over a large adult age span qualify it as a major advance. The study assumes that homosexuals vary considerably in most dimensions of their lives. The title of their book encapsulated their major conclusion, i.e., *Homosexualities: A Study of Diversity*. Beyond the shared attraction and preference for members of the same sex, few scientifically based generalizations could be made. Anyone who has more than a passing interest in the subject is urged to read this study.

Bell and Weinberg divided male homosexuals into the following groups. It is clear from their nonpsychiatric perspective that about 60% are socially well-adjusted; some, however, have serious problems.

Close-coupled: people who were closely bound to one another. Close-coupled individuals tended to look to each other, rather than to outsiders, for sexual and interpersonal satisfactions. They had the smallest number of sexual problems and were unlikely to regret their homosexuality. They seldom cruised. They were rarely arrested, in trouble at work, or involved in assault and battery. They were less tense and paranoid and more exuberant than others.

Open-coupled: Although living with a special partner, these individuals tended to seek sexual satisfaction elsewhere. They cruised a lot and engaged in a great deal of sexual activity. Their psychological adjustment was intermediate.

Functionals: "swingers"—Their lives are organized around sexual activity. They were most likely to have been arrested, booked, or convicted for a "homosexual" offense. They are energetic, self-reliant, cheerful, and optimistic. They are also described as more tense, unhappy, and lonely than the close-coupled.

Dysfunctionals: "tormented homosexuals"—Troubled people whose lives offer little gratification. They have trouble managing their existence. They have poor sexual, social, and psychological adjustment in comparison to other homosexuals.

Asexuals: Lack of involvement with others. They had the least sexual activity, fewest partners, and most narrow sexual repertoires. They had trouble finding partners and were less interested in sex. They had fewer friends and were less overt about their homosexuality. Despite complaints of loneliness and unhappiness, these people are not very interested in establishing a special partner relationship. They are often described as apathetic.

The American Psychiatric Association's deletion of homosexuality as a disease was based on the review of numerous studies which failed to show any consistent or clear-cut differences in the psychological adjustment of homosexuals and heterosexuals.

FEMALE HOMOSEXUALITY

Introduction

The word "homosexual" has only recently begun to lose its automatic male association. Female homosexuality, or lesbianism, may be as common as the male counterpart, but has been even more cloaked in mystery and less adequately studied.

Fewer female homosexuals have availed themselves of psychiatric care and there are fewer nonpatient studies about this group. (Those interested in exploring this topic from a personal perspective should read Abbott and Love's *Sappho Was A Right-On Woman* [23].)

Analogous Categories

Tomboy or Boy-Like Syndromes. Both the tomboy and the sissy share persistent aversions to associations and activities usually thought of as typical for their genders. In boys, this behavior elicits isolation, teasing, and pressure from parents to modify preferences and activities. Tomboys, in contrast, are often warmly accepted and quite popular with boys; they are not a source of parental gloom and apprehension. The 3–5% prevalence of sissiness in grade schools approximates the prevalence of adult male homosexuality. The prevalence of tomboyism has not been determined in random samples. Sixteen percent of the controls and 70% of the 57 homosexuals in Saghir and Robins' study met criteria for tomboyism (14). There was some suggestion that tomboys who developed into heterosexuals had some interest in dolls. Homosexuals were exclusively interested in trucks, footballs, guns, etc.

The notion that tomboyism is an innocuous developmental phase is supported by the 16% prevalence of boylike syndrome among the heterosexual group. Some tentative concern about the ultimate outcome of tomboyism is generated, however, by the 70% prevalence among homosexual women.

A majority (63%) of homosexual women had repeated wishes to be boys and regretted being born female. Eleven percent repeatedly fantasized having a penis, and 6% desired a sex change operation at some point in their lives. The desire to become a boy involved fantasized male occupational choices and was related to the woman's ability to excel in "male" activities. Only a very small number of homosexual women reported ever dressing in male clothing—although a great majority displayed tastes for tailored or masculine-oriented clothing, shunning makeup and "feminine" accessories. A repetitive conscious wish to be a boy was not invariable in tomboys who became homosexual.

Development of Sexual Psychological Responsiveness

The development of sexual psychological responsiveness is strikingly similar in male and female homosexuals. Awareness of homophilic interests begins for both groups in preadolescence, earlier than in heterosexuals. The sexualization of romantic responses tended to occur in later adolescence in female homosexuals. A large proportion of homosexual women reported early romantic attachments to female teachers. Females experienced homosexual arousal for the first time in the context of nongenital relationships.

Many homosexual women displayed the potential for heterosexual responsiveness for a short time during adolescence. Most involved themselves in heterosexual genital activities, either because of social pressure or the desire to experiment. Their conscious response was indifference and they subsequently avoided heterosexual contacts because they provided little arousal and gratification.

Homosexual Practices

Sexual practices among homosexual women include self-stimulation, mutual masturbation, full body contact with orgasm, and object-genital contact. Every adult homosexual had experienced manual genital stimulation, about half before the age of 20. Only one-third of the women practiced full body contact to orgasm, and in most this was an adult experience. Only one-fourth ever experienced vaginal object insertion, and this too was an adult experience. Cunnilingus was almost universal among homosexuals, although many did not begin until adulthood. Only about one-fourth of the homosexual women became involved sexually prior to age 15. Female homosexuals tend to do a lot of necking and manual genital stimulation prior to adulthood; other techniques are added later.

Bell and Weinberg found that black homosexuals had more extensive sexual repertoires (22). The favorite sexual activity *for both races* was receiving cunnilingus.

Relationships Involving Genital Contact

Lasting less than four months. 82% of homosexual women have experienced these. These relationships occurred less frequently than among male homosexuals, but more so than among experienced heterosexual women.

Lasting 4 to 12 months. 70% of homosexual women have fewer than four such relationships. Male homosexuals displayed similar patterns. Heterosexual females formed such relationships significantly less often.

Lasting over a year. 93% of homosexual women, 61% of homosexual men. Eighteen percent of heterosexual women had such affairs with men. Most of the long-term relationships lasted up to three years.

Bell and Weinberg found that the majority of homosexual women had fewer than ten partners throughout their lives; about a quarter had fewer than five; about a third had between ten and fifty partners. Most women said none of their partners were ever seen again after sex. Most respondents were monogamous. Almost the entire sample reported never having paid a partner for sex. Responses to the question, "What kinds of physical characteristics do you most desire in a partner?": Those who mentioned any at all were most frequently concerned with body type or frame. Face, hair, or eyes were important to some. Few had special interest in breast size.

On the average, the women were 22 at the beginning of a first affair. They tended to be younger than the partner and thought they were in love with her. Many were very upset when the affair ended, but were able to acknowledge gains in insight, maturity, and feelings of peace and happiness.

Social Consequences

Awareness of being different often occurs by late adolescence, a bit later than males.

"Coming out"—The majority come out between the ages of 21 and 29.

"Cruising" is almost nonexistent among females. Overt sexual behavior is usually preceded by weeks or months of relationships.

Heterosexual Practices of Female Homosexuals

A vast majority of homosexuals engage in dating; many marry and establish a heterosexual relationship which lasts over a year. This heterosexuality is in response to family, social, and personal pressures to try the traditional female role. It is not quite accurate to think of these women as bisexual just because they are sexually responsive to men.

Bell and Weinberg found that more than one-third of white, and almost one-half of black, lesbians had been married at least once. They had intercourse less frequently than heterosexual women. Many didn't consider themselves homosexual when they married. Homosexuality and homosexual affairs were the most common reasons for breaking up marriages. Half of the white, and three-quarters of the black, women bore children—generally fewer than heterosexual women.

Mental Health of Homosexual Women

Saghir and Robins. Twenty-five percent were excessive or problem drinkers, as compared with 4–8% in the general population and 5% in the control group; 10% were alcoholics. The prevalence of parental alcoholism is higher for homosexuals than for heterosexual controls. Like the homosexual man, the homosexual woman is likely to drop out of college. (This is the peak period of conflict for homosexuals.) Female homosexuals consider themselves to be less feminine and more masculine than heterosexuals. While female homosexuals have a higher prevalence of alcohol problems than heterosexual controls, their resultant functional disability is not greater.

Bell and Weinberg.

1. *Happiness.* The close-coupled were the happiest. Homosexuals as a group, however, were less happy than heterosexuals.

2. *Suicidal Feelings.* About one-third had imagined committing suicide; 16% of the whites and 8% of the blacks had seriously considered it. Homosexuals demonstrated more suicidal ideation than heterosexuals—most strikingly among the asexual group. Most cited reasons other than their homosexuality. About 25% of the whites and 16% of the blacks had actually attempted suicide. There were no differences between homosexual and heterosexual women.

3. *Professional Help.* About two-thirds of the whites and one-half of the blacks had sought help for emotional problems—mostly from the dysfunctional, asexual, and open-coupled groups. Less than one-fifth of those who sought help were motivated by a desire to give up their homosexuality. The vast majority felt the contact had been beneficial; the most common benefit was "insight."

4. *Black vs. White.* Black lesbians reported poor health, more frequent feelings of loneliness, and more psychosomatic symptoms. They displayed more tension and paranoia, but were less suicidal.

Siegelman. Siegelman's carefully controlled questionnaire studies have consistently revealed that there are more similarities than differences in the mental health of female homosexuals and heterosexuals (24).

The Family of the Female Homosexual

Saghir and Robins were unable to clearly define the mother-daughter or father-daughter relationship in a way which significantly differed from those of the controls (13). Siegelman reviewed other recent data on parental background and concluded that both psychoanalytic and nonanalytic studies produced inconsistent and contradictory findings. His attempt to make an objective comparison of the backgrounds of nonpatient homosexual and heterosexual women led to the following limited conclusions (25). The fathers of homosexual women were less loving and more rejecting; their mothers were less loving and more demanding. There was less closeness to either parent and more friction between parents.

CONCLUSION

Bell and Weinberg's study demonstrates the possibility of male and female homosexuals being mentally healthy, productive, and friendly. The failure of some homosexuals to display these characteristics can no longer be used to justify the conclusion that homosexuality is a developmental tragedy. It should, rather stimulate the helping professions to investigate the personal, familial, and social forces which facilitate mental health, productivity, and the capacity to develop interpersonal relationships.

REFERENCES

1. Freud S: Three essays on the theory of sexuality (1905), in Strachey J (trans): *The Complete Psychological Works of Sigmund Freud, st'd ed. London, Hogarth Press, 1953, vol 7, pp 125-243.*
2. Bayer R: *Homosexuality and American Psychiatry: The Politics of Diagnosis.* New York, Basic Books, 1981.
3. Spitzer RL: The diagnostic status of homosexuality in DSM-III: A reformulation of the issues. *Am J Psychiatry* 1981;138:210-215.
4. Pattison EM, Pattison ML: "Ex-gays": Religiously mediated change in homosexuals. *Am J Psychiatry* 1980;137:1553-1562.
5. Kinsey AC, Pomeroy WB, Martin CE: *Sexual Behavior in the Human Male.* Philadelphia, WB Saunders, 1948.
6. Salzman L: "Latent" homosexuality, in Marmor J (ed): *Sexual Inversion The Multiple Roots of Homosexuality.* New York, Basic Books Inc, 1965, pp 234-247.
7. Meyer-Bahlburg HFL: Hormones and homosexuality. *Psychiatr Clin North Am* 1980; 3:349-364.
8. Masica DN, Money J, Ehrhardt AA: Fetal feminization and female gender identity in the testicular feminizing syndrome of androgen insensitivity. *Arch Sex Behav* 1971;1:131-142.
9. Money J, Ehrhardt A: *Man and Woman Boy and Girl: Differentiation and Dimorphism of Gender Identity.* Baltimore, Johns Hopkins University Press, 1972.
10. Diamond M: Sexual identity, monozygotic twins reared in discordant sex roles and the BBC follow-up. *Arch Sex Behav* 1977;6:477-481.
11. Sipova I, Starka L: Plasma testosterone values in transsexual women. *Arch Sex Behav* 1982;11:181-186.
12. Gartrell NK, Loriaux DL, Chase TN: Plasma testosterone in homosexual and heterosexual women. *Am J Psychiatry* 1977;134:1117-1119.
13. Thomas A, Chess S: *The Dynamics of Psychological Development.* New York, Brunner/Mazel Publishers, 1980.
14. Saghir M, Robins E: *Male and Female Homosexuality. A Comprehensive Investigation.* Baltimore, Williams & Wilkins Co, 1073.
15. Whitham FL: Childhood indicators of male homosexuality. *Arch Sex Behav* 1977; 6:89-96.
16. Whitham FL: The prehomosexual male child in three societies: U.S. Guatemala, Brazil. *Arch Sex Behav* 1980;9:87-99.
17. Bieber I, Dain HJ, Dince PR, *et al.: Homosexuality: A Psychoanalytic Study.* New York, Basic Books Inc, 1962.
18. Zuger B: Effeminate behavior present in boys from early childhood: I. The clinical syndrome and follow-up studies. *J Pediatr* 1966;69:1098-1107.
19. Green R: Childhood and cross-gender behavior and subsequent sexual preference. *Am J Psychiatry* 1979;135:692-697.
20. Bell AP: Research in homosexuality. Back to the drawing board. *Arch Sex Behav* 1975; 4:421-431.

21. Hobson LZ: *Consenting Adult.* New York, Warner Books, 1975.
22. Bell AP, Weinberg MS: *Homosexualities: A Study of Diversity Among Men and Women.* New York, Simon & Schuster, 1978.
23. Abbot S, Love B: *Sappho Was A Right-on Woman.* New York, Stein & Day, 1972.
24. Siegelman M: Adjustment of homosexual and heterosexual women: A cross-national replication. *Arch Sex Behav* 1979;8:121–125.
25. Siegelman M: Parental backgrounds of homosexual and heterosexual women: A cross-national replication. *Arch Sex Behav* 1981;10:371–378.

Chapter 32

THERAPIES

**MARVIN WASMAN, Ph.D., STANLEY E. ALTHOF, Ph.D.,
ROBIN N. MOIR, M.D., and ELIZABETH A. KLONOFF, Ph.D.**

Individual Psychotherapy

MARVIN WASMAN, Ph.D.

INTRODUCTION

Definitions of psychotherapy vary according to theoretical orientation, goals, and technique. Indeed, the diversity is so great that it may be difficult to view the psychotherapies as a single treatment modality. According to Redlich and Freedman (1), however, most definitions include certain common elements: an effort to produce some type of behavioral or psychological change; a relationship between a patient or client who is suffering or seeking change and a designated professional who attempts to facilitate change or alleviate distress; the use of verbal or other forms of symbolic communication.

Within this framework, the specific goals of psychotherapy depend upon its conceptualization as a treatment for mental disorders, a method for achieving behavioral change, an experience enhancing self-awareness and personal growth, a process for improving interpersonal relationships, or a means of promoting a more adequate adjustment to society. For example, types of therapy which emphasize either treatment for a diagnosed mental disorder or behavior modification, generally aim toward symptomatic improvement and anxiety reduction. On the other hand, approaches which emphasize growth and self-awareness usually aim toward greater self-actualization or personal fulfillment. Many types of therapy are defined broadly enough to include all of the above goals. The priority of these aims for any given case would depend upon the patient's reasons for seeking help and his or her own goals for treatment, as well as other factors, such as diagnosis, defenses, time and money available for therapy, etc.

Psychotherapy is generally classified into the following broad categories: individual psychotherapy, group psychotherapy, marital and family therapy, and behavior therapy. The first two categories simply refer to whether patients are seen individually or in groups, regardless of the techniques employed. Marital and family therapy focuses on a marital or family unit as a problem and is structured so that marital partners or family members are seen together, either regularly or at some time during treatment. Although behavior therapy, a therapeutic approach derived from principles of behavioral psychology, is generally classified separately, it may be utilized with individuals, groups, or families. Within these broad categories, there are a myriad of types or schools of therapy, such as the psychoanalytic therapies, Gestalt therapies, cognitive therapies, etc. These schools can further be subdivided so that it is estimated that well over a hundred identified forms of therapy are in current practice.

Psychotherapy generally begins with some form of evaluation, in which the patient's suitability for psychotherapy is assessed. The evaluation typically involves several sessions in which the therapist formulates a picture of the patient's conflicts, symptoms, defenses, and interpersonal relationships. The therapist examines these issues in the context of the patient's current life and past history. In addition, the therapist observes the patient's self-understanding, ability to communicate that understanding, and the nature of the therapist-patient relationship which emerges during the initial evaluation.

PSYCHOANALYTIC PSYCHOTHERAPY

Psychoanalytic psychotherapy is probably the most widely practiced form of therapy. It is sometimes referred to as analytically oriented therapy, dynamic psychotherapy, or insight therapy. It is based upon psychoanalytic theory in terms of its conception of personality development and pathogenesis of neurotic symptoms. It also utilizes many psychoanalytic techniques which are appropriately modified according to the needs of the patient and the dimensions of the treatment situation. Treatment is generally based upon the premise that therapeutic change can be achieved by understanding how unresolved childhood and adolescent conflicts continue to cause distress in the patient's current life. This insight is achieved through an examination of the present, the past, and the patient's relationship with the therapist.

Psychoanalytic therapy usually involves once or twice weekly, face-to-face sessions with the therapist. The patient is encouraged to express thoughts and feelings as they occur. At the beginning of treatment, it is important to establish an atmosphere and relationship in which the patient feels secure enough to express conflicts, emotions, and ideas about himself which may be difficult to share with another person. In the opening phase of psychotherapy, the therapist usually listens, in an attempt to understand the patient and his problems, and to develop a strategy or treatment plan. At the same time, the patient learns about therapy and how to engage in the process of self-observation through an intimate relationship with another person.

Although increased autonomy and independence are frequently stated goals of therapy, the process itself is structured to facilitate a regressive experience, in which many of the feelings and conflicts of the patient's childhood may emerge. The patient initially views the therapist as a doctor from whom he seeks help. The therapist encourages the free expression of feelings even to the point of abreacting or reexperiencing an intense emotional experience from the past. The therapist seeks the expression of childhood needs and conflicts, but withholds gratification of these needs. For example, the patient may want the therapist to become a lover or parent who will provide the love and protection which the patient wanted as a child. Rather than assuming such a role, the therapist attempts to increase the patient's understanding of the nature of these wishes and their manifestations in his current life relationships.

In all forms of therapy, it is important for the therapist to maintain some control over the degree and intensity of regression. All patients must maintain some adult judgment and intellectual capacity to work through such conflicts. They have to leave the therapy hour and function as adults in their work and family environments. Patients with weak ego strength or borderline conditions may be especially disturbed by regressive feelings. In such instances, the therapist attempts to limit regression or provide additional support, through extra sessions or even hospitalization, when necessary.

According to Freud's conception of psychoanalytic theory, symptoms or defenses constitute a partial resolution of an unconscious conflict which inhibited the expression of an unacceptable wish or feeling. In order to resolve symptoms or conflicts, he believed that the forbidden impulses must be brought into conscious awareness. However, the ego provides a series of barriers aimed at prohibiting the acknowledgment of forbidden impulses; Freud termed such barriers "resistances."

Much of the work in psychotherapy involves the working through or removal of resistances. The therapist frequently confronts the patient with his defenses and methods for protecting himself from the acknowledgment and expression of threatening issues. Resistances frequently take the form of silence, avoidance of topics, withholding of feelings, or even missed appointments. Other forms of more subtle resistance include intellectualization, denial, displacement, and other defenses. "Acting-out" is a type of resistance in which the patient repeats or reports an earlier conflict in current relationships or activities outside the therapy hour rather than verbally communicating the issue to the therapist. Thus, the therapist must repeatedly confront and work through a variety of resistances which constitute the patient's typical methods of dealing with stress and conflict. As part of the process of uncovering the neurotic conflict, the patient learns about his mechanisms for self-protection.

The patient's relationship with the therapist is one of the most important factors in the therapeutic process. Indeed, the patient-therapist relationship is frequently viewed as the primary factor in facilitating both personal growth and symptom relief in all forms of psychotherapy. Considerable benefit is frequently derived from expressing and sharing intimate feelings with another person. The patient begins to successfully experience a sense of closeness and understanding which he never achieved in previous relationships.

Psychotherapy also involves a special kind of relationship, which Freud (2,3) described and termed "transference." Freud observed that the patient's attitudes and feelings towards the therapist often constituted a repetition of past feelings and impulses which were displaced on to the therapist. These feelings from the past were frequently directed toward parental figures, and played an important role in the development of the patient's character and neurosis. Freud noted that transference occurred spontaneously in all relationships, and is not created by psychotherapy; however, the conditions of psychotherapy, i.e., the patient is given little information about the therapist and tends to view him as an authority figure—facilitate the development of intense transference reactions. Through transference, conflicts of early childhood emerge in therapy as real and immediate feelings which can be examined and understood. This process may have a much greater impact than the simple recollection of early childhood experiences. All patients develop some form of transference reaction. The extent to which transference is actively explored varies somewhat depending upon the treatment goals, type of patient, and the orientation of the therapist.

Freud noted that transference included both positive and negative feelings toward the therapist. The positive transference can involve erotic feelings which the patient may find disturbing and embarrassing to express. In less intensive forms of therapy, these feelings may be left unexplored, unless they become an obstacle or resistance to treatment. Negative transference, in the form of angry or hostile feelings, must be confronted and understood if therapy is to proceed effectively. Negative transference may frequently be expressed through missed appointments, late payment of bills, arguments with other people, etc. In such instances, the transference is repeated in the patient's behavior rather than in his verbal response to the therapist and is termed "acting-out" (4). The goal in such cases is to have the patient recognize the message in his behavior and deal with it verbally in the therapeutic relationship.

In addition to erotic elements, the positive transference includes friendly or affectionate feelings which enable the patient to form an effective working relationship with the therapist. This aspect of the relationship is sometimes referred to as "rapport;" more recently, it has been termed the "therapeutic alliance" or "working alliance" (5,6). In general, it refers to the rational, non-erotic aspect of the relationship which enables the patient to work toward the goals of treatment. The therapeutic alliance enables the patient to sustain his relationship with the therapist, in spite of the anxiety and negative feelings which he may experience during the course of therapy. It also enables the patient to take distance from the therapeutic process and view himself as if he were another person. The inability of some patients to develop a therapeutic alliance—such as those with paranoid or borderline pathology—may preclude the use of psychotherapy as a treatment modality.

Therapeutic change may also be facilitated by the repetition of early childhood conflicts within the context of therapy. By assuming a neutral attitude which is strikingly different from that of authoritative persons of the past, the therapist gives the patient an opportunity to face stressful and emotional situations with someone who does not resent his aggression or overindulge him to the point of seductiveness. Alexander (7) stressed this view in his description of therapy as a "corrective emotional experience," in which the patient learns that he is no longer a child and that the persons in his life are not his parents. Most therapists reject Alexander's suggestion that the therapist play out transference roles to "correct" original parental attitudes.

The final or ending phase of therapy is usually referred to as "termination." It constitutes a very special part of the therapeutic process and has been described in detail by Dewald (8) and Storr (9). Optimally, termination is based upon a mutual decision by therapist and patient about ending therapy. The decision should be made in advance, so that it can be worked through in a meaningful fashion. The decision to end therapy rarely results from a dramatic improvement in symptoms; instead, there is a mutual recognition that most, or many, of the goals or objectives of therapy have been at least partially fulfilled. These goals usually include either reduction in symptoms or better management of those symptoms which do persist, improved interpersonal relationships, enhanced self-esteem, and increased insight into the role of childhood and unconscious factors in determining one's behavior. The patient may also come to recognize and accept those aspects of himself and his life situation which cannot be changed. In a sense, the patient is now able to continue the process of therapy on his own.

The working through of termination is an intense emotional experience for most patients. The process involves giving up a relationship which has come to represent intense childhood feelings toward parental figures. In particular, ending psychotherapy may arouse earlier conflicts over dependency and autonomy characteristic of stages of childhood and adolescent development. The process involves painful feelings of loss and separation which may be especially difficult for patients who have experienced previous losses of parents or other significant relationships. Patients gain an understanding of such feelings in the context of their very real emotional responses to separating from the therapist or analyst. Indeed, some forms of brief or time-limited psychotherapy specifically focus on autonomy and separation as basic issues which need to be resolved for almost all individuals.

PSYCHOANALYSIS

Historically, many analysts drew sharp distinctions between psychoanalysis and psychoanalytic psychotherapy as treatment modalities. In recent years, however, there has been increasing recognition of the common elements in many types of individual psychotherapy. Many therapists now see the boundaries between psychoanalytic psychotherapy and psychoanalysis as either distinct or blurred depending upon the individual case (10). In general, psychoanalysis involves more comprehensive goals aimed at changes in personality structure, defenses, and resolution of character problems and neurotic conflicts. A greater degree of regression is facilitated by frequent sessions (4–5 times per week), minimal face-to-face contact (patient lies on a couch with the analyst sitting behind him), and an emphasis on free association—in which the patient is encouraged to explore his internal psychological life through images, fantasies, and dreams, as well as more organized thought processes. The analyst provides understanding, rather than gratifying the patient's infantile wishes by giving advice or support. While transference may be dealt with in a limited manner in psychotherapy with some patients, it is always a primary focus of psychoanalysis. Indeed, the development and understanding of the transference is sometimes regarded as the defining characteristic of psychoanalysis (11). Thus, the process involves the interpretation and understanding of the dynamics of childhood conflicts through their repetition in the immediate analytic situation. Since the demands of the analytic situation require a relatively high degree of ego strength, this technique is usually reserved for patients with neurotic or character problems. It is used less frequently with borderline patients, and rarely utilized for major affective or psychotic disorders. The time and cost of treatment place further limitations on the utilization of classical psychoanalysis.

Most psychoanalysts in this country conduct psychoanalysis in accord with Freud's basic formulations. A number of Freud's students and other analysts have introduced certain modifications of Freud's theory and methods, which have come to constitute various schools of psychoanalytic theories and practice. However, classical or Freudian psychoanalysis itself has continued to evolve and build upon Freud's basic concepts. Developments include a greater emphasis on analysis of character rather than neurosis, a greater emphasis on recognition and analysis of preoedipal conflicts, and increasing acceptance of the notion that techniques may have to be modified in order to reach a wider range of patients. In the past few years, object relations theory, which stresses the importance of early mother-child relationships in the development of self and subsequent interpersonal relationships, has had a major impact upon analytic theory. There has also been increasing debate about the analyst-patient relationship, particularly regarding the issue of the optimal degree of neutrality which the analyst should strive to maintain. Perhaps the most significant controversy and debate in recent years surrounds the criticism that Freud's thinking reflected the values and cultural stereotypes of the Victorian society in which he lived and worked; this society especially influenced his views concerning the psychology of women. Psychoanalytic theory and practice have had to deal with the dramatic changes in women's roles in virtually all aspects of society.

SUPPORTIVE THERAPY

Supportive therapy is a widely practiced form of psychotherapy in which the therapist plays an active, directly supportive role in helping an individual cope with stressful life situations and restore psychological equilibrium. Supportive therapy is frequently utilized to deal with an acute life crisis such as death, divorce, or chronic illness; to aid reconstitution following a psychiatric illness, especially one which involved hospitalization; or to help those who are unable to deal with internal conflicts, either because of intellectual limitations or an inability to observe and understand their own behavior (12).

Supportive therapy is frequently regarded as distinctly separate from insight-oriented psychotherapy. However, it is probably more accurate to view these forms of therapy as representing points on a continuum. All forms of therapy contain some elements of support, and most supportive therapy involves at least a limited focus on internal issues. Many therapists who conduct psychodynamic therapy provide considerable support during periods of crisis, while continuing to analyze the patient's feelings and behavior.

Supportive therapy utilizes a wide variety of techniques to restore psychological equilibrium, provide symptom relief, and resolve problematic life situations. The therapist is likely to be fairly active in structuring the content and focus of therapy. He may offer advice, reassurance, and information. The therapist may utilize the authority associated with the doctor's role as a powerful suggestive tool. The therapist is also prepared to utilize adjunctive supports when necessary, such as seeing family members, prescribing medication, and recommending hospitalization when indicated. Behavioral approaches, such as relaxation training or biofeedback, are sometimes employed for symptom reduction and tension control.

The patient-therapist relationship constitutes an important factor in supportive therapy (8). In contrast to insight-oriented therapy, however, it is less frequently explored or allowed to become the primary focus of the therapeutic experience. Instead, the therapist may attempt to maintain a positive relationship and encourage the patient to see him as a real person, rather than a neutral transference object. With highly disturbed patients, the therapist may actually interpret and support reality as a substitute for impaired ego functions. In a sense, the therapist gratifies a variety of childhood feelings, especially those involving dependency, which in an insight-oriented approach are frustrated and interpreted.

Termination of supportive therapy is frequently initiated by extending the interval between appointments. The patient is encouraged to try out new behaviors and then report his experiences. The duration of treatment may range from a few visits, in an acute life crisis, to several years with individuals who have chronic psychiatric disorders. Supportive therapy is sometimes considered a lesser form of treatment for both patient and therapist, especially by beginning therapists. Treatment effectiveness appears limited by the lack of emphasis on personal growth and self-understanding. In reality, supportive therapy requires a high level of skill, and frequently results in significant, sustained therapeutic benefits.

EFFICACY OF PSYCHOTHERAPY

In recent years, psychotherapy has enjoyed increasing popularity and acceptance, to the point where therapies and therapists have become a part of the popular culture through the media. At the same time, most forms of psychotherapy are a medical procedure, reimbursable through private insurance and public health support systems. Thus, psychotherapy is also a part of the problem of burgeoning health care costs, and practical, as well as scientific, issues are involved in questions about its efficacy.

Challenges of the efficacy of psychotherapy began with Eysenck's (13) appraisal of psychotherapy research studies up to the early 1950s. He concluded that the literature failed to demonstrate that psychoanalytically-oriented psychotherapy and psychoanalysis yielded benefits beyond those attributable to spontaneous recovery. Eysenck's appraisal was challenged as biased and inaccurate but had the sanguine effect of stimulating a number of studies with more adequate design and better controls.

Meltzoff and Kornreich (14) have described the complex methodological problems inherent in psychotherapy outcome research. Beyond a description of general principles and concepts, the process itself is difficult to define. Estimates of the number of types or schools of psychotherapy range from 90 to over 200. Even therapists, within the same school may differ in technique, experience, or in other ways which influence the treatment process. The measurement of behavioral and psychological changes constitutes another formidable problem. The investigator must decide when to assess change, what measures to utilize, and who should be responsible for their administration. Patient selection represents still another problem since the treatment group must be defined in terms of diagnosis, age, chronicity, and other important variables. However, the most difficult methodological issue involves the problem of selection of an untreated control group to provide a baseline for assessing spontaneous recovery. The use of random and matched controls is complicated by the extensive list of relevant treatment variables. Since there is no placebo for psychotherapy, the use of waiting lists to provide untreated controls is limited by patient frustration, tendencies to seek help elsewhere, and an increasing dropout rate if the study extends beyond a few months.

Despite these methodological problems, several hundred studies of treatment effectiveness have been conducted utilizing adequate controls and satisfactory outcome measures. The results of these studies have been widely reviewed and analyzed by Luborsky *et al.* (15), Smith & Glass (16), Bergin & Lambert (17), and Parloff (18), among others. All of these surveys conclude that the vast majority of studies show that groups treated with psychotherapy show more improvement than an untreated control group. Parloff notes that, "There is now overwhelming evidence that a broad spectrum of psychotherapies are effective." However, there is little or no evidence to date, of differences in efficacy among various forms or types of psychotherapy. A high percentage of patients generally improve, regardless of the specific form of psychotherapy utilized. Reported results are generally based on behavioral and time-limited approaches, since treatment duration and other factors virtually preclude studies on outcome of psychoanalysis and other long-term therapies. Research also indicates that psychotherapy alone is not the treatment of choice for major affective disorders or schizophrenia, although a combination of psychotherapy and pharmacotherapy may be of significant benefit.

In summary, the literature shows that the psychotherapies are of benefit but the question of what kind of therapy works best for specific patients remains unanswered. Indeed, Rosenzweig (19), Frank (20), and others have suggested that different types or systems of psychotherapy are all effective because they share major common elements. Most important, all therapies are based upon a helping relationship with a caring, empathic therapist. Other elements include the expression of intense emotional feelings and the view of the therapist as an authoritarian figure who can relieve distress. Since these factors are also important aspects of the doctor-patient relationship, they indicate the potential effectiveness of internists, pediatricians, and other physicians in treating the emotional and physical symptoms associated with a variety of psychiatric disorders.

Group Psychotherapy
STANLEY E. ALTHOF, Ph.D.

INTRODUCTION

Psychoanalysis and biological psychiatry focus on understanding the forces within individuals, whether they are psychodynamic or biochemical. Yet, people do not develop in isolation; they are shaped by powerful group forces—e.g., nuclear and extended families; school; religion; peer groups. One derives a sense of belonging and identity from group affiliation. Groups define codes of behavior and influence attitudes, values, emotions, and what we call "sense of self." Groups protect, nurture, educate, pleasure, punish, and foster survival and change. Group treatment attempts to combine the effects of individual therapy with the formidable forces that operate when people meet together regularly.

DEFINITION

Group psychotherapy constitutes a specialized and select type of group meeting. It is a form of treatment in which persons who are psychologically distressed and amenable to a shared therapeutic setting are placed in groups guided by trained therapists, for the purpose of effecting personality change. "By means of a number of technical maneuvers and theoretical constructs, the leader uses the group members' interactions to bring about this change" (21).

SOME CONTRASTS BETWEEN INDIVIDUAL
AND GROUP THERAPIES

In individual therapy, the patient is the sole recipient of the therapist's attention. He/she is responsible for what is discussed and is the only one receiving help. In group therapy, other patients may be the focus of the therapist's and other group members' attention; other patients may direct the flow of conversation. The patient may act as a helper to another member, or be the recipient of help.

Individual therapy allows the patient to analyze his feelings toward the therapist (transference). Although the presence of five to eight other people may dilute the intensity of the patient-therapist relationship, it enables the formation of important relationships with several other people. The development of these multiple transferences provides a richer medium for observing interpersonal styles and understanding interpersonal and intrapsychic dynamics.

Individual therapists generally do not reveal information about themselves. Patients are not aware of the therapist's struggles, dilemmas, and current life conflicts. In a group, patients are exposed to the achievements and difficulties of other members. This serves to reduce their sense of isolation and broaden their perspective on the uniqueness of others' lives.

CONCEPTS UNDERLYING GROUP THERAPY

Modern group therapy has its roots in two distinct schools of thought: 1. group as a whole; 2. individual psychotherapy.

Group As A Whole

The group as a whole approach is an outgrowth of social/group psychology. Kurt Lewin's field theory states that:

> "An individual's acts cannot be explained on the basis of individual psychodynamics but must be explained on the basis of the nature of the social forces of the field to which he is exposed. Similarly, in group therapy, group pressure is brought to bear on a particular member of the group to the extent that his behavior can be altered. In turn, this individual influences the group and together they form a Gestalt or whole" (21).

English psychoanalysts like Bion, Ezreil, and Foulkes began to study the "group as a whole." Groups were organized and run solely for the purpose of studying the phenomonology of group life. These studies enabled the development of theories of group formation and a new language for describing group dynamics.

The studies on the "group as a whole" phenomenon taught group therapists to focus on issues beyond the problems that any one individual brings to the group. Examples of "group as a whole" issues include: what is the task of the group; how does a group begin to work; how does it react to group trauma; how does it deal with sub-grouping; how does a group handle termination of members.

Individual Psychotherapy Within the Context of a Group

The pioneers of group treatment began by treating individuals within a group context. The group served as a non-participatory, quiet, listening audience as the therapist(s) worked individually with each group member. There was no member-to-member feedback or communication. It was believed that listening to other group patients would show members that they were not alone in their suffering. Also, hearing these dialogues might engender and accelerate the production of new patient material. It became clear that listening to others was helpful to some patients.

A Combined Approach

In the 50s, clinicians began to integrate the "group as a whole" approach with the treatment of individuals within the context of a group. The combined treatment approach emphasizes the important relationships among group members, as well as the relationship of each group member to the therapist. The group therapist also monitors the development and conflicts of the group as a whole. Patients in the group are likely to reenact with other members the behaviors resulting from their intrapsychic conflicts, as well as interpersonal difficulties which create problems for them outside of the group. For example, concerns with intimacy will be evident in their relationships to other group patients. Also, the group situation allows patients to reenact the problems they experienced with their original families. Sibling rivalry is commonly encountered. Group members must share the attention of the therapist, as well as divide the therapy time among themselves. At this point, the therapists and group members can clarify, confront, and attempt to understand the dynamics of these interactions. Over time, the interpretation of these past and present conflicts leads to interpersonal and intrapsychic change; members are more inclined to try new solutions/styles in relating to others.

Newer forms of group psychotherapy are called "encounter groups." These differ from traditional group treatment in that they lessen the psychological distance between leader and members, incorporate a greater number of structured exercises, and emphasize emotionality (22).

GROUP PSYCHOTHERAPY OUTCOME RESEARCH

Psychotherapy outcome studies are plagued by numerous methodological difficulties—i.e., how to assess and control for the multiple confounding interactions between patient, therapist, and treatment variables. Ideally, one would want to be able to determine the specific treatment conducted by a specific therapist which is most helpful to a specific patient suffering from a specific problem. Bednar and Lawlis (23) reviewed over 30 group psychotherapy outcome studies. The vast majority of these studies suggested that group psychotherapy improved patients' self-adjustment, environmental adjustment, and mental functioning. Group treatment was most helpful to patients with mood disorders, anxiety states, and somatic complaints. It was least helpful to those with more severe thought disorders and marked interpersonal withdrawal.

The most comprehensive group psychotherapy outcome study was undertaken by Lieberman, Miles, and Yalom (22), who report on the outcome of 250 persons participating in 17 encounter groups. Highly experienced clinicians of diverse theoretical orientations led each group. Data were derived from: 1. pre- and post-tests of group members; 2. interviews with friends of the subjects; 3. group members' observations of fellow participants; 4. leaders' ratings of group members; 5. trained observers' ratings of leaders and group members.

The results indicated that 38% of the participants benefited, 44% were unchanged, and 19% were harmed by therapy. The most significant positive changes occurred in participants' values, attitudes, and sense of themselves. Subjects described themselves as more open and change-oriented. They felt there was an increased congruency between their ideal and actual selves.

Eight percent of participants were judged to be casualties—that is, they were clearly harmed psychologically by the group experience. There was one suicide. The following mechanisms accounted for most of the negative outcome: 1. attack or rejection by the leader or group; 2. failure of members to obtain unrealistic goals; 3. coercive expectations; 4. sensory or emotional overload.

This study suggests that group leaders' behavior did influence patient outcomes. Therapists who were more caring and who provided a cognitive framework for patients' emotional experiences seemed to have positive outcomes. Leaders who encouraged emotionality without creating a cognitive framework, or those who excessively employed structured exercises, were less effective. Leaders' theoretical orientations were unrelated to positive or negative outcomes.

Participants felt that universality (a sense of others having similar feelings, thoughts, and conflicts), feedback, and emotional expression were the most salient mechanisms of change. Investigators felt the best outcomes were achieved by those patients who were able to share details of their lives and express emotion, thus integrating what they shared with how they felt.

Irvin\ Yalom's *The Theory and Practice of Group Psychotherapy*\ (24) is recommended to readers interested in specific techniques employed in group psychotherapy.

Family Therapy
ROBIN N. MOIR, M.D.

INTRODUCTION

The term "family therapy" refers to the psychotherapy of the whole family—that is, those members of a family group who either live in the same household or have a sufficiently intense and continuing involvement with one another that they comprise an enduring, interacting, and mutually influencing group. Introduced and popularized within the last few decades (25,26), family therapy represents a reaction to the frustrations and limitations of other forms of therapy. Time after time, clinicians would observe that patients had profited from individual therapy or in-hospital care, only to regress rapidly when returned to the family environment (27). Similarly, apparently concerned and well meaning families would abruptly withdraw their support for therapy or engage in behaviors that undermined or sabotaged the treatment. Perplexingly, they would become distraught when the disturbed member was improving or present another member for treatment. Observations such as these led clinicians to conclude that the families of their patients were unwittingly involved in the problems they wished to have resolved; perhaps, they even had a need for the problem's continuing existence (27–29).

FAMILY CONCEPTS

Comprehensive theories of psychopathology increasingly attempt to integrate biological, psychological, and sociological influences on human behavior, particularly through their effects on development. The family plays a central role in transmitting and modulating each of these broad influences; it is, of course, also the setting in which the most critical stages of development occur. The family is the group in which we experience our strongest loves and our strongest hates, our deepest satisfactions and most painful disappointments. As such, the family is a crucial mediator between the individual and society at large. An understanding of the family has long been recognized as fundamental to an understanding of individual psychology (30). Until recently, however, psychology has been primarily interested in the effects of family patterns upon the individual. In this perspective, the individual was perceived as the main actor—internalizing and incorporating family experiences in egocentric and idiosyncratic transformations and distortions, playing out multiple dramas against the shadowy backdrop of the family. As more attention has focused on the family as an interacting entity with its own charcteristics, rules, needs, and demands, a new dimension in psychological thought has gradually been defined.

Psychoanalysis, sociology, and psychology—especially social learning theory and small group theory—have all made major contributions to the development of family therapy (25,31-33). These diverse influences are reflected in the different orientations to theory and practice espoused by the several schools of family therapy. Common to all family therapy orientations, however, is an emphasis on systems concepts, derived from General Systems Theory (34). General Systems Theory is the science of "wholeness," i.e., what comprises the "thingness" of things. The essential quality of a system is that it is an organization of things or objects so related or interconnected as to form a unity or organic whole. Atoms, molecules, cells, organs, organisms, groups, societies, planets, and galaxies are all examples of systems. Systems may be biological, psychological, or social, living or non-living. Systems have the following characteristics: 1. the system as a whole is greater than the sum of its parts; 2. anything that affects the system as a whole affects each individual unit within the system; 3. a disturbance or change in the state of one part of a system is reflected in changes in other parts of the system and the system as a whole.

A systems perspective leads us to examine the whole family for dysfunction when we encounter symptomatic behavior in one member (35,36). For example, if a youngster presents with school avoidance, we look to see whether this behavior reflects problems in the family system. These problems could include discord in the parents' marriage, pervasive anxiety in the family unit about the dangers of the extrafamilial world, or intergenerational transmission of specific fears and concerns, e.g., children in our family are at risk of early death. The symptomatic behavior of the troubled family member may be seen as both reactive to family system dysfunction and serving a system maintenance function—that is, behavior which is maladaptive for the individual may serve the greater good of the family. The school phobic youngster may remain restricted and fearful, having little interpersonal involvement with peers, and interrupted educational goals; nevertheless, parental focus on this youngster's "problems" may successfully divert them from the problems of their marriage, or give others in the family a sense of being competent and strong.

A system may be open or closed. An open system is influenced by interaction or exchange with other systems, as well as interaction within its own system. The family is an excellent example of an open system in dynamic interchange with other systems—particularly those social institutions serving educational, economic, political, and religious functions. This recognition of the family as an open system is important from both theoretical and daily clinical problem-solving perspectives. In the situation of a school-avoidant youngster, one would need to evaluate the family system, as well as the educational system, and economic and social factors impinging on the child, school, or family. The nature of the problem will be very different if the youngster is found to be reacting to neurotic fears or to realistic dangers, e.g., if guns, knives and threats of violence are endemic to the school settings. While the focus of this discussion is on the family system, it should always be remembered that other systems are interacting with the family; particular attention should be paid to biological, intrapersonal (psychology of the individuals), and extrafamilial interpersonal systems.

Another systems concept of considerable utility in family therapy is that of homeostasis (29,31). Homeostasis is the tendency of a system to maintain itself in a relatively stable condition. This concept has often been misunderstood and applied too rigidly to family systems. The concept is based on observed resistance to those changes which would throw the family into severe disequilibrium, rather than resistance to any change. Indeed, some of the most important human activities are characterized by constant change, e.g., spontaneous activity; the processes of growth, development, and creativity (34). The only truly homeostatic human activities are those which are essential to survival and self-preservation. The homeostatic model is applicable in psychopathology, however, because non-homeostatic functions decline in the presence of psychiatric disorder (34). This is readily seen by comparing well-functioning families with those that are functioning poorly. In dysfunctional families, there is a decline in the occurrence of spontaneous and creative activities for both the family as a whole and individual family members. Attempts are made to deal with tension and conflicts by avoidance, rigid authoritarianism, repeated patterns of maladaptive behavior, and so forth. Any change in one member's pattern of activities or interests —such as a young adult seeking to be independent and leave the family—is met with resistance, opposition, or sabotage by other members.

Another important systems concept is that of boundaries. "Any system as an entity which can be investigated in its own right must have boundaries, either spatial or dynamic. Strictly speaking, spatial boundaries exist only in naive observation, and all boundaries are ultimately dynamic" (34). The family system's boundaries are both fundamental and precarious. Boundary disturbances may be manifested through retreat from exchange with the extrafamilial environment (e.g., friendless, isolated, or even paranoid and seclusive families), inappropriate exchange (e.g., seeking of the primary affectional relationship outside of the couple relationship), or a fragmentation and diffusion of the family into a loosely tied grouping of individuals whose interrelationships are barely distinguishable from those of transient groups. The boundaries of the family system vis-a-vis the outside world, and those of each of the family subsystems, must be clear and well-defined, but flexible enough to change as needed. If the members of the family are disengaged, the boundaries between individuals or subsystems are overly rigid. While this allows for individual variation and independence, it makes it too difficult for the members to support one another and be interdependent. In an enmeshed system, the boundaries between systems or subsystems are diffuse. It is difficult to tell who or what is autonomous, making it hard for the family system and individual members to handle problems that arise. There is less distance between family members (high interdependence) than there is in a disengaged system. However, an enmeshed system may be essentially feeding on itself. It may not have developed the internal and external resources needed to adapt and change under stressful conditions.

Boundaries between family subsystems are equally important. The integrity of the family system is dependent upon the integrity of the alliance between the parents, i.e., the development and maintenance of a parental coalition (30,37). The allegiance between the partners has to replace, or at least be superordinate to, the allegiance each marital partner has to his or her own parents. The marital relationship has to become the primary affectional relationship for each partner. Similarly, the addition of children to a family optimally results in the deepening and strengthening of the affectional bonds between the parents, rather than a displacement in the allegiances and affectional ties from the husband-wife to the parent-child relationship.

It is also necessary for the family to maintain generational boundaries by making a clear delineation between the responsibilities and authority assigned to the parents and to the children. Parents who are tyrannized by their child's every wish and fail to utilize appropriate guidelines and controls in regulating impulsive, greedy, and aggressive behaviors deprive their children of appropriate reality experiences and opportunities for ego and superego development.

Parents may also place children in roles in which they are expected to perform tasks and assume responsibilities that are age-inappropriate, and properly belong to the parental generation. Conversely, harshly disciplinary, authoritarian parents with little empathy for the feelings and immature development of young children may create boundaries between the generations which are too rigid. A final kind of family boundary is the maintenance of sex-linked roles. Gender role is learned within the family matrix by imitation of, and identification with, the parenting adult of the same sex. In addition, parents and others provide information about the customs, interests, attributes, privileges, and constraints associated with the respective roles of the sexes. If these role models significantly vary from societal norms and mores, the child is presented with a difficult task of adaptation—to which he or she may or may not be equal.

FAMILY ASSESSMENT

An assessment of the family should be included in any thorough psychiatric evaluation. Traditionally, this has been obtained by interviewing the presenting patient, spouse, or parent. These approaches can yield extremely important information regarding biological, developmental, and dynamic influences deriving from the patient's family of origin; sources of stress existing within the current family are also delineated. There are, however, significant limitations to these methods. Most importantly, the patient is limited by his or her own awareness. This limitation results in major gaps in historical information. Direct assessment is also necessary in order to evaluate methods of communication, interpersonal interaction, and affect, which are important clues to underlying family dynamics (37). Thus, in the context of family therapy, family assessment includes direct assessment of the whole family.

Requesting the participation of the whole family when one of the members presents with psychological difficulties is an important intervention in itself. Implicit in the request is the statement that there is some significant relationship between family functioning and the troubles of the individual member. A second implication is that the solution of the individual's problems requires the involvement of other family members (37). The context is very different from the usual methods of assessment, in which scrutiny of the individual reinforces the view that the person's troubles arise from within. While it is important to maintain a focus on the family system, every care should be taken to diminish the sense of guilt and blame that families often experience; in fact, family members may perceive the request for their involvement as a confirmation of their guilt.

The major task of family assessment is to delineate the relationship between the troubled person's presenting problems and the functioning of the family as a system. The following diagnostic scheme outlines some of the most important areas for assessment:

A. Structure

How is the family organized and structured—as demonstrated in the interview, at home, and by history? How cohesive is the family as a group, in terms of sense of closeness, family unity, loyalty, shared values, and goals? What is the nature of the leadership and power within the family that oversees the realization of family goals, maintenance of order and control, discipline, decision-making, etc.? Does the family have appropriate, well-functioning, effective boundaries between individuals, generations, and sex roles; between family and community?

Consider the clarity vs. diffuseness and flexibility vs. rigidity of these goals. What are the subsystem characteristics? In particular, what types of alliances, coalitions, family triangles, and splits exist? One should especially study the marital coalition for overt or covert conflict.

B. Roles

What are the role patterns, and how do they enable the performance of basic functions, such as protection from danger, provision of basic resources (food, shelter, clothing, and other necessities), meeting of basic nurturant and affectional needs? Especially in families with children, evaluate the effectiveness of the roles in insuring adequate development.

One needs to assess the means by which the family provides conditions for adequate psychosocial and psychosexual development, including a satisfactory sense of self, and the capacity to love and work. Role function is assessed according to its clarity and consistency. In addition to the affectional and instrumental roles described above, one needs to look for specific family roles, such as "scapegoat," "caretaker," "good guy," "bad guy," "sick one," "strong one," "weak one."

C. Communication

Communication is an interactional dimension whereby the family performs the family functions, solves problems, copes with crises, negotiates roles, conveys rules, etc. In addition to assessing the content of the communication, attention should be paid to the process and its effectiveness.

Note the pattern of verbal communication for clarity and organization, goal directedness or confusion, interruptions, supportive vs. threatening aspects, etc. Also note who talks to whom, who doesn't talk, who listens, who doesn't listen, who the spokesperson is, who controls communications.

Observe the non-verbal communication, such as seating, touching, gestures, eye contact, and the congruency between verbal and non-verbal messages.

Communication may be clear or masked, direct or indirect. The most effective type of communication is direct; the most ineffective is masked and indirect.

D. Relationships

This term particularly refers to the quality of feeling and regard among family members. Healthy relationships are empathic, need-satisfying, reciprocal, and mutually pleasurable. Unsatisfactory relationships may be characterized by lack of involvement, exploitation, over-protectiveness, dependency, ambivalence, inconsistency, hostility, or sadism.

In assessing relationships, one needs to particularly focus on how family members manage attachment, separation, loss, commitment, sustainment, and consistency in their relationships. It is important to identify assets, strengths, and growth-promoting and gratifying aspects.

E. Affect

Note the basic mood of the family and the individuals within it, including the degree of expressivity and tolerance of feelings, range of emotions, i.e., openness vs. subdued vs. covert or absent, level of tension, conflict, and anger.

How are mood and affect communicated and shared? Are certain moods dominating or missing? Do particular affects, such as sadness or anger, create difficulty?

F. Themes

These will be the answers to the question, "What does the behavior say?" That is, how do verbal and non-verbal behaviors express attitudes, ideas, and beliefs that have persistent, unifying, recurring qualities? These themes represent the crystallization of intergenerational issues, interpersonal defenses, etc., into a cohesive system of dynamics. Possible themes include: people outside the family are untrustworthy, persecutory, dangerous, or unworthy; emotional expression is risky, especially the expression of anger; one of the children is going to turn out bad, sick, etc.

Family secrets, such as a child being illegitimate or someone being fatally ill, have major impact on family communications.

G. Identification

It is often extremely useful in family assessment to look for identifications —not only with stereotyped roles, but with actual individuals, usually figures from previous generations. "Whom does that remind you of?" is a potent question. Not uncommonly, children will be identified with abusive ex-spouses or parents, deceased and idealized brothers or sisters, former lovers, disowned aspects of self, etc. The family members identified in such ways may enact self-fulfilling prophesies, in which the active participation of all family members results in bringing about feared or undesirable situations.

THERAPEUTIC APPROACHES

There are a number of schools of family therapy that reflect different theoretical and therapeutic orientations (25,31). These different approaches emphasize interventions at varying levels within the family. The communications school of family therapy, for example, places emphasis on improving family communicational patterns, i.e., allowing them to become clear and direct; making overt what has been covert (29). This approach will focus on improving the family's problem-solving, often using a very explicit, didactic, educational approach.

Therapists who utilize psychoanalytic concepts tend to emphasize themes and identifications within families, particularly issues dealing with separation and attachment. They endeavor to help the family discover the underlying basis for conflict avoidance, role distortions such as scapegoating, etc. (33,36,38). In this school, the focus is often on intergenerational issues, and the need to deal with the unfinished business of parental families of origin.

Other theorists are guided by structural viewpoints (37). System and subsystem disturbances of power, boundaries, alliances, and coalitions are seen as pathogenic. Emphasis is placed on bringing about changes in family structure. For example, a disturbance in the marital or parental coalition may result in an overly involved, conflicted relationship between parent and child. This interferes with the child's normal developmental needs, and may show up in symptomatic behaviors, such as school phobia, somatic symptoms, etc. The structural therapist would attempt to block the overinvolvement between the parent and symptomatic child, on the presumption that this will make the marital conflict overt and accessible to therapy and change.

A number of other approaches to family therapy have evolved. Behavioral family therapy has been quite successful in dealing with aggressive and delinquent children. Modern outgrowths of communications theory have been embodied in strategic and paradoxical family therapy approaches which have intriguing theoretical implications (39,40).

Despite their diversity, all approaches to family therapy share the common goal of bringing about change in the system as a whole (36). Individual dysfunction is seen as a reflection of family group dysfunction, and/or as negatively affecting family function. Unfortunately, this important concept has often been applied simplistically, as though it were a sufficient and complete explanation for all disorders. When genetic, biological, developmental, intrapsychic, and sociocultural influences are integrated into a family systems orientation, however, the clinician has powerful conceptual tools with which to address a broad range of clinical problems. Being alert to family disturbances can be a very important aspect of the treatment of diverse medical, surgical, and psychiatric problems. In the treatment of schizophrenia, for example, it has been found that outcome is highly dependent upon the nature of family support and involvement. The family approach, therefore, becomes an important orientation to all clinical work, rather than something which should be regarded solely as a specific treatment modality.

CASE ILLUSTRATION

Mrs. Jones felt considerably improved after 2 months of treatment in the psychiatric unit. As she made plans to return home, however, she felt there was one further matter that needed attention. Her ten-year-old son, John, had been the source of a great deal of concern because of obstinance, disobedience regarding assigned chores, and annoying mannerisms, such as tongue clicking, that she felt were directed at her.

In the first meeting with the family—attended by Mrs. Jones, Mr. Jones (John), the 13-year-old daughter, and "little John"—the mother declared that she could not tolerate her son's presence, either at the interview or at home. Her intense hostility toward her son was manifested by angry glances, interruptions when he was speaking, and belittling or dismissing comments.

John Jr., a good-looking boy, conducted himself well during the interview. Far from being aggressive or out of control, he was extremely polite and well-mannered. He was obviously distressed by his mother's attitudes toward him, and seemed very apprehensive when she spoke or looked in his direction. The father, John, was a quiet, passive man who minimized any concerns about "little John." At the same time, however, he failed to support his son against his wife's onslaughts. The daughter also conducted herself very carefully and politely. She clearly allied herself with the mother, joining in the latter's complaints about "little John."

Prior to the mother's admission, she had become desperately depressed and suicidal. When she declared her feelings to her husband, he failed to show any response, saying only, "People say things like that— I'm not a psychiatrist." She had also been increasingly losing control of her anger toward her son. She would "beat him nightly," and even locked him in a bedroom to protect him from her own attacks. She had called the child abuse line, but received no assistance. Her husband dismissed any basis for her fury by saying young John was "just going through a phase" even though John had set some fires and once sprayed some insecticide in his mother's drinking mug.

The mother stated that the only problems were those between John and herself. She and her husband specifically denied any marital difficulties. It rapidly became apparent, however, that there were enormous covert marital problems which were very actively avoided by both parents. The mother declared, for example, that for a number of years they had arranged to work at different hours, "because if we saw too much of each other, we would have broken up." By the end of the first interview, it was not difficult to recognize John Jr.'s difficulties as a manifestation of a broad family system dysfunction, in which intense marital conflict was being detoured onto the son. The working hypothesis was that John Jr.'s scapegoated role served to stabilize the marital subsystem. At the same time, the fury of the mother's attack upon him was based on projective identifications. She was able to see that she had always "had difficulties with little boys," acknowledging that this also extended to "big boys."

In the course of several months of family therapy, the above hypotheses were confirmed even more dramatically than had been anticipated. It was learned that the mother had been in a state of depression shortly after John Jr.'s birth. During this time, the father became involved in an affair with the young babysitter who came to care for the children. The babysitter became pregnant and subsequently gave birth to a child, who was raised in their community. The mother was devastated by her husband's infidelity. Together, they experienced enormous shame and guilt, and isolated themselves and their children from social contact. The mother was able to say that she had never forgiven her husband. He guiltily tried to make retribution, and felt unjustified in intervening with the anger his wife directed toward her son. As these marital conflicts were addressed in therapy, the mother was gradually able to relinquish her anger toward John Jr., while the father became more actively supportive and constructively involved with his son.

Several additional months of therapy were spent in addressing issues from the parents' families of origin that were being repeated in this family, and the rigid boundaries which had been established between this family and the community. Therapy resulted in marked improvements. The parents were able to resume a satisfactory marital relationship, and even renewed their marital vows and commitments in a "marriage ceremony" that was part of a Marriage Encounter program. They renewed their involvement with friends, church, and other social activities. The mother's hostilities toward her son were considerably resolved, and John Jr. lost his symptomatic behavior.

INDICATIONS, LIMITATIONS, AND OUTCOME OF FAMILY THERAPY

The most obvious indications for family therapy are relationship problems between family members, particularly parent-child conflicts, and problems in the conduct of regular family life, such as discipline. An ideal referral might involve family members' recognition of a lack of satisfaction and pleasure in their relationships, but such insight is rare. Rather, one tends to see troubled families who present with concerns about a child. Family therapy has become established as one of the most important treatment modalities in child psychiatry; it has also been increasingly applied in the therapy of troubled adults. The most exciting, though less obvious, indications for treatment include conditions which were formerly thought to require extensive individual therapy. These conditions range from phobias and other neurotic problems to psychophysiologic disorders, and even such exotic conditions as anorexia nervosa (37). Family therapy is often the only effective way of addressing the issues of multi-problem families; it is also particularly effective for handling crises in healthy families. It may be an important adjunct to an overall program for the treatment of medical disorders, mental retardation, or the psychoses.

Family therapy can be extremely powerful and effective, even in cases which may be resistant to other psychotherapeutic approaches. Because of this, it was initially hailed by some as a revolutionary treatment which promised to supplant other forms of therapy. A more moderate viewpoint is that family therapy is an important theoretical development, and an invaluable addition to the repertoire of psychological treatments. Unfortunately, little systematic work has been done to delineate the types of conditions or problems which are more responsive to family therapy than to other approaches. There is a virtual absence of randomized controlled studies which would help to answer such questions. There are, however, an increasing number of uncontrolled outcome studies which offer preliminary encouragement (41).

In the enthusiasm which greets a new field, family therapy has been applied to conditions that are not likely to be amenable to change with psychological approaches. Family systems theorists need to recognize the existence of other important systems, especially biological and sociocultural systems, and choose the most effective level at which to intervene.

Behavior Therapy
ELIZABETH A. KLONOFF, Ph.D.

INTRODUCTION

Behavior therapy refers to a relatively recent theoretical perspective on the conceptualization and treatment of psychiatric problems. Although originally derived from the work of learning theorists in the field of experimental psychology, modern behavior therapy is based on a wide range of theoretical underpinnings. In the late 1970s, a group supported largely by the Foundations Fund for Research in Psychiatry met to evaluate the status of behavior therapy. Many of the conceptualizations presented here derive from reports of that group's meetings (42).

The application of behavioral principles to clinical problems began with three major events during the 1950s. Skinner's 1953 publication, *Science and Human Behavior* (43), presented a reconceptualization of psychotherapy in behavioral terms. It was viewed as an educational, rather than a medical, endeavor, and emphasized the importance of symptomatic behavior in its own right. Eysenck (44), in a 1959 critique of psychotherapy, argued that it was more scientific and efficacious to look at behavior. Finally, Wolpe (45) presented the results of his research on the elimination of experimentally-induced neurotic reactions in cats; this text, *Psychotherapy by Reciprocal Inhibition,* included a number of treatment techniques for working with neurotic patients. Since that time, the clinical application of behavioral approaches has grown exponentially. By 1972, there were more citations in *Psychological Abstracts* about behavioral treatments than there were about psychoanalytic approaches. Thus, behavior therapy is now considered both a major psychotherapeutic approach and the subject of numerous attempts at empirical validation.

This section is an introduction to behavior therapy from its broadest perspective. The four major components of modern behavior therapy will be presented, along with the derived treatments. The underlying concepts and the integration of behavioral and traditional psychotherapeutic orientations will also be discussed.

APPLIED BEHAVIORAL ANALYSIS

Commonly referred to as *"behavior modification"* or *"behavior therapy,"* this approach involves the modification of personal and social behaviors. The emphasis is exclusively on overt, observable behaviors in applied settings. This approach is best exemplified by B.F. Skinner's philosophy, "A person does not act upon the world, the world acts upon him" (46).

Applied behavioral analysis is based on techniques derived from *operant conditioning* theory; the fundamental assumption is that behavior is a function of its consequences. Thorndike's Law of Effect (47) states that a behavior which is followed by a pleasure will tend to be strengthened; behavior which is followed by an unpleasant consequence will be weakened. Thus, in operant terms, pleasant or unpleasant consequences are deemed, respectively, positive or negative *reinforcers.* Operant conditioning is probabilistic in nature, i.e., reinforcers increase the probability, or likelihood, of recurrent behavior. Another aspect of operant conditioning is *shaping*. Shaping involves the reinforcement of each successive approximation to the desired target behavior; careful attention to this progression of small steps enables the teaching of new behaviors. Finally, the ways in which a person is affected by reinforcing and punishing contingencies are intensively evaluated. This aspect of operant conditioning has led to the development of a number of single-case experimental designs in which each subject serves as his or her own control.

The focus in applied behavioral analysis is on powerful environmental variables that produce clinically obvious, important changes; this precludes the need for statistical analysis. Related techniques, based on the operant approach, include: reinforcement; punishment; extinction; stimulus control; other laboratory-derived procedures. These techniques can be applied to both individuals and groups, e.g., chronic psychotic patients; the severely mentally retarded; the token economy. Interventions can occur in institutional, rehabilitation, and educational settings, as well as in the community, the home, and out-patient treatment facilities.

In summary, applied behavioral analysis represents the stereotype of the "behavior modifier." It focuses on environmental effects on behavior, and utilizes an operant approach. Since it cannot be used with many presenting psychiatric problems, however, newer behavioral approaches have been developed.

THE NEOBEHAVIORISTIC MEDIATIONAL
STIMULUS-RESPONSE MODEL

The concept of *classical conditioning* forms the theoretical basis for this approach. As best exemplified by Pavlov and his dogs, classical conditioning involves the use of an unconditioned stimulus to elicit an unconditioned, or reflexive, response, e.g., the smell of meat powder elicits the dog's salivation. The unconditioned stimulus is then paired with a conditioned stimulus, e.g., the ringing of a bell. By repeatedly presenting both the unconditioned and the conditioned stimuli simultaneously, the unconditioned response will eventually be elicited by the conditioned stimulus alone. At this point, the unconditioned response becomes a conditioned response. A number of empirical investigations have called into question the role of classical conditioning in intervention techniques; therapeutic techniques themselves, however, are widely used.

Eysenck (44), Rachman (48), and Wolpe (45) have all contributed to this methodological approach. The behavioral approach is based on the learning theories of Pavlov (49), Guthrie (50), Hull (51), Mowrer (52), and Miller (53); the use of interventions incorporates the concept of private events or imagery. The rationale is that covert processes follow the laws of learning that govern overt behaviors. In other words, an imaginary anxiety-eliciting event can be associated with both antecedent and consequent operant referents. Since imaginary and actual anxiety-invoking situations precipitate similar psychophysiologic responses, this is actually a "deconditioning" approach.

Systematic desensitization is the major treatment paradigm derived from this theory. It has been demonstrated in several laboratories over the past ten years that systematic desensitization is perhaps the most effective treatment for phobic-like disorders. The approach to the phobic stimulus is broken down into a series of small, graduated steps; this is called "development of the hierarchy." While the patient maintains a state of relaxation, each of these small steps is presented through imagery. The patient does not move on to the next item until the less threatening situation can be imagined without any physiologic or psychologic discomfort. Breaking down the feared stimulus and presenting it in a slow, comfort-inducing, systematic way is crucial to the success of systematic desensitization.

While therapeutic techniques, such as systematic desensitization, have proven very useful for treating phobias and phobic-like conditions, they do not explain the genesis of phobias, or the therapeutic mechanism of systematic desensitization itself. Behavior therapy theorists have, therefore, developed additional approaches which can also be used with other types of disorders.

SOCIAL LEARNING THEORY

The social learning approach, first introduced by Bandura (54), presumes that human behavior is developed and maintained via three separate, but interacting, systems. Psychological functioning involves behavior, cognitive processes, and environmental factors. A person is not driven by internal forces; nor is he a passive reactor to external events. A person is both the agent and the object of environmental influence.

The social learning approach emphasizes the role of cognitive processing, the person's thoughts about what is happening, in influencing behavior. Other people are also important, since social learning theory was initially derived from work with modeling. In modeling, an individual learns a behavior or sequence of behaviors from watching another person. The positive or negative events that follow the model's experience will affect the onlooker's decision about imitating the behavior. Thus, learning probably occurs through coding of representational processes, based on exposure to instructional, observational, or imagined material. Because learning can occur through observation alone, without any reinforcement, modeling is also called vicarious learning.

The idea that the person is an agent of change—that is, has the capacity for self-directed behavioral change, is another key aspect of social learning theory. A traditional operant conditioning approach denies the notion of self-control, and emphasizes the importance of external environmental events. By assuming that the individual must interpret environmental events, social learning theory states that behavior change is an individual responsibility. Bandura (55) has introduced the notions of *self-mastery* and *self-efficacy* as possible explanations for behavior change in psychotherapy, regardless of theoretical orientation. Psychotherapy is conceptualized as a means of returning control to the individual. As the patient gains a sense of control, he is able to give up his past neurotic, self-defeating behaviors. Social learning theory also represents behavior therapy's first attempt at rapprochement with other forms of psychotherapy. By emphasizing the universal underlying causes of behavior change, e.g., self-control, cognitive interpretation of events, social learning theorists have produced a form of behaviorism that is more in keeping with traditional theoretical orientations. Behavioral rehearsal, i.e., imagining a potentially stressful event to decrease the associated anxiety, communication skills training, and modeling are derived from this approach.

COGNITIVE BEHAVIOR THERAPY

Cognitive behavior therapy is the most recently developed behavior therapy. This approach shifts the therapeutic focus from external environmental events to internal thoughts and feelings. This technique encompasses a number of diverse procedures, many of which were developed outside the mainstream of behavior therapy; the basic assumption is that clinical disorders are the result of maladaptive or faulty thought patterns. The identification and replacement of these faulty thought patterns with more adaptive cognitions is the therapeutic task. Once this is accomplished, the maladaptive behavior will, presumably, cease.

Ellis (56), Meichenbaum (57), and Beck (58) are the three major theorists initially associated with cognitive behavior therapy. Ellis developed a system called rational-emotive therapy. This involved the identification of patients' presumed maladaptive beliefs and an attempt to facilitate change. Meichenbaum's self-instructional training uses the therapist as a model of appropriate behavior. The therapist verbalizes constructive problem-solving self-instructions; he assists the client in imitating the appropriate behavior and repeating these self-instructions. Eventually, the self-instructions are internalized. The third major variation is Beck's cognitive therapy. Beck considers both cognition and behavior as important in altering faulty thought patterns. He gives depressed individuals specific task schedules, aimed at providing successful coping experiences, and other individually-tailored homework assignments. He also assists patients in changing their maladaptive cognitions. All of these approaches emphasize procedures that facilitate a more objective, detached view of emotion-arousing events.

Other techniques of cognitive behavior therapy include problem-solving skills, stress inoculation, coping skills training, thought stopping, and attribution therapy. These techniques often utilize unique procedures. Despite their demonstrated therapeutic efficacy, many of these procedures have little theoretical basis; cognitive behavior therapy has thus been the subject of a great deal of research.

Biofeedback is a relatively new intervention strategy that has developed within the behavioral tradition. Biofeedback uses psychophysiological measuring instruments to provide the patient with information about his/her internal states; by having access to this information, patients are able to learn to control certain parameters (e.g., muscle tension, surface skin temperature) that were once believed to be outside of volitional control. This treatment modality, often used in combination with interventions deriving from cognitive behavior therapy, has been used successfully in treating a wide range of psychophysiological disorders.

THE COMMON CORE OF THE BEHAVIOR THERAPIES

There are a number of fundamental assumptions underlying all approaches to behavior therapy. Behavior therapy can be defined in terms of two basic characteristics: 1. It is a psychological model of human behavior that is fundamentally different from the traditional intrapsychic, psychodynamic, or quasi-disease models of mental illness. 2. The commitment to scientific method, measurement, and evaluation emphasizes the empirical basis of any intervention. These basic assumptions have given rise to a number of corollaries (42):

1. Abnormal behavior that is not due to a specific brain dysfunction or biochemical disturbance is assumed to be governed by the same principles that regulate normal behavior.
2. Many types of abnormal behavior that were previously regarded as either illnesses in themselves or indicative of illness, can be alternatively construed as pathological "problems of living." Thus, the belief that psychiatric problems represent illness per se is de-emphasized.

3. Since abnormal behavior is assumed to be acquired and maintained in the same manner as normal behavior, it can be treated through the application of behavioral procedures.

4. Assessment should focus on current determinants of behavior, rather than on post-hoc analyses of possible historical antecedents. This presumes an emphasis of specificity, i.e., a person can be best understood and described by what he or she does in any given situation.

5. Treatment strategies are individually tailored.

6. Understanding the development or etiology of a problem is not essential to its amelioration. Conversely, the ability to change a problematic behavior does not imply knowledge of its etiology.

7. Since behavior change occurs in a specific social context, it may result in side-effects (e.g., changes in behaviors that were not the focus of treatment); many changes embody more broadly-based, positive outcomes than were anticipated.

8. Behavior therapy is committed to an applied science approach. There must be an explicit, testable, conceptual framework. Treatment techniques must be suitable for objective measurement and replication. Lastly, treatment methods and concepts must be subjected to ongoing empirical evaluation.

Behavior therapy is not the mechanized, rigid, stereotypic administration of punishments and reinforcers. It is a psychotherapeutic enterprise. As in all psychotherapy, it must include concern for the patient's feelings and attention to the psychotherapeutic relationship. As practitioners with diverse theoretical orientations begin to communicate and influence each other, we may perhaps discover more similarities than differences among these approaches.

REFERENCES

1. Redlich FC, Freedman DX: *The Theory and Practice of Psychiatry.* New York, Basic Books, 1966, pp 268–305.
2. Freud S: Fragment of an Analysis of a Case of Hysteria, in *The Complete Psychological Works of Sigmund Freud,* st'd ed. London, Hogarth Press, 1953, vol 7, pp 3–122.
3. Freud S: The Dynamics of Transference, in *The Complete Psychological Works of Sigmund Freud,* st'd ed. London, Hogarth Press, 1958, vol 12, pp 99–108.
4. Freud S: Remembering, Repeating and Working Through (Further Recommendations on the Technique of Psychoanalysis, II), in *The Complete Psychological Works of Sigmund Freud,* st'd ed. London, Hogarth Press, 1958, vol 12, pp 147–156.
5. Greenson RR: *The Technique and Practice of Psychoanalysis.* New York, International Universities Press, 1967, pp 190–216.
6. Sandler J, Holder A, Dare C: Basic psychoanalytic concepts: II. The treatment alliance. *Br J Psychiatry* 1970;116:555–558.
7. Alexander F, French TM: *Psychoanalytic Therapy, Principles and Application.* New York, Ronald Press, 1946.

8. Dewald PA: *Psychotherapy: A Dynamic Approach,* ed 2, New York, Basic Books, 1971.
9. Storr A: *The Art of Psychotherapy.* New York, Methuen, 1980.
10. Paolino TJ: Some similarities and differences between psychoanalysis and psychoanalytic psychotherapy: An unsettled controversy. *J Oper Psychiatry* 1981;12:105-114.
11. Gill MM: Psychoanalysis and exploratory psychotherapy. *J Am Psychoanal Assoc* 1954; 2:771-797.
12. Meissner WW, Nichol AM: The psychotherapies: Individual, family, and group, in Nicholi AM (ed): *The Harvard Guide to Modern Psychiatry.* Cambridge, Belknap Press, 1978, pp 357-386.
13. Eysenck HJ: The effects of psychotherapy; An evaluation. *J Consult Psychol* 1952; 16:319-324.
14. Meltzoff J, Kornreich M: *Research in Psychotherapy.* New York, Atherton Press, 1970.
15. Luborsky L, Singer B, Luborsky L: Comparative studies of psychotherapies: Is it true that "everyone has won and all must have prizes"? *Arch Gen Psychiatry* 1975; 32:995-1007.
16. Smith ML, Glass GV: Meta-analysis of psychotherapy outcome studies. *Am Psychol* 1977;32:752-760.
17. Bergin AE, Lambert MJ: The evaluation of therapeutic outcomes, in Garfield SL, Bergin AE (eds): *Handbook of Psychotherapy and Behavior Change,* ed 2. New York, Wiley, 1978, pp 139-189.
18. Parloff MB: Psychotherapy and research: An anaclitic depression. *Psychiatry* 1980; 43:279-293.
19. Rosenzweig S: Some implicit common factors in diverse methods of psychotherapy. *Am J Orthopsychiatry* 1936;6:412-415.
20. Frank JD: *Persuasion and Healing: A Comparative Study of Psychotherapy.* Baltimore, John Hopkins Press, 1965.
21. Sadock B: Group psychotherapy, in Freedman A, Kaplan H, Sadock B (eds): *Comprehensive Textbook of Psychiatry,* ed 2. Baltimore, Williams & Wilkins, 1979, pp 1850-1876.
22. Liebermen M, Yalom I, Miles M: *Encounter Groups: First Facts.* New York, Basic Books, 1973.
23. Bednar R, Lawlis F: Empirical research in group psychotherapy, in Garfield SL, Bergin AE (eds): *Handbook of Psychotherapy and Behavior Change.* New York, John Wiley & Sons, 1971, pp 812-838.
24. Yalom I: *The Theory and Practice of Group Psychotherapy,* ed 2. New York, Basic Books, 1975.
25. Ferber A, Mendelsohn M, Napier A: *The Book of Family Therapy.* New York, Jason Aronson, 1972.
26. Beels CC, Ferber A: Family therapy: A view. *Family Process* 1969;8:280-332.
27. Bell NW, Vogel EF (eds): *A Modern Introduction to the Family.* Glencoe, IL, Free Press, 1960.
28. Grotjahn M: *Psychoanalysis and the Family Neurosis.* New York, WW Norton, 1960.
29. Satir V: *Conjoint Family Therapy: A Guide to Theory and Technique.* Palo Alto, CA, Science and Behavior Books Inc, 1967.
30. Parsons T, Bales RF: *Family: Socialization and Intervention Process.* Glencoe, IL, Free Press, 1955.
31. Stein JW: The Family as a Unit of Study and Treatment. Monograph One, Rehabilitation Research Institute, University of Washington.
32. Flugel JC: *The Psychoanalytic Study of the Family.* London, Hogarth Press, 1921.
33. Stierlin M: *Psychoanalysis and Family Therapy.* New York, Jason Aronson, 1977.

34. von Bertalanffy L: *General Systems Theory: Foundation, Development, and Applications*. New York, George Brasiller, 1968.
35. Erikson GD, Hogan TP: *Family Therapy: An Introduction to Theory and Technique*. Monterey, CA, Brooks/Cole, 1972.
36. Skynner ACR: *Systems of Family and Marital Therapy*. New York, Brunner/Mazel, 1976.
37. Minuchin S, Fishman HC: *Family Therapy Techniques*. Cambridge, MA, Harvard University Press, 1981.
38. Boszormenyi-Nagy I, Framo JL: *Intensive Family Therapy: Theoretical and Practical Aspects*. New York, Harper & Row, 1965.
39. Watzlawick P: *The Language of Change: Elements of Therapeutic Communication*. New York, Basic Books, 1978.
40. Rabkin R: *Strategic Psychotherapy: Brief and Symptomatic Treatment*. New York, Basic Books, 1977.
41. Gurman AS, Kniskern DP: Research on marital and family therapy: Progress, perspective, and prospect, in Garfield SL, Bergin AE (eds): *Handbook of Psychotherapy and Behavior Change: An Empirical Analysis*, ed 2. New York, John Wiley & Sons, 1978, pp 817–902.
42. Agras WS, Kazdin AE, Wilson GT: *Behavior Therapy: Toward an Applied Clinical Science*. San Francisco, WH Freeman & Co, 1979.
43. Skinner BF: *Science and Human Behavior*. New York, MacMillan, 1953.
44. Eysenck HJ: Learning theory and behavior therapy. *Br J Ment Sci* 1959;105:61–75.
45. Wolpe J: *Psychotherapy By Reciprocal Inhibition*. Stanford, CA, Stanford University Press, 1958.
46. Skinner BF: *Beyond Freedom and Dignity*. New York, Knopf, 1971.
47. Thorndike EL: *Animal Intelligence: Experimental Studies*. New York, MacMillan, 1911.
48. Rachman S: The conditioning theory of fear-acquisition: A critical examination. *Behav Res Ther* 1977;15:375–388.
49. Pavlov IP: *Conditioned Reflexes: An Investigation of the Physiological Activity of the Cerebral Cortex*. New York, Oxford University Press, 1927.
50. Guthrie ER: *The Psychology of Learning*. New York, Harper, 1952.
51. Hull C: *Principles of Behavior*. New York, Appleton-Century-Crofts, 1943.
52. Mowrer OH: A stimulus-response analysis of anxiety and its role as a reinforcing agent. *Psychological Review* 1939;46:553–565.
53. Miller NE: Studies of fear as an acquirable drive: I. Fear as motivation and fear reduction as reinforcement in the learning of new response. *J Experimental Psychology* 1948;38:89–101.
54. Bandura A: *Social Learning Theory*. Englewood Cliffs, NJ, Prentice-Hall, 1977.
55. Bandura A: Self-efficacy: Toward a unifying theory of behavior change. *Psychological Review* 1977;84:191–215.
56. Ellis A: *Reason and Emotion in Psychotherapy*. New York, Lyle Stuart, 1962.
57. Meichenbaum D: *Cognitive-Behavior Modification*. New York, Plenum Press, 1977.
58. Beck AT: *Cognitive Therapy and the Emotional Disorders*. New York, International Universities Press, 1976.

Chapter 33

PSYCHOPHARMACOLOGY

GLENN C. DAVIS, M.D.

INTRODUCTION

The availability of relatively specific chemotherapeutic agents for the management of behavioral disorders has been a rather recent development in the history of psychiatry.

Psychotropic drugs have three types of therapeutic effects on psychiatric disorders: disorder-specific effects; symptom-specific effects; symptom-amelioration effects. For example, the tricyclic antidepressants have disorder specific effects, i.e., the entire depressive syndrome will respond to the agent. Neuroleptics have target symptom-specific effects, e.g., to eliminate hallucinations and delusions. Anxiolytics tend to attenuate anxiety without restoring the individual to a normative state.

Rational pharmacotherapy depends upon proper diagnosis, the appropriate selection of target symptoms, selection of an appropriate medication, a weighing of adverse effects to determine the risk-to-benefit ratio, assessment of compliance, evaluation of concomitant medical disorders, drug-drug interactions, accurate assessment of response, and determination of dose adequacy and duration (see Flow Chart, Figure 1).

The psychiatrist must be familiar with the pharmacology of a wide range of compounds, e.g., neuroleptics; antidepressants; lithium; anxiolytics; sedatives; anticholinergics; antihistaminics; drugs of abuse. Psychopharmacological agents share a number of properties. They are generally lipid soluble, a requirement for brain access. The more potent the drug, the more clearly its effects are mediated through specific synaptic mechanisms. Many psychotropic drugs have the potential for abuse. Since most of these drugs affect mood and cognition, this is not such a surprising fact; most substance users initially seek mood or cognitive effects. This chapter will focus on: 1. neuroleptics; 2. antidepressants; 3. anxiolytics; 4. lithium.

FIGURE 1
THE LOGIC OF PHARMACOTHERAPY

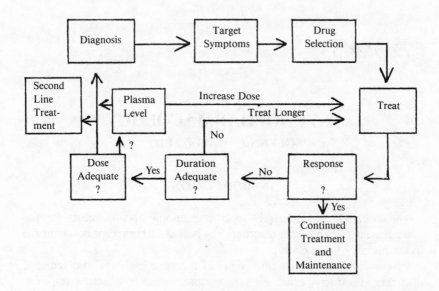

NEUROLEPTICS

Neuroleptics have been available in the United States since the introduction of chlorpromazine in the 1950s. Their initial use had an enormously beneficial impact on psychiatric patients hospitalized throughout the country. Table I lists only a few of the many neuroleptics available to the practitioner.

The Effects of Neuroleptics

Neuroleptics are also called antipsychotics and major tranquilizers. Neuroleptics influence: 1. arousal; 2. affect; 3. motor activity; 4. disorders of reality testing, such as hallucinations and delusions; 5. disorders of communication (formal thought disorder); secondarily, they may reduce social stigmata, such as withdrawal and isolation. Neuroleptics are not specific for given disorders, though they are most commonly prescribed in schizophrenia. They exert both symptom-specific effects, such as eliminating hallucinations and delusions, and ameliorative effects on selected symptoms. Neuroleptics do not cure diseases, but are quite effective in reducing the morbidity associated with acute psychotic illness. It is important to learn the target symptoms of neuroleptics so that one will not confuse the treatment of a disorder (e.g., schizophrenia) with the specific treatment effects of neuroleptics on selected symptoms (e.g., hallucinations associated with schizophrenia).

TABLE I
NEUROLEPTICS

Generic	Commercial	Equivalent Dose (mg)
Phenothiazines		
Aliphatic		
Chlorpromazine	Thorazine	100
Piperidine		
Thioridazine	Mellaril	100
Mesoridazine	Serentil	50
Piperazines		
Trifluoperazine	Stelazine	5
Perphenazine	Trilafon	10
Fluphenazine	Prolixin	2
Thioxanthenes		
Aliphatic		
Chlorprothixene	Taractan	65-100
Piperazine		
Thiothixene	Navane	5
Butyrophenones		
Haloperidol	Haldol	2
Indolones		
Molindone	Moban, Lidone	8-10
Dibenzazepines		
Loxapine	Loxitane	10-15

Arousal. Patients experiencing acute psychoses present to the physician with enormous levels of arousal. The arousal may be exhibited by autonomic nervous system signs and symptoms, such as increased heart rate, tachypnea, and elevated blood pressure. Subjectively, the patient appears hypervigilant, and may report bombardment by sensory stimuli. Neuroleptics may improve this group of symptoms the most quickly. Improvement may appear to occur within the first several doses of sedating neuroleptics, such as chlorpromazine. The hyperaroused state will usually improve within three days of the initiation of an effective neuroleptic dose.

Affective Symptoms. Neuroleptics constrict or flatten affect. Suspicious, paranoid, and grandiose affects are often selected as target symptoms for neuroleptics. Affective symptoms are closely tied to elevated arousal. Nevertheless, significant improvement in arousal may reduce the vigilance and external manifestations of fearfulness, without reducing the patient's subjective awareness of fear or suspicion. A typical response in an acute schizophrenic psychosis would be a reduction in arousal with persistence of the suspicious affect, this may later be followed by a reduction in suspicious affect but a persistence in the suspicious content. When the arousal and affect have improved, the verbalized content may seem almost inappropriate. That is, the patient may state that the FBI is following him, but not seem concerned about it. This seemingly inappropriate behavior results from pharmacologic reduction of only one group of symptoms.

Psychotic confusion, perplexity, and anxiety may also improve. The affective improvement associated with neuroleptic use may not be disorder-specific.

Psychomotor Symptoms. The reduction in excited psychomotor behaviors caused by neuroleptics is, at least in part, a dose-dependent phenomenon. Again, the reduction in motor behaviors is not disorder-specific; normals also demonstrate a reduction in total body movements. Since extrapyramidal motor function is greatly influenced by neuroleptics (via effects on nigrostriatal dopaminergic tracts), treatment causes both motor improvement and adverse effects (see the "adverse effects" section of this chapter). The development of extrapyramidal adverse effects poses a major problem in assessing psychomotor improvement. Neuroleptics produce minimal improvement in patients with a paucity of movement or catatonic symptoms.

Psychotic Thought Content. Thought disordered behavior has two components—psychotic thought content (sometimes called speech content) and formal thought disorder. Neuroleptics appear to produce symptom-specific improvement in psychotic thought content. Hallucinations and delusions improve, and ideas of reference and bizarre ideation may disappear. However, there are several major problems with the pharmacologic management of these symptoms. Chronic psychotic thought content tends to become refractory to treatment. Thus, the degree of improvement in hallucinations is often a function of the number of prior episodes, the duration of untreated episodes, and the degree of prior responsiveness. Hallucinations in the first psychotic episode may respond within several weeks and completely remit. The hallucinations of the third episode may require a full month for significant reduction. The tenth episode may involve persistent, residual hallucinations that appear refractory to neuroleptic management.

Formal Thought Disorder. Disordered communication may also improve with neuroleptic treatment. Some aspects of formal thought disorder present between acute schizophrenic episodes may be resistant to treatment—for example, poverty of speech and content of speech. On the other hand, derailment, incoherence, tangentiality, loss of goal, and pressure of speech may improve dramatically. The former symptoms are often called "negative" symptoms of schizophrenia; the latter have been called "positive" symptoms.

Social Stigmata. The social impairment found in schizophrenic patients is largely a secondary consequence of this demoralizing disorder. The degree to which social impairment will improve with neuroleptics depends upon the extent of primary symptom response, family network, social supports, careful social work, and education.

It is important to emphasize the fact that the above groups of symptoms are overlapping. An understanding of these target symptom groups enables the physician to grasp the scope of the illness and highlight the differing time course of responses. Arousal and affect improve first, and overlap with psychomotor response; attenuation of thought disorder follows. A gradual improvement in social functioning is the final response.

Spectrum of Use

Neuroleptics are primarily used in the management of schizophrenia— i.e., acute schizophrenic psychoses, chronic management of residual symptoms, and prophylaxis of acute episodes.

Manic states also improve with neuroleptics, though the primary benefit appears to be a reduction of arousal and a flattening of affect. Neuroleptics do not seem as specific as lithium in the overall management of the manic episode. Currently, neuroleptics only play a major role in the acute management of deleriform, or so-called third degree, mania.

The use of neuroleptics in the treatment of depressive illness remains somewhat controversial. Most commonly, neuroleptics are used in combination with a standard antidepressant to treat delusional or hallucinating depressed patients. A major short-term goal in such patients should be the reduction and elimination of neuroleptics; they flatten affect and reduce psychomotor behavior, making it difficult to determine whether the antidepressant is working. Furthermore, the concomitant use of neuroleptics may hasten catabolism of antidepressants.

Neuroleptics are commonly used to treat psychotic behaviors associated with organic injury to the brain, drug-induced psychotic states, such as amphetamine psychoses and hallucinogenic states, and Gilles de la Tourette's disorder. While neuroleptics are not effective analgesics, they are purported to enhance the pain reducing properties of standard analgesics. A number of physicians use low dose neuroleptic regimens for the management of anxiety; in general, however, the risk-to-benefit ratio does not seem to justify this course of action.

Adverse Effects

Adverse effects may be classified according to the involved organ system or their presumed etiology. Neuroleptics appear to have antidopaminergic, antiadrenergic, anticholinergic, and antihistaminic effects (for a more extensive review of side effects of their treatment, see [1]).

A host of dyskinesias including acute dystonic syndromes; akathisias; parkinsonism; bradykinesia; and tardive dyskinesia are a consequence of antidopaminergic effects of neuroleptics. Several dyskinesias respond to the addition of anticholinergic medications, while others require a reduction in the dose of neuroleptics. Since the presumed antipsychotic effects of neuroleptics are thought to be antidopaminergic, it appears unlikely that the biochemical pharmacologist will be able to separate their beneficial effects from their dyskinesia-inducing side effects. Antidopaminergic and antiadrenergic effects produce several endocrine abnormalities. Galactorrhea and gynecomastia may result from the increase in prolactin, secondary to antidopaminergic mechanisms. Amenorrhea, weight gain, and the syndrome of inappropriate ADH may also result from neuroleptic effects on neurotransmitter systems in the brain and pituitary.

Anticholinergic effects occur throughout the length of the gastrointestinal tract. Dry mouth, delayed stomach emptying, and slowed bowel function with constipation are common problems. The combination of anticholinergic and antiadrenergic side effects produces sexual dysfunctions and pupillary problems with accommodation. Cardiotoxicity may be primarily a function of the anticholinergic effects of neuroleptics.

Antiadrenergic effects cause postural hypotension, a common problem in psychiatric patients. The antihistaminic and antiadrenergic effects of neuroleptics may produce sedation.

Other effects include hepatotoxicity (a cholestatic jaundice), leukopenia, corneal lenticular opacities, photosensitivity, and allergies. There appears to be a .05% incidence of agranulocytosis.

Mechanism of Action

For the past 20 years, dopamine receptor blockade has been the proposed therapeutic mechanism of action for neuroleptics. The most convincing evidence supporting this hypothesis is a strong relationship between the clinically-demonstrated potency of neuroleptics and their affinity for the dopamine receptor (2,3). Several other hypotheses have been recently suggested. Neuroleptics also bind to a calcium binding protein called calmodulin (4). Calmodulin is associated with the dopamine receptor complex in the neuronal cell membrane. Several neuroleptics which do not bind avidly to the dopamine receptor do appear to bind to calmodulin. Furthermore, several drugs which bind to the dopamine receptor but do not have clinical efficacy do not bind to calmodulin. Thus, in a preliminary way, this hypothesis explains data which are not accounted for in the dopamine receptor antagonism hypothesis.

Blood Levels

Therapeutic plasma or serum levels have been defined to some extent for a variety of neuroleptics (5). The major problems in monitoring blood levels include: the host of active metabolites of most neuroleptics (6); the presence of several catabolic pathways; the wide range of levels found to be effective in treating disorders such as schizophrenia (5). Blood level monitoring currently remains a research tool. It may be clinically useful to detect extremely low levels, suggesting poor compliance or rapid catabolism.

Common Problems with Neuroleptic Use

Neuroleptics have adverse effects, some of which may be irreversible. They also produce cognitive slowing and a subjective sense of "mental constraint." It is extremely important for the physician to educate the patient involving him as an active participant in the treatment. (See [7] for a review of general principles of treatment integrating patient education, rapport, and psychotherapy.)

It is difficult to determine an individual's optimum minimal dose. Many physicians prescribe higher doses of neuroleptics than are necessary to ensure adequate levels; this is an attempt to avoid the severe morbidity which accompanies prolonged psychosis.

Some psychotic patients respond minimally to neuroleptics. The clinical profiles of many psychotic patients who are refractory to neuroleptics do not differ from those of treatment-sensitive patients—making it difficult to predict the efficacy of treatment.

There is excellent evidence that neuroleptic maintenance therapy reduces the intensity and frequency of acute exacerbations of schizophrenia. On the other hand, there are little scientific data on the clinical pharmacology of maintenance therapies. It is difficult to determine when, and by how much, to reduce neuroleptic doses in chronic patients. Many physicians systematically reduce doses over several months after the successful management of an acute episode. Often the goal is to maintain the patient with a low to moderate dose of neuroleptic (e.g., 10–20 mg/day of haloperidol). Other physicians artificially target maintenance, e.g., at ½ of acute treatment requirements.

ANTIDEPRESSANTS

Like neuroleptics, antidepressants have been available since the early 1950s. Both monoamine oxidase inhibitors (MAOI) and tricyclic antidepressants (TCS) dramatically reduce the mortality and morbidity of affective illness. The beneficial impact of specific antidepressants has continued to increase as the diagnosis of affective syndromes has become much more accurate. Table II lists a few representative MAOI and tricyclic antidepressants.

TABLE II
ANTIDEPRESSANTS

Tricyclics	
Tertiary Amines	
Amitriptyline	Elavil
Imipramine	Tofranil
Doxepin	Sinequan
Secondary Amines	
Nortriptyline	Aventyl
Desipramine	Norpramine, Pertofrane
Protriptyline	Vivactil
MAO Inhibitors	
Phenelzine	Nardil
Tranylcypromine	Parnate

While there are several classes of antidepressant compounds, when they are effective they reverse the entirety of the selected depressive syndromes. Not all depressive states are reversible with antidepressants. Thus, the recent evolution of the major affective illness diagnoses (DSM-III), which respond extremely well to antidepressant drugs, lends credibility to the notion that these disorders are diseases.

Spectrum of Use

Antidepressants do not persistently elevate mood in those who are not suffering from depressive disorders. Whether due to life circumstances or the consequences of maladaptive behavior, simple unhappiness will not improve with antidepressant treatment.

Of the affective disorders, bipolar disorder, depressed episode, and major depressive disorder demonstrate the most clear-cut antidepressant responses. Studies demonstrate a 70% average antidepressant response rate for these diagnostic categories (8). Dysthymic disorder, cyclothymic disorder, atypical bipolar disorder, and atypical depression respond much more sporadically to this class of compounds. Many investigators believe that these depressive syndromes are etiologically heterogeneous. That is, some dysthymic individuals really have "subaffective" expressions of major depressive disorders; the depressive symptoms of other dysthymic individuals are associated reactions and accommodations to life circumstances (9).

Tricyclic antidepressants are also used in the management of chronic pain, both alone and in combination with other analgesics (10). Tricyclic antidepressants and MAOI are also used in agoraphobia, and selected anxiety disorders (11). The beneficial effects of imipramine on agoraphobic symptoms may not be the result of the mechanisms responsible for antidepressant effects.

Target Symptoms and Time Course of Response

Neurovegetative symptoms include appetite and sleep disturbances, changes in libido and sexual performance, energy impairment, loss of interest, and gastrointestinal problems. This group of symptoms responds most promptly to proper doses of antidepressants. It is important to realize that improvement in sleep, which ordinarily heralds improvement in the depressive process, may be due to the sedating side effects of certain drugs, e.g., tertiary tricyclic antidepressants such as amitriptyline, rather than a specific antidepressant effect.

Psychomotor symptoms also tend to show some improvement in the early phases of treatment. Psychomotor retardation may persist as a subjective complaint while the ward staff observes that the patient is more active. Both groups of symptoms may improve within 7–14 days of achieving of the proper dose.

Both psychomotor and neurovegetative symptoms may improve several weeks before the lifting of gloom, despair, and depressive thought content. Nursing staff may report that the patient now comes into the dayroom voluntarily, has more facial mobility, and is sleeping well—but continues to complain of depressive thought content. The first mood improvement may not be noticeable as mood elevation or "good" mood, but may be a return to a variety of moods. The presence of expressed anger in a retarded or depressed patient may often represent the beginning of the recovery of mood regulation.

Improvement in mood precedes progress in the cognitive aspects of depression. The patient's formulation of "incompetence" or elaborate explanations for decreased self-esteem may take months to disappear; they may even remain as part of his sense of self. The impact of depressive episodes on the sense of self is a major contributor to the morbidity of these illnesses. Cognitive impairment in thinking, concentration, and attention may improve somewhat earlier than actual thought content.

A small percentage of major affective syndromes are associated with psychotic symptoms of hallucinations and delusions. Antidepressants are generally effective in treating these symptoms. When significant agitation and arousal accompany hallucinations and delusions, early treatment with neuroleptics may be necessary. The presence of such psychotic symptoms complicates management, but does not reduce the antidepressant outcome if diagnosis is clear. Psychotic symptoms often require several weeks at effective doses of medication before recovery begins. The presence of psychotic symptoms often indicates that ECT is the treatment of choice.

Social stigma and demoralization are also consequences of affective illness. Recovery from these secondary effects often takes a year.

Adverse Affects

As with neuroleptics, the specific side effects of tricyclic antidepressants may be classified according to the effects on neurotransmitter function, i.e., adrenergic, anticholinergic, serotonergic, and antihistaminic effects. (See [12] for a more extensive review of side effects of tricyclic antidepressants.)

Anticholinergic problems—ranging from dryness of the mouth to constipation—are perhaps the most disturbing and common side effects. Because antidepressants are more potent anticholinergics than neuroleptics, cardiovascular risk and genitourinary effects, such as urinary retention, are more common. Impairment of sexual function and risk of exacerbating narrow angle glaucoma are also significant problems.

The adrenergic and the serotonergic effects are thought to relate to the therapeutic mechanism of antidepressant action (see chapter on Affective Illnesses). Adrenergic side effects, including orthostatic (postural) hypotension, also contribute to sexual dysfunction, cardiovascular risk, and tremor. Serotonergic and antihistaminic effects produce sedation.

Overdose with tricyclic antidepressants may be fatal. Ingestion of 1.5 to 2 grams produces serious intoxication; greater than 2 grams produces agitation, delirium, hyperreflexia, rigidity, and seizures. The anticholinergic overdose effects also include severe tachycardias, urinary retention, and paralytic ileus. Management of overdose should take place in an intensive care setting in which arrhythmias may be monitored and treated. Prompt lavage and plasma drug level monitoring should also be accomplished.

Mechanisms of Therapeutic Action

It is believed that the therapeutic actions of all classes of antidepressants can be traced to their effects upon adrenergic and serotonergic neurotransmission (13). Early biogenic amine hypotheses (see chapter on Affective Illness) proposed that the blockade of norepinephrine (NE) re-uptake by these drugs resulted in a functional increase in NE at the synapse. Current amine hypotheses focus on receptor mechanisms, rather than presynaptic effects. (See [14] for a review of the role of biogenic amines in the pathogenesis of depression.) Receptor changes induced by antidepressants are sub-acute, and are more consonant with the long latency of antidepressant effects. Antidepressants appear to reduce the sensitivity of adrenergic receptors for their agonists.

Plasma Levels

Analytic assays for the tricyclic antidepressants are well established. While there are a number of active metabolites of these drugs, many of them may be measured in the same assay system. Research has established threshold levels for antidepressant effects (15). A rather wide definition of a therapeutic range for the tricyclic compounds is also rather well established. Plasma levels can be used with unresponsive patients to determine whether the level is in the rather broad therapeutic range. If the level is quite low, tricyclic doses should be raised above the commonly used upper limits (e.g., 300 mg/day for amitriptyline, imipramine, desipramine, doxepin; 150 mg/day for nortriptyline).

Monoamine Oxidase Inhibitors (MAOIs)

In the 1950s and 60s, the toxicity of the early monoamine oxidase inhibitor compounds severely limited their use (16). Nevertheless, monoamine oxidase inhibitors have had an interesting role in the treatment of depression in recent years. While they are less effective than tricyclic antidepressants in patients suffering from major affective illnesses, investigators have suggested that they are more effective than TCAs in certain diagnostic subgroups of affectively ill patients, e.g., atypical depressions; somatic depressions; hysteroid dysphoria (16).

MAOIs are also used for a number of anxiety disorders such as agoraphobia, agoraphobia with panic attacks and panic disorder. MAOIs may also alleviate some symptoms of post-traumatic stress disorder.

Side effects include hypotension, jaundice, anorexia, nausea, and vomiting. MAOIs potentiate the cardiovascular toxicity of aminergic agents, ranging from dietary amines such as tyramine and tyrosine to amines used in management of hypertension or cold symptoms. Combinations of such drugs with MAOIs may produce hypertensive crises. (See [16] for a more extensive review of side effects.)

Overdose is associated with agitation, hallucinosis, hyperpyrexia, hypertension, convulsions, and even death.

Treatment with MAOIs may be monitored with assays of platelet MAO inhibition. A baseline MAO function must be done if platelet MAOI is to be used as an indicator of treatment progress. After medication is initiated, the subsequent reduction in platelet MAO function is expressed as a percentage of baseline. A number of studies suggest that 80% inhibition of platelet MAOI function is associated with therapeutic effects (17).

MAOI is often used as a secondary treatment in patients who appear resistant to tricyclic therapy. There is little controlled research to indicate the percentage of TCA-resistant depression that responds to MAOIs.

TABLE III
"SECOND" GENERATION ANTIDEPRESSANTS

Generic	Commercial
Maprotiline	Ludiomil
Trazodone	Desyrl
Bupropion	Wellbutrin
Nomifensine	Merital
Amoxapine	Asendin
Mianserin	Tolvin
Zimelidine	

Second Generation Antidepressants

The so-called "second generation" antidepressants (Table III) have not proven superior to tricyclic antidepressants in controlled clinical trials. Because several of these compounds have fewer anticholinergic side effects, they are prescribed for elderly patients who are more vulnerable to the cardiovascular risks.

ANXIOLYTICS

Whether the anxiolytic effects of drugs are different from their sedative properties is still being disputed among pharmacologists. It appears, however, that the "separatists" are developing stronger arguments. Recent research has demonstrated that benzodiazepines act at specific sites (called diazepam receptors) (18). Scientists are seeking endogenous compounds (e.g., neurotransmitters) that act at these brain receptors. A number of sedative drugs, such as the barbiturates, do not act at diazepam receptors. Thus, if both drugs are anxiolytics by virtue of sedating properties, they at least act at different sites. Teleologically speaking, it is clear that anxiety and sleep-wake arousal mechanisms have different purposes. Anxiety often serves a learning function, whereas sleep-wakefulness is a neurovegetative function.

In any case, most sedatives have been used as anxiolytics by giving lower doses than are required for sleep-induction. Prior to the synthesis of benzodiazepines (BDZs), barbiturates were the primary anxiolytics (discounting alcohol). A host of other compounds (See Table IV) have also been used as both sedatives and anxiolytics. Almost all these drugs demonstrate cross tolerance, may be used to suppress abstinence, and have other therapeutic uses in common (e.g., as anticonvulsants).

With the exception of benzodiazepines, anxiolytics have a great deal of mortality associated with accidental and intentional overdose, as well as accidental or intentional abstinence.

TABLE IV
ANXIOLYTICS
(Sedative Hypnotics)

Generic	Trade Name
Benzodiazepines	
Chlordiazepoxide	Librium
Diazepam	Valium
Oxazepam	Serax
Clorazepate	Tranxene
Lorazepam	Ativan
Flurazepam	Dalmane
Prazepam	Verstran
Barbiturates	
Phenobarbital	
Butabarbitol	
Antihistaminic	
Diphenhydramine	Benadryl
Diphenylmethane antihistamines	
Hydroxyzine	Atarax
	Vistaril

FORMERLY USED, NO LONGER INDICATED

Glycol Esters	
Meprobamate	Miltown
Tybamate	Solacen
Cyclic Ether	
Paraldehyde	
Piperidinediones	
Glutethimide	Doriden
Methyprylin	Noludar
Quinazalines	
Methaqualone	Tuazolene

The high therapeutic ratio of benzodiazepines (therapeutic/lethal dose) make them extremely effective in the management of anxiety (19). There is little pharmacological rationale for using any compound other than a benzodiazepine for the management of anxiety.

Effects

All benzodiazepines function as anxiolytics at certain doses and sedatives at higher doses. In most cases, BDZs attenuate anxiety symptoms without eliminating them. When BDZs are discontinued, anxiety usually returns. Thus, they do not treat the etiology of the anxiety. Their effects are confined to temporary reduction of this unpleasant affect.

Spectrum of Use

Indications for the use of BDZs are controversial because they do not specifically treat anxiety disorders. Their use is often tied to the physician's metapsychological assumptions. Thus, from the psychoanalyst's perspective, anxiety is the primary expression of an underlying psychological conflict. The analyst uses the patient's anxiety in the therapeutic setting, and is often reluctant to pharmacologically reduce the anxiety. A learning theorist may believe that suppressing anxiety will only augment its underlying biology; therapy will depend upon the extinction of anxiety, e.g., through a procedure called systematic desensitization. Regardless of theoretical background, most therapists agree that there is such a thing as "too much" anxiety, some of which must be reduced if other therapies are to be effective. Thus, when anxiety rules the patient's life, often impairing vocational, social, and family function, medications are usually recommended for a brief period of time.

Target Symptoms

Subjectively experienced anxiety, even without peripheral manifestations of increased autonomic nervous system function, will respond to BDZs. It is common for anxiety to be accompanied by a host of peripheral symptoms which will improve with treatment (e.g., tachycardia; tachypnea; diaphoresis; flushing).

Time Course of Response

Anxiolytic response is dependent upon appropriate dose selection: a single adequate dose will attenuate anxiety. Oral doses usually produce peak blood levels within an hour and promptly reduce anxiety.

Adverse Effects

The BDZs have few adverse effects. A few individuals experience paradoxical excitement with BDZs. Exceptionally high doses are required for toxicity. No clear-cut case of a BDZ overdose death has been reported, except in patients with pre-existing medical disorders or those who were also receiving other drugs.

Mechanism of Action

BDZs act at specific neuronal receptor sites in the brain; these are thought to be neurotransmitter receptor sites, though an endogenous substance has not been clearly identified (20). Methylxanthines (e.g., caffeine) and other compounds have an affinity for these sites. BDZs appear to be antagonists at this receptor.

LITHIUM CARBONATE

Effects and Spectrum of Use

Lithium carbonate is used to treat bipolar disorder, and has few effects upon normal individuals. It is most effective in treating manic episodes in bipolar disorder. The antimanic effects of the drug appear to be quite specific—that is, when used alone, the drug will terminate all the symptoms attributable to the acute episode (21). The efficacy of lithium in mania (perhaps as high as 95%) is greater than that of antidepressants in major affective disorders (21). In the early stages of severe mania, sometimes called "deliriform" or "tertiary" mania, neuroleptics may also be required.

Lithium has prophylactic effects for both manic and depressive episodes in bipolar patients. With compliance and the maintenance of therapeutic levels, lithium can sometimes prevent subsequent manic and depressed episodes. The major prophylactic effects are the reduction of the frequency and intensity of subsequent episodes (21). Reducing the intensity of symptoms in a given episode is important, since intensity is frequently related to morbidity, e.g., degree of judgment loss. Lithium appears to be more effective in reducing the frequency of manic, rather than depressive, episodes. Lastly, it has been demonstrated that bipolar depressive episodes will occasionally respond to lithium. Lithium has also been used in major depressive disorders which have been refractory to treatment. Some psychiatrists feel that refractory patients who respond to lithium have a bipolar vulnerability, though they may not have experienced a manic episode.

Target Symptoms

The target symptoms of lithium are those of mania or depression. Rate aspects of both psychomotor and verbal behaviors will improve with treatment. Arousal and lability of mood also respond. As with depression, the therapeutic mood effects occur after some reduction in arousal and activity level. Mood elevation or paranoid hostility will improve gradually, as will thought content and flight of ideas. Impairment of judgment and grandiose thoughts recover slowly.

The antidepressant effects of lithium when present are similar to those of previously-discussed antidepressants.

Time Course of Response

Improvement in manic symptoms usually occurs within 10 to 14 days in the patient treated with lithium alone. The improvement continues for several weeks and is more rapid than that seen in most depressive episodes. Rapid improvement in the manic patient may, however, be accompanied by a shift into depressive symptoms.

Adverse Effects

The most frequent complaints are dry mouth, thirst, increase in liquid intake, polyuria, and tremor. A small proportion of the population (about 5%) find these symptoms severe. Although memory impairment is also a frequent complaint, affectively ill patients treated with antidepressants also complain of memory loss. (See [21] for a more extensive description of adverse effects.)

Therapeutic plasma levels of lithium inhibit thyroid hormone release, which leads to an initial decrease of the free thyroxine (T4) and triiodothyronine (T3). After 3 to 4 months of treatment, TSH increases and T4 and T3 levels return to baseline levels. Some patients develop a transient, persistent hypothyroidism as a consequence of lithium therapy (21).

There is little evidence to suggest that creatinine clearance is affected by long-term lithium use, in spite of early unfounded claims of renal damage. An increase in urinary volume is probably a key renal effect to monitor.

Mechanisms of Action

While lithium has a variety of effects on biogenic amine synapses, including membrane stabilization (which tends to reduce amine discharge), blockade of amine re-uptake, and MAO inhibition, current thinking attributes its therapeutic effect to post-synaptic effects (22). Lithium appears to decrease fluctuations in biogenic amine receptor sensitivity.

Blood Levels

Lithium has established therapeutic and toxic serum and plasma levels. (For a description of the kinetics of lithium and clinical response see [23].) The range of effective plasma levels is .8–1.2 mEq/liter. The physician strives to maintain levels in this range during treatment of an active episode. Occasional patients will respond at levels below or above these limits.

Toxic symptoms usually occur at levels of 1.5 mEq/liter or above. Levels in the therapeutic range can produce the adverse effects listed above, but rarely produce neurotoxic effects. Levels above 2.5 mEq/liter have been associated with severe morbidity and occasional mortality.

Problems with Use

Some patients are quite sensitive to unpleasant or disabling side effects of lithium, such as tremor. This is a particularly difficult problem since neuroleptics are the second choice for the treatment of mania. Neuroleptics are not nearly as efficacious, and are associated with a series of adverse effects not present with lithium.

While lithium may be helpful during the depressed phases of many bipolar patients, it appears to impair the management of depression in others. Decreasing lithium dose and/or adding tricyclic antidepressants is frequently necessary for management of the bipolar depressed individual.

REFERENCES

1. Klein DF, Gittelman R, Quitkin F, *et al.: Diagnosis and Treatment of Psychiatric Disorders: Adults and Children.* Baltimore, Williams & Wilkins, 1980, pp 174–214.
2. Snyder SH, Banerjee SP, Yamamura HI, *et al.:* Drugs, neurotransmitters and schizophrenia. *Science* 1974;184:1243–1253.
3. Seeman P, Lee T, Chau-Wong M, *et al.:* Antipsychotic drug doses and neuroleptic/ dopamine receptors. *Nature* 1976;261:717–718.
4. Weiss B, Sellinger-Barnette M: Effects of antipsychotic dopamine antagonists and polypeptides hormones on calmodulin, in Gessa GL, Corsisi GU (eds): *Apomorphine and Other Dopaminomimetics: Basic Pharmacology.* New York, Raven Press, 1981, vol 1, pp 179–192.
5. Morselli PL: Clinical significance of neuroleptic plasma level monitoring, in Usdin E, Dahl, SG, Gram LF, *et al.* (eds): *Clinical Pharmacology in Psychiatry.* London, MacMillan, 1981, pp 199–210.
6. Dahl SG: Active metabolites of phenothiazine drugs, in Usdin E, Dahl SG, Gram LF, *et al.* (eds): *Clinical Pharmacology in Psychiatry.* London, MacMillan, 1981, pp 125–138.
7. Strauss JS, Carpenter WT Jr: *Schizophrenia.* New York, Plenum, 1981, pp 137–161.
8. Klein DF, Gittelman R, Quitkin F, *et al.: Diagnosis and Drug Treatment of Psychiatric Disorders: Adults and Children.* Baltimore, Williams & Wilkins, 1980, pp 276.
9. Akiskel HS: Dysthymic disorder: Psychopathology of proposed chronic depressive subtypes. *Am J Psychiatry* 1983;140:11–20.
10. Houde RW: Clinical pharmacology (opiates and other compounds), in Ng, LKY, Bonica JJ (eds): *Pain, Discomfort, and Humanitarian Care.* New York, Elsevier/North-Holland, 1980, pp 191–203.
11. Klein DF, Gittelman R, Quitkin F, *et al.: Diagnosis and Drug Treatment of Psychiatric Disorders: Adults and Children.* Baltimore, Williams & Wilkins, 1980, pp 548–557.
12. Klein DF, Gittelman R, Quitkin F, *et al.:* Side effects of mood stabilizing drugs and their treatment, in *Diagnosis and Drug Treatment of Psychiatric Disorders: Adults and Children.* Baltimore, Williams & Wilkins, 1980, pp 449–492.
13. Frazer A: Tricyclic antidepressants—basic considerations, in Palmer G (ed): *Neuropharmacology of Central Nervous System and Behavior Disorders.* New York, Academic Press, 1980, pp 73–91.
14. van Praag HM: Central monamines and the pathogenesis of depression, in van Praag HM, Lader MH, Rafaelson OJ, *et al.* (eds): *Handbook of Biological Psychiatry.* New York, Marcel Dekker Inc, 1981, vol 4, pp 159–205.
15. Gram LF, Kragh-Sorensen P: Pharmacokinetics and plasma level/effect relationships of tricyclic antidepressants an update, in Usdin E, Dahl SG, Gram LF, *et al.* (eds): *Clinical Pharmacology in Psychiatry.* London, MacMillan, 1981, pp 241–251.

16. Nies A, Robinson DS: Monamine oxidase inhibitors, in Paykel ES (ed): *Handbook of Affective Disorders.* New York, Guildord Press, 1982, pp 246–261.
17. Robinson DS, Nies A, Ravaris CL, *et al.:* Clinical pharmacology of phenelzine. *Arch Gen Psychiatry* 1978;35:629–635.
18. Squires RF, Braestrup C: Benzodiazepine receptors in rat brain. *Nature* 1977; 266:732–734.
19. Lader MH: Clinical anxiety and the benzodiazepines, in Palmer G (ed): *Neuropharmacology of Central Nervous System and Behavioral Disorders.* New York, Academic Press, 1981, pp 225–241.
20. Speth RC, Guidotti A, Yamamura HI: The pharmacology of benzodiazepines, in Palmer G (ed): *Neuropharmacology of Central Nervous System and Behavioral Disorders.* New York, Academic Press, 1981, pp 244–283.
21. Coppen A, Metcalf M, Wood K: Lithium, in Paykel ES (ed): *Handbook of Affective Disorders.* New York, Guilford Press, 1982, pp 276–285.
22. Gerbino L, Olesnansky M, Gershon S: Clinical use and mode of action of lithium, in Lipton MA, DiMascia A, Killam KF (eds): *Psychopharmacology: A Generation of Progress.* New York, Raven Press, 1978, pp 1261–1275.
23. Cooper TB, Simpson GM: Kinetics of lithium and clinical response, in Liptom MA, DiMascio A, Killam KF (eds): *Psychopharmacology: A Generation of Progress.* New York, Raven Press, 1978, pp 923–931.

SELECTED REFERENCE TEXTS

DiMascio A, Shader RI: *Clinical Handbook of Psychopharmacology.* New York, Aronson, 1970.

Fann WE, Karacan I, Pokorny AD, *et al.: Phenomenology and Treatment of Anxiety.* New York, Spectrum Publications, 1979.

Jefferson JW, Greist JH, Ackerman DL: *Lithium Encyclopedia for Clinical Practice.* APA Press, 1983.

Klein DF, Gittelman R, Quitkin F, *et al.: Diagnosis and Drug Treatment of Psychiatric Disorders: Adults and Children.* Baltimore, Williams & Wilkins, 1980.

Lipton MA, DiMascio A, Killam KF (eds): *Psychopharmacology: A Generation of Progress.* New York, Raven Press, 1978.

Schoolar JC, Claghorn JR (eds): *The Kinetics of Psychiatric Drugs.* New York, Brunner/ Mazel, 1979.

Usdin E, Dahl SG, Gram LF, *et al.: Clinical Pharmacology in Psychiatry.* London, MacMillan, 1981.

Chapter 34

ELECTROCONVULSIVE THERAPY

GLENN C. DAVIS, M.D.
DODI FOSTER, PA-C
ZIPORA ARISON, M.D.

INTRODUCTION

Electroconvulsive therapy (ECT), a major somatic therapy in psychiatry, was introduced by Cerletti and Bini in 1937. ECT is only one of several types of convulsive therapies that have been used in psychiatric treatment though it is the only convulsive therapy used in the United States today. Even before 1937, the therapeutic effects of convulsions on depressive illnesses were known; 25% camphor in oil or metrazol was used to induce therapeutic seizures. Controlled scientific research on ECT has demonstrated that the therapeutic effects are dependent upon the convulsions, not the passage of electrical current across the brain per se.

DIAGNOSTIC INDICATIONS FOR ECT

ECT is not a treatment for depressed or unhappy feelings. ECT has beneficial effects upon a limited group of syndromes: the major affective disorders, both manic and depressed episodes; some schizophrenic symptoms, particularly catatonic behavior. ECT is also used as a last resort in drug-resistant schizophrenic or depressive episodes characterized by persistent suicidal or homicidal behavior. Nevertheless, the major indications for ECT are major depressive disorder and manic depressive disorder, depressed episode.

The efficacy of ECT is not altered by age; in fact, it seems to be enhanced in the elderly. ECT is also used as a treatment for postpartum depressions, and may even be used during pregnancy, though special care is necessary. ECT is especially indicated for depressions that accompany certain medical conditions, such as parkinsonism, hypothyroidism, and systemic lupus erythematosus. Brain tumors and other causes of increased intracranial pressure pose specific dangers for ECT. Nevertheless, there are no absolute contraindications to ECT since there is an unacceptably high mortality from untreated depressive episodes.

TREATMENT COURSE

The number of ECTs required to bring about remission of depressive episodes varies from patient to patient. Treatment is usually given 2 or 3 times a week; some improvement is often observed after 3 or 4 treatments. Eight to 12 treatments are usually necessary for significant, long-term symptomatic improvement. Fewer treatments may produce significant improvement, but the depressive symptoms often recur. As with the use of antidepressants, improvement in vegetative symptoms is a particularly useful indication of the patient's progress. If signs of organicity, such as amnesia and confusion, persist for a one- or two-day period, the treatment is often discontinued. After ECT, many physicians will initiate maintenance doses of antidepressants to prevent relapse. Maintenance ECT, e.g., once a week to once a month for several months, is occasionally used for prophylaxis of depression in patients who cannot be treated chemically. In patients with recurrent depressions, a second course of ECT may require more treatments than the first.

PRE-ECT WORK-UP

Prior to ECT, a complete medical history, family history, especially of complications during anesthesia, and a complete physical examination should be recorded (Table I); emphasis should be placed on the evaluation of the cardiovascular and neurological systems. Because the principal risk in ECT is cardiovascular, special attention should be paid to evidence of recent myocardial infarctions, arrhythmias, or vulnerability to malignant hypertension. The neurological exam should concentrate on orientation and memory. Increased intracranial pressure should be ruled out (e.g., by fundoscopic examination for papilledema). History of seizures, headache, and memory difficulties should be obtained. Illnesses such as diabetes, glaucoma, porphyria, renal or bone disease should be explored; these conditions or their management may interfere with the anesthetic, thus creating additional risk. The pre-ECT work-up (Table I) should be included as a progress note in the patient's chart.

TABLE I
WORK-UP FOR ELECTROCONVULSIVE THERAPY

Indications for ECT:

Failure to respond to antidepressants
Suicide risk
Prior good response to ECT
High risk for chemotherapy

Identifying Data:

Age, sex, race, handedness, diagnosis, and prior history of ECT.

History:

(1) Cardiovascular: MIs, arrhythmias, hypertension
(2) Neurologic: seizures, headache, memory difficulty
(3) Illnesses: glaucoma, diabetes, porphyria, renal, bone

Medications:

List current medications, sensitivities, and allergies.
Specific questions about anesthesia reactions.

Physical Examination:

Vital Signs, dentures, memory tests, fundoscopy,
Thorough cardiovascular and neurologic exam.

Laboratory:

EKG; chest x-ray; selected blood chemistries, such as electrolytes, glucose, and creatinine;
other relevant studies—e.g., thoracic and lumbar spine x-rays in vulnerable individuals.

Progress Notes:

Note that the procedure and adverse effects have been explained to the family and that all
questions have been answered.

MEDICATIONS

The ECT procedure usually requires an anticholinergic premedication, an anesthetic agent, and a neuromuscular blocker (Table II). Atropine, the usual anticholinergic premedication, is often given intramuscularly 30 minutes prior to treatment to decrease tracheobronchial secretions and block vagal discharge, thus reducing the risk of aspiration and cardiac arrhythmia. An ultra-short acting barbiturate, such as sodium methohexital (® Brevital), is administered intravenously for anesthesia. The anesthetic is followed by the neuromuscular blocker, e.g., succinylcholine (® Anectine), also given intravenously. Succinylcholine acts at the myoneural junction to block neural transmission thus briefly paralyzing all muscles. The use of succinylcholine prevents the motor manifestations of the seizure. Secobarbital (® Seconal) is occasionally used to pretreat the patient who experiences significant anxiety.

TABLE II
MEDICATIONS USED IN ECT

Medication	Dose	Action
Atropine	1.0 to 2.0 mg. I.M. 30 min prior to treatment	decreases secretions, blocks vagus
Methohexital (® Brevital)	60–200 mg. I.V. push at time of treatment	anesthesia
Succinylcholine (® Anectine)	10–50 mg. I.V. push at time of treatment	muscle relaxant
Optional: Secobarbital (® Seconal)	50 mg. p.o. elixir 30 min to 1 hr prior to treatment	allay anxiety

PROCEDURE

The patient should not eat or drink after 10 PM the night before the treatment. The anticholinergic drug is given in the morning prior to treatment to reduce secretions (Table III). ECT may be performed in the patient's room, a treatment room, or a recovery room. Wherever ECT is performed, personnel and necessary equipment should be available to handle emergencies, such as the loss of spontaneous respiration, airway obstruction, arrhythmias, hypertension, or hypotension. An anesthetic is administered through an intravenous line. A blood pressure cuff is inflated on the arm contralateral to the IV in order to occlude arterial flow prior to administration of succinylcholine. This procedure allows visual monitoring of the seizure in one extremity. An electroencephalogram (EEG) and electromyogram (EMG) may also be used to monitor the seizure. Modern ECT devices contain direct monitoring equipment for observing the EEG which can routinely indicate the presence and time course of the seizure. An oral airway is inserted and the succinylcholine adminstered. After paralysis, the patient is manually ventilated until spontaneously respiration returns.

The electrodes are placed bilaterally over the scalp area, or unilaterally over the non-dominant hemisphere. Good contact between the electrodes and the skin is essential. Prior to induction of the seizure, a bite-block is inserted in the patient's mouth to protect the teeth and tongue. A brief electrical current is then administered with insulated paddles in a manner similar to cardioversion. After the seizure, the bite-block is removed, the teeth are checked

```
┌─────────────────────────────────────────────────┐
│                   TABLE III                       │
│                 ECT PROCEDURES                    │
├─────────────────────────────────────────────────┤
│ Transport patient to ECT location                 │
│ Administer anticholinergic and anesthetic         │
│ Inflate BP cuff on arm without I.V. line          │
│ Administer muscle relaxant (succylcholine)        │
│ Insert airway and ventilate patient               │
│ Place electrodes                                  │
│ Insert bite-block                                 │
│ Induce seizure (Time)                             │
│ Remove bite-block                                 │
│ Check teeth                                       │
│ Suction secretions                                │
│ Ventilate until voluntary respirations resume     │
│ Monitor until fully conscious                     │
└─────────────────────────────────────────────────┘
```

and secretions are removed by suction. Immediately after the ECT, the patient requires careful monitoring since he may be confused and mildly ataxic.

ECT MYTHS

There are many myths and prejudices about ECT, most of which arise from a lack of understanding of this procedure. In the early years of ECT's use, the seizure was induced without the use of neuromuscular blocking drugs or sedation. Patients frequently experienced anxiety, and even panic. Today the patient is anesthetized and thus does not experience respiratory distress or the convulsion.

Memory impairment is a common patient complaint. Acute organic brain symptoms, such as confusion, disorientation, and memory loss, do accompany each ECT treatment. However, these organic symptoms are short-lived and gradually improve after the last treatment. Most patients regain pretreatment cognitive function within several weeks. Nevertheless, memory loss is the most commonly reported concern after ECT. Drugs and ECT evoke equal numbers of complaints about memory impairment. Careful experimental studies do not reveal persistent memory deficits following ECT.

EFFICACY

ECT has been shown to be superior to both chemotherapy and psychotherapy in treating major affective disorders. ECT brings about a remission in 60–90% of the major depressive disorders and mania. Depression in the geriatric population responds particularly well. Several studies indicate that ECT is associated with a shorter hospital stay and decreased risk of suicide. Its other advantages include avoidance of the cardiovascular risk associated with most antidepressant medications, and the fact that it is a simple, easily monitored procedure with short-term risks.

MECHANISM OF ACTION

Like all somatic therapies in psychiatry, the therapeutic mechanism of action of ECT remains unknown. The effects of convulsions on central nervous system neurochemistry are extensive, and include an increase in biogenic amines and endorphins. It is known that the therapeutic effects of ECT are dependent upon the induction of the seizure; subthreshold shocks do not bring about therapeutic antidepressant effects. Furthermore, as we have already discussed, the mode of the seizure's induction has little effect upon its efficacy.

The antidepressant effects of ECT do not appear to be altered significantly by the administration of anesthesia, neuromuscular blockade, or oxygen. Confusion and immediate memory loss may be minimized by proper placement of electrodes, choice of current strength, and duration of treatment.

RISKS OF ECT

Patients commonly complain of headaches and temporary memory loss. Rare adverse effects include fractures and spontaneous seizures. Although deaths have been reported with ECT, they have usually been due to anesthesia complications. Studies suggest that the mortality rate associated with the ECT procedure is approximately .06%, with the major cause being cardiovascular complications.

ETHICAL ISSUES

The use of ECT is controversial, perhaps because of its apparent physical invasiveness, earlier unrestricted use in benign and inappropriate conditions, and earlier administration without anesthesia.

ECT is particularly beneficial to patients who have been unresponsive to other forms of treatment, and those whose suicidal behavior is difficult to manage. It may also be preferred by patients whose financial and family obligations preclude prolonged hospitalization. It is the safest, most rapid antidepressant therapy. However, ECT cannot be forced on a competent, non-consenting patient. In some states, public law requires that several physicians agree to the necessity of ECT.

CONCLUSIONS

ECT is a specialized procedure. Information about its effectiveness and risks should be communicated early in the hospital course. Education of both patient and family is essential. Treating the depressed and suicidal patient with ECT often reduces the cardiovascular risk associated with large doses of antidepressant drugs. It may shorten hospitalization, and decrease the need for dehumanizing security measures, such as the use of physical restraints.

REFERENCES

1. Avery D, Winokur G: Mortality in depressed patients treated with electroconvulsive therapy and antidepressants. *Arch Gen Psychiatry* 1976;33:1029-1037.

RECOMMENDED READING ON ECT

Kalinowsky LB, Hippius H, Klein HE: *Biological Treatments in Psychiatry.* New York, Grune & Stratton, 1982, pp 217-271.

Small JG, Small IF, Milstein V: Electrophysiology of ECT, in Lipton MA, DiMascio A, Killam KF: *Psychopharmacology: A Generation of Progress.* New York, Raven Press, 1978, pp 759-769.

INDEX

Gould, Roger, 167, 170
Grade school state, 127–130
Graham, D.T., 277
Green, Hannah, 76
Grief, management of, 13, 48, 97
Group psychology, 3
Group psychotherapy, 412–416
    outcome research, 415, 416
Group therapy, 13, 50, 210, 255
"Growth curve," 134
Guardian, in forensic psychiatry, 265
Gustatory hallucinations, 57
Guthrie, E.R., 429
Gynecological surgery, sex after, 340, 341
Gynecology, in adolescence, 138

H

Habits of thought, in grade school stage,
    127
Haldole, 437
Hallucinations, 19, 26, 27, 36–39, 41, 43,
    44, 50, 57, 60, 62, 64, 65, 73–75, 86
Haloperidol, 40, 50, 150, 255, 437
Handicapped children, educational impli-
    cations for, 161
Handicapped, mental–myths about, 162–
    164
Harry Benjamin Gender Dysphoria Associ-
    ation, 372
Hebephrenic psychoses, 52, 73
Hecker (1871), 52
Hellerstein, H.K., 362
Hepatic failure, 47
Hepatic or renal disease, 38
Hermaphroditic disorder, 371
Heroin abuse, 244, 246, 252, 260
Heston, J.J., 67
Heteroerotic behavior, 311, 312
Hirsutism, 375
Histronic personality disorder, 201, 202,
    215
    diagnostic criteria for, 202
Hollingshead, A.G., 73
Holmstrom, J.J., 347, 350
Homeostasis, in concept of family therapy,
    418, 419
Homicidal impulses, 26, 184–186, 453
Homoerotic
    behavior, 311, 312

pattern, consequences of, 393, 394
    special difficulties in, 394, 395
Homosexual
    impulses, 54, 60, 62
    phenomena, types of, 384
Homosexuals
    adults, hormonal levels in, 386
    females, suicidal feelings in, 400
    males, 387–393
        behavior of, 391–393
        social structure of, 392, 393
        specific sexual behavior of, 391, 392
Homosexuality, 317, 323, 326, 347, 371,
    374, 376, 382–401
    in adolescense, 317
    biological basis for, 384–387
    classification and definition, 383
    different biological perspectives on,
        386, 387
    differences in mental health, according
        to race, 400
    "episodic," 384
    "facultative," 384
    family dynamics in, 389, 391, 400, 401
    in females, 386, 397–400
        analogous categories of, 397
        development of sexual psychology,
            398
        family dynamics in, 400, 401
        homosexual practices, 398
        mental health status of, 398–400
        social consequences of, 399
    interactive model of, 387
    "latent," 384
    male, influence of psychological forces
        on, 387–391
    prejudice against, 382, 383
Human behavior, psychiatric approach to,
    3, 4
Human sexuality, through the life cycle, 3
Huntington's chorea, 45, 47
Hydroxyzine, 437
Hyperactivity, 144, 145
Hyperkinetic syndrome, 145
Hyperpyrexia, 60
Hypnosis, 180, 190, 228
Hypnotics, 40, 50, 248
    abuse of, 248
    barbiturate-like, 40

Normal behavioral landmarks and charac-
teristics, 4
Normal pressure hydrocephalus, 45–47
Nortriptyline, 445
Note-taking, in evaluation session, 16

O

Oedipal conflict, 189, 196
Oedipal phase, 188
"Oedipus complex," 118, 135, 188–190
Object relations theory, 101
Obsessive-compulsive
neuroses, 12, 176
personality, 4, 26, 48, 297, 323
traits, 48
Offer, D., 133, 315
Offer, J.L., 315
Old age, 166–172, 355–360
affective illness in, 172
dementia in, 172
depression in, 172
in females, 357–359
importance of sexuality in, 355–360
in males, 356
"paraphrenia" in, 172
psychopathology in, 172
schizophrenia in, 172
Olfactory hallucinations, 57, 239
Opiates, abuse of, 243–245, 247, 254
Oppositional disorder, 148
Oral period, 10, 11
Organic affective syndrome, 85
Organic brain syndrome, 34, 46, 56, 86,
100, 197, 218, 272
Organic formulation, in eitology of schizophrenia, 65
Organic mental disorders, 35, 42, 52, 61,
62, 143, 152
in childhood and adolescence, 143, 152
Organic psychoses, 73, 182
differential diagnosis in, 73
Organic states, 25, 27
Orgasm,
in adolescence, 314, 315
in sexual response, 280–284, 314, 315,
335
Orgasmic problems
primary, 337, 338
secondary, 337

Orgastic phase dysfunction, 284
Orientation, in mental status examination,
27
Orthopaedics, in adolescence, 138
Osmond, H., 68
Over-anxious disorder, 146, 147
Over-the-counter medication, abuse of,
249, 250
Oxman, T.E., 63

P

Palilia, 150
Paraldehyde, 447
Paranoia, 26, 48, 50, 51, 61, 62
Paranoid delusions, 50, 63, 238
Paranoid disorders, 52, 53, 61–63, 172
associated features, 61
diagnostic criteria for, 62
differential diagnosis, 61
etiology of, 62
Paranoid ideation, 51
Paranoid personality, 62, 63, 198–200, 296
disorder, 198–200
diagnostic criteria for, 199, 200
style, 296
Paranoid psychoses, 52, 67, 247, 255, 376
drug-induced, 247
Paranoid schizophrenia, 53, 61–63, 172,
238
Paraphilias, 326
"Paraphrenia," 172
Parental development, in adolescence, 138
Parkinson's disease, 45
Parkinsonism, 454
Parloff, M.B., 411
Passive aggression, 197
Passive-aggressive personality disorder,
208, 209
diagnostic criteria for, 209
Passive-dependent character, 323
Past psychiatric history, 21
Pathological states, in medicine and
psychiatry, 5
"Patienthood," in psychiatry, 5
Pauling, Linus, 69
Pavlov, I.P., 428, 429
Pavor nocturnus, 151
Peer group acceptance, in adolescence, 314
Peer relations, 127, 138